Against the Odds

Against the Odds

New Zealand's First Women Doctors

CYNTHIA FARQUHAR & MICHAELA SELWAY

MASSEY UNIVERSITY PRESS

Contents

Forewords

In 1891 Emily Siedeberg became Otago's first female medical student and New Zealand's first female medical graduate in 1896. A year later Dr Siedeberg set up private practice in Dunedin.

That same year, 1897, Margaret Cruickshank became the second woman to complete a medical course at Otago. Dr Cruickshank was the first female doctor registered in New Zealand. She practised in Waimate, South Canterbury, until her untimely death in 1918 from influenza.

These two incredible women became role models for the generations of women who succeeded them. Their stories represent many early pioneers in medicine who pushed the boundaries of societal norms of their times. Through their passion for medicine, through sheer determination and perseverance, they overcame formidable personal and professional obstacles that are hard for us to imagine today. They went on to leave an indelible mark on the medical profession while blazing a trail for the generations of women who followed.

Now, women comprise more than half of medical students and nearly half of the physician workforce. I am sure that, if alive today, the doctors featured in this book would be proud of the progress that has been made. The tremendous collective contribution of women over the decades to medicine and healthcare is tribute to the enduring legacy of the early trailblazing women in medicine.

Grant Robertson
Vice-Chancellor
University of Otago
May 2025

The story of both the women graduates of the early decades of Otago Medical School and the practice of medicine in New Zealand over that period needed to be recorded and has now developed from an oral history and an online site into this book.

It is also the story of the further emancipation of women, New Zealand being the first self-governing country in the world to give women the vote in 1893. About the same time, New Zealand women wanted not only to vote but also to have access to higher education with science and mathematics included. Otago Girls' High School was the first public high school for girls in Australia and New Zealand and provided an education to the girls along academic lines similar to the high school for boys. Founded in 1871, it had an enlightened curriculum and encouraged girls to pursue an academic education. It is not surprising that New Zealand's first three medical women graduates — starting with Miss Emily Siedeberg, later Dr Emily Siedeberg-McKinnon, the first woman to be admitted in 1891 — went to Otago Girls' High School.

This is a history of women entering the medical profession, but men must have had a part to play in assisting them to achieve their goals. Some were vigorously opposed to having women in their classes but others, perhaps the less vocal majority, supported the women students and helped them to succeed.

This book is being published in time for Otago Medical School's 150th anniversary, celebrated in Dunedin in late May 2025. Professor Cindy Farquhar and her team are to be congratulated for their efforts and as a graduate I am pleased to see the stories of fellow graduates in print, and proud to be associated with this endeavour and to support it.

Dr Wendy Hadden (1968)
Auckland
May 2025

Preface

In 2011 my father, Dr Bryce Gunn, died aged 87. He had been a popular general practitioner in the Waikato town of Cambridge for 53 years. Following his death the *Waikato Times* ran a full-page feature about him, and the editor of the *New Zealand Medical Journal* (*NZMJ*) wrote to me asking for an obituary, which was published a few months later.

In 2014 my mother, Dr Meredyth Gunn (née Wilson), died aged 89. Meredyth was also a medical practitioner, and apart from the time she spent bringing up four children and a period of ill health she worked for most of her life. She had worked for the School Medical Service when she first graduated and then part-time in general practice with my father. After they divorced, she worked for 15 years as a medical officer at Tokanui Hospital. The *Waikato Times* did not publish the news of her death and nor did the *NZMJ* write to me asking for an obituary. I wrote one anyway and it was published a few months later.

In 2011, with my niece Tracey Gunn, I recorded an oral history with Meredyth. Her story was one of 'overcoming the odds'. She grew up in the small town of Te Kūiti, and from the age of 15 travelled each week to Hamilton by train to attend Hamilton High School, where she studied Latin, physics and chemistry. These subjects were important in order to pass the intermediate year for medical school entry and not available at Te Kuiti High School. She was a national scholarship winner (ranked ahead of my father in the same year) and was accepted into Otago Medical School in 1944.

The journey from Te Kūiti to Dunedin took two days and involved two train trips and an overnight ferry. When she failed her second year after missing two months when her appendix ruptured, she had to repeat the year. She subsequently passed her second and then her third year. During her third year she developed a relationship with my father and when she returned to Dunedin in February 1947 to start her fourth year, she was pregnant. She had told no one. They were married within the week, and informed their parents afterwards.

Their son Graeme was born on 13 September 1947. At the end of October, her mother-in-law came to Dunedin from Wellington and took Graeme, who was only seven weeks old, back to Wellington so that Meredyth could sit her end-of-year exams. This separation was not easy for Meredyth. She failed. After the summer break in Te Kūiti and Wellington, Meredyth returned to Dunedin in January 1948 to sit 'specials', which fortunately she passed.

Her mother-in-law cared for Graeme in Wellington for all of her fifth year (1948) and then in 1949 Meredyth went to live in Wellington with Bryce's parents so she could complete her sixth year while Bryce worked as a first-year house officer in Palmerston North. Graeme went to a day nursery while Meredyth was at Wellington Hospital. She did not pass that year and had to repeat it in 1950. Her second baby, Diana, was born in January 1950, and she finally graduated in 1952.

It was difficult to work as a house surgeon with two children and so Meredyth took a position with the School Medical Service. In 1954 Bryce and Meredyth moved to Coromandel township, where Bryce ran the Coromandel Hospital and a general practice that looked after the population north of Thames. They had two more children: David in 1954 and me, Cynthia (Cindy), in 1956. In 1958 they moved to Cambridge, where they set up a new general practice.

My parents' marriage was not a happy one. Family violence marred our home life and my mother became increasingly dependent on alcohol. My parents separated in 1973, after 27 years of marriage, and divorced in 1976. After a few years of treatment, including in-patient care, for alcohol addiction and depression, Meredyth worked as a medical officer at Tokanui Hospital, where she remained until her retirement in 1991. By all accounts, her patients (and their families) appreciated her efforts on their behalf. In her later years, she was a very good bridge player, a breeder of lovely Burmese cats, and generous to her family.

My relationship with my mother was never simple. One might think that the child of two doctors would have a privileged upbringing. While I do have some good memories of my parents talking about their patients and problem-solving together at mealtimes, mostly my memories are of disharmony.

By the time I was at high school, my mother was well into a downward spiral of alcohol addiction and depression. After the divorce and treatment, she seemed to me to be mostly sad.

+++

As I reflected on her life after she died, I considered (not for the first time) the trajectory that her life had taken. I had never seen the happy, smiling Meredyth of her medical school photos. So I asked myself: How had she gone from that happy medical student to her later persona? Was it simply bad luck? Had she made poor decisions? Was it that the abusive relationship with my father was never acknowledged? Or was it that access to contraception, abortion and paid maternity leave, let alone the supports that would allow her to navigate single motherhood, were almost non-existent and the circumstances were always stacked against her as a young female student in the 1940s?

The burden of an unplanned pregnancy had initially fallen solely — and unevenly — on my mother. My father's medical studies and career progressed without interruption while my mother had to re-sit exams, repeat a year and was never able to be a house surgeon, a role considered an important step in clinical training. Despite supportive parents, the disapproval of both families would have been palpable. And the disapproval would not have ended there. It is also likely that her fellow medical students, her teachers and hospital staff would also have disapproved.

After writing her obituary, and thinking about her struggles, I marvelled that she had got through at all. Although her parents encouraged her studies, there was little practical support for Meredyth: no one accompanied her at the start of the course to help her settle in, her parents never came to Dunedin in the years she was there, and there was no easy means of communication — weekly letters had to suffice. And certainly there were no mid-year trips home or holidays visiting the beauty spots of the South Island. When she became pregnant, her parents could not travel down to support her.

The fact that she completed her studies when other students in the same circumstances usually left the course is admirable and speaks to her motivation to become a doctor. And after the travails of completing medical school, raising four children in an increasingly abusive relationship and a slow recovery from depression and addiction, it is remarkable that she managed to return to useful work at all. At her funeral, I told everyone that I was proud of her and her recovery to health. At the same time, I privately wondered what might have been had the circumstances been different.

Finally, after all this introspection, I decided it was important to tell Meredyth's story, even though some would say that her career was not particularly notable. What stood out, at least to me, was that she had overcome those many adversities. At the same time, I wondered whether other medical women had similar stories, and so I conceived the idea of collecting as many biographies as possible of women who graduated from Otago Medical School between 1896 — the year the first woman was accepted — and 1967, after which a second medical school opened in Auckland.

This project started in 2016 with initial funding from the Maurice and Phyllis Paykel Trust. Over the next nine years we were told remarkable stories. Many women both faced and overcame great adversity, and it came in so many guises. My mother certainly was not alone. By mid-2025 we had published the biographies of 150 of the 400 women graduates. Only women who graduated were included. We do not know the numbers who enrolled and then left the course without graduating, or why they did not graduate, but marriage, children, disenchantment and the hostility of teachers, hospital staff and students would be some of the reasons.

Special thanks are due to Dr Wendy Hadden, a graduate from 1968, whose generous donation made this book possible. Wendy would have graduated in 1967 but was selected to tour England with the New Zealand women's cricket team in 1966. I am also very grateful to my co-editor Michaela Selway, who has worked on the project with me over the past nearly five years with enthusiasm and commitment.

Finally, a very big thank you to all the medical women who agreed to be interviewed, and to their extended families and colleagues who provided information and photographs. Without their input this project would have been very difficult, if not impossible. Hearing all these stories has been both delightful and humbling. There were sometimes tears, and often sadness, but mostly admiration at what these women achieved.

Cindy Farquhar
Auckland
May 2025

The third-year Otago Medical School class of 1946. Front row, from left: Beryl Howie (graduated in 1949), Miss Nicholson, Noeline Burn (née Clemens; 1949), Rosemary Faull (née Clendon; 1949), Beverley Luke (née Brown; 1949), Kathleen Wake (née Brown; 1950), Stella Johnstone (née Horwell; 1949), Miss Lindsay, Marjorie Young (1951), Meredyth Gunn (née Wilson; 1952), Jane Munro (née Aylward; 1950), Noeline Walker (1960), Mrs Salas, Marie Simpson (1951), Margaret Tennent (née Andrews; 1949), Thelma Becroft (1949). The women for whom no date is recorded either did not graduate or were members of staff. *Otago Medical School Archives*

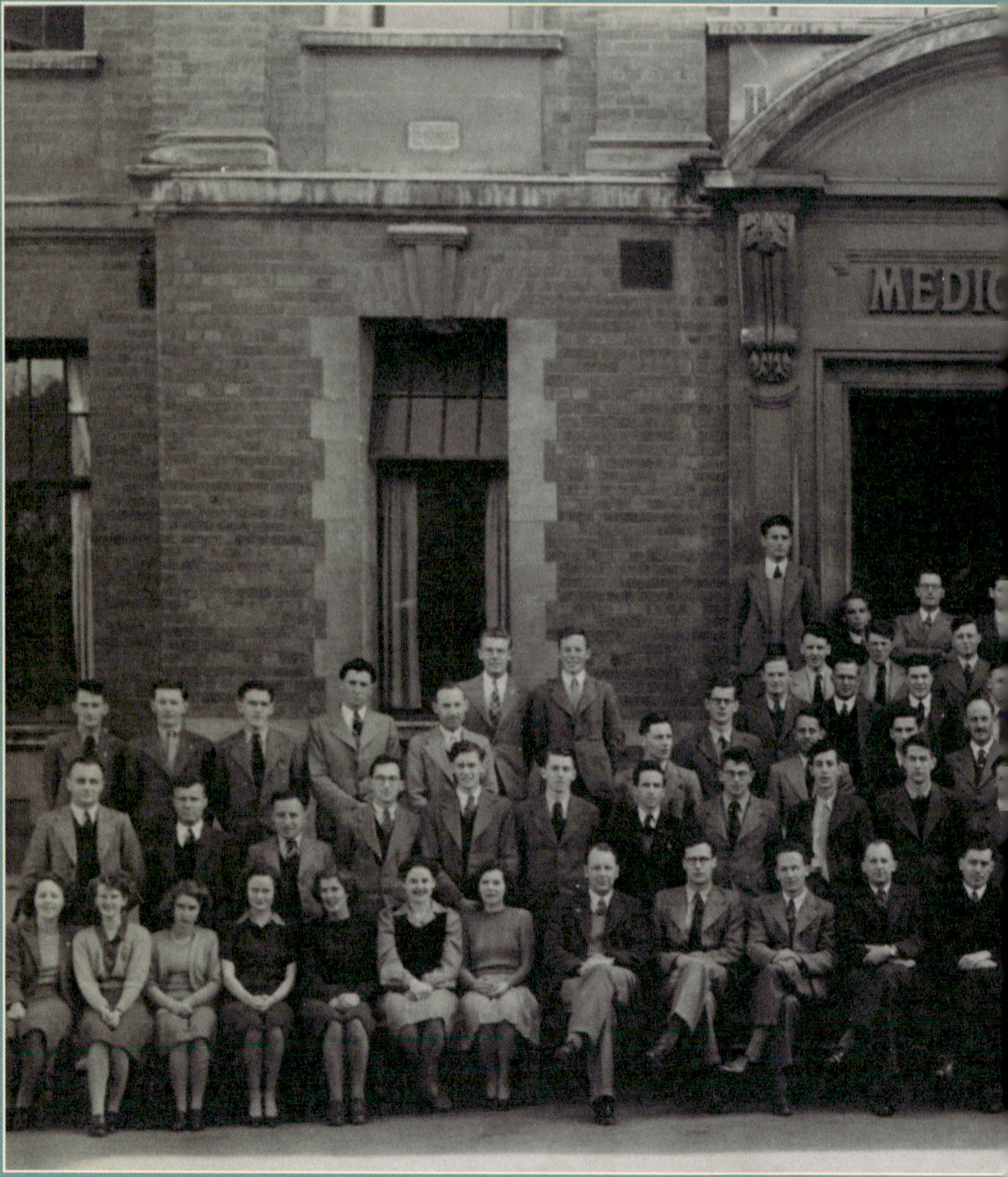

Introduction

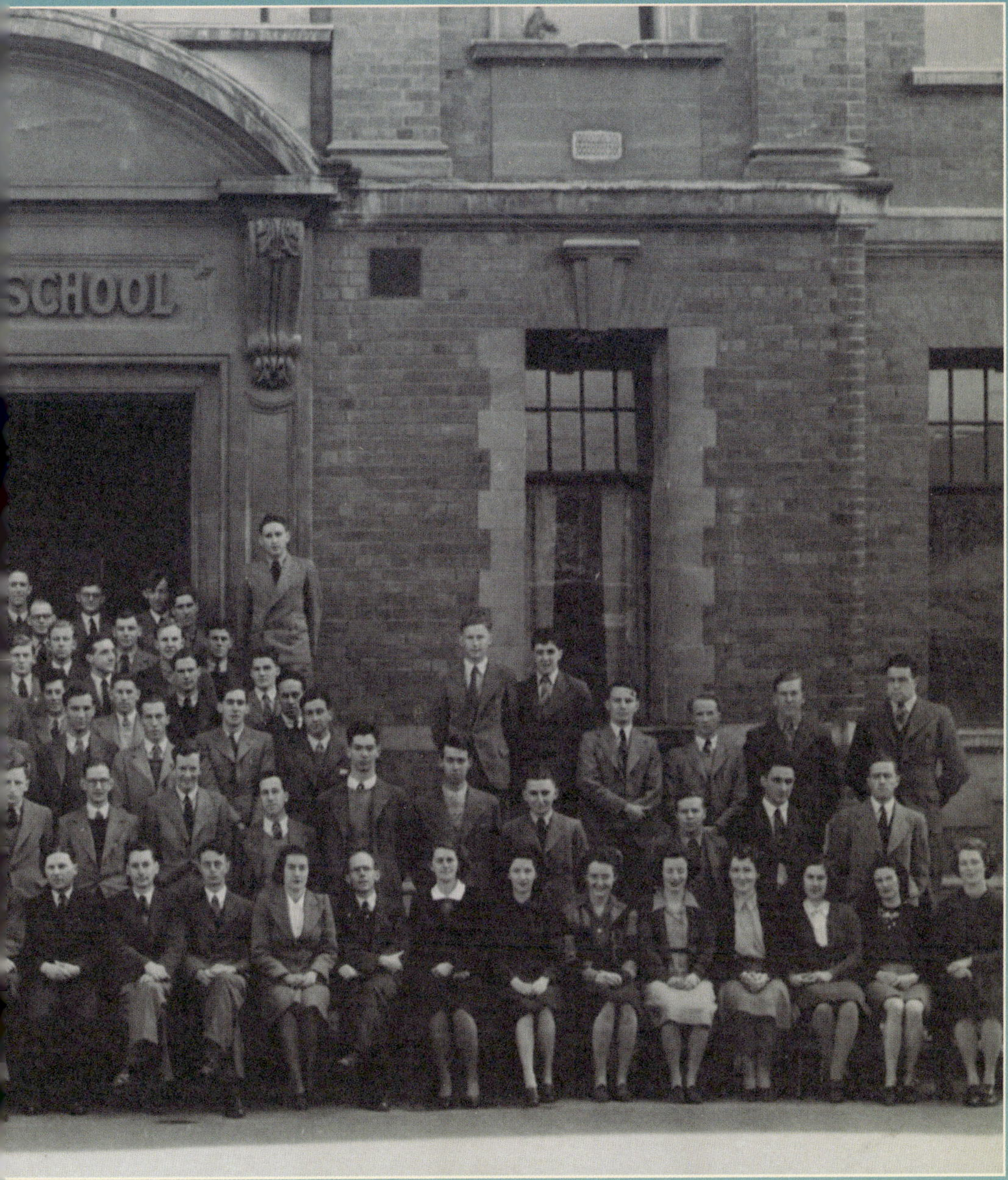

Until the 1960s, this is how the first day of lectures at Otago Medical School began for first-year women students: as they took their places in the front row of the lecture theatre — as they had been advised to do by women students in the years ahead of them — they were greeted with boos, whistles and stomping from the young men in the back rows.[1] Some noticed the words 'Women's place is in the home' engraved into their desks.[2] Some professors stood at the lectern and declared, 'I see we have females. You have taken a male's place and will waste it . . . You are all going to get married and have children and it will have been a waste of time training you.'[3]

Having worked so hard to get into medical school, this first belittling introduction was a precursor to the obstacles they would face in the coming years. It might be a laboratory session, as happened in 1964, in which a professor announced, 'We are going to be listening to hearts today. I want three volunteers to strip to the waist', and the male students turned to the women and demanded they strip.[4] It might be professors ignoring them or calling them 'chaps' and addressing the whole class as 'gentlemen'.[5]

It might be midway through the academic year, when it was time for lectures on reproductive organs and contraception, and a professor would declare, 'I now come to the part of my lectures I refuse to give before women. Therefore, the women must leave the room, or I will leave.'[6]

It might be that in the anatomy dissection rooms, pieces of flesh would be slid into their lab coat pockets,[7] or that male students and lecturers would make inappropriate comments in sessions on the female anatomy. It might be, as happened in the mid-1910s, that when a lecturer tried to kiss a woman student and she objected, her marks for the rest of the year plummeted.[8] Many had to make a rapid adjustment in the face of these pressures. Some considered it was their responsibility to not give any cause for offence or criticism; they kept their heads down and worked hard.

Experiences such as these, or variations of them, have been recounted by many of the women who studied at the Otago Medical School across the seven decades covered by this book.[9] Not every woman experienced such hostility and, indeed, many were adamant that they did not ever encounter sexism or discrimination, either during their studies or throughout their careers. Others said that at that point in their lives they 'hadn't heard of the word "harassment". We didn't know about that. We just felt we weren't fitting in well enough.'[10]

The underlying issue, however, was not the women or their predominantly male teachers. It was the social mores of those times. New Zealand society, in all spheres, was highly gendered over these seven decades. The prevailing opinion in the wider community was that working mothers who did not prioritise their families above all else were selfish. This changed slowly in the face of the manpowering of women into the workforce in wartime, and the various feminist and socialist movements of the first half of the twentieth century, but medicine continued to be considered a man's domain. On the other hand, nursing, where the primary purpose was to care for and serve patients, was considered an extension of a woman's sphere. Women seeking more than that — to train and work equally with men as doctors — were not readily accepted. Many medical men did not consider women equal to the 'higher calling' of medicine, and some women doctors were in conflict with nurses who thought that they were stepping beyond the accepted boundaries.

It was against this background that a small group of women persisted in their desire to be doctors and went on to carve out successful and impactful careers. Societal pressures may have resulted in some women who qualified in medicine but did not go on to practise. A study of the first 50 women medical students reported that just over half married and did not start working as doctors.[11] However, when the entire period between 1896 and 1967 is considered it shows that the majority did go on to have successful and influential careers. Even those who left formal practice (whether they were expected to or chose to) continued to be actively

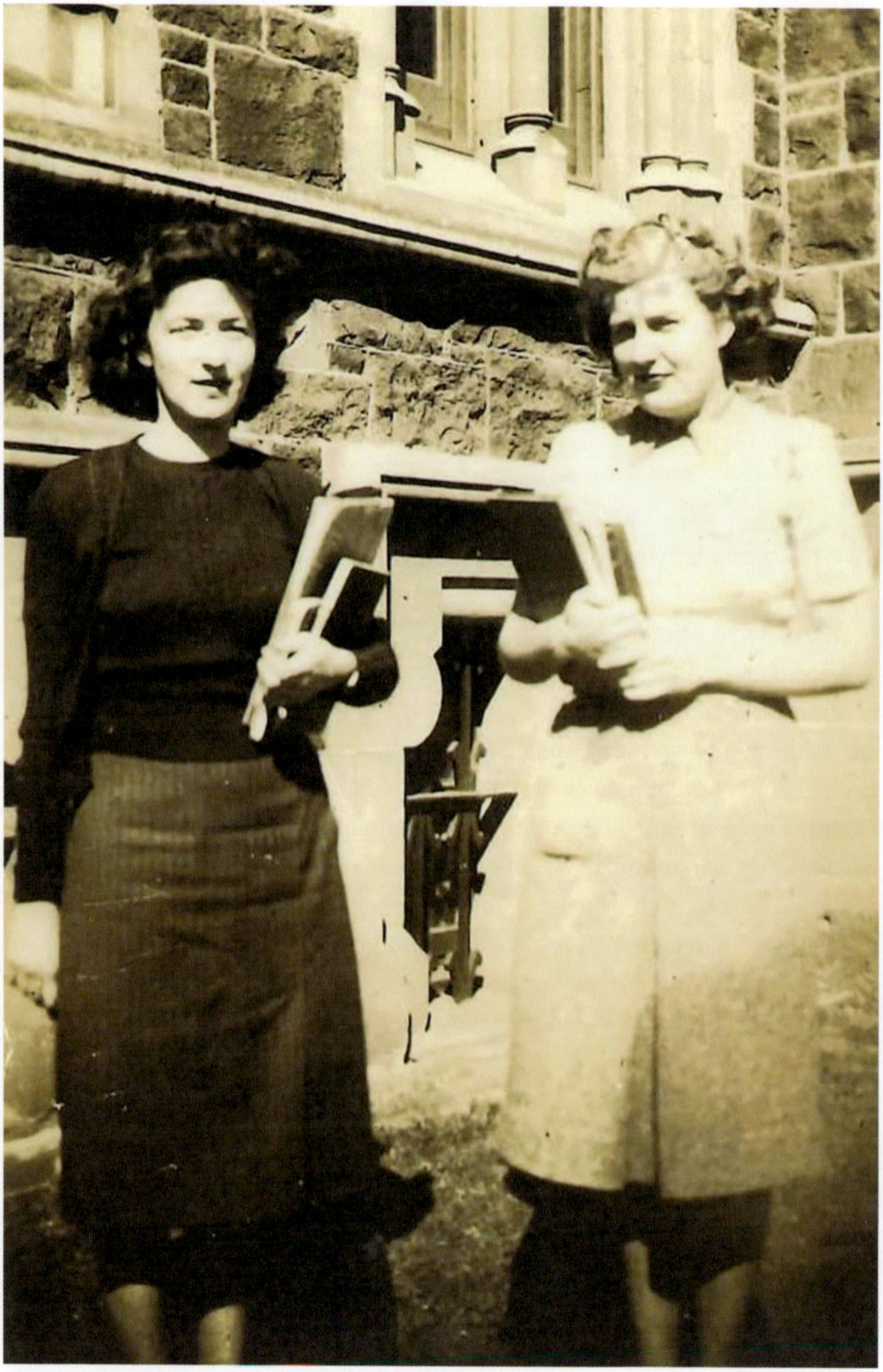

Meredyth Gunn (née Wilson; 1952), at left, and Anne McKinnon (née Pearson; 1951) on their way to a lecture in October 1944. *Courtesy Priscilla Gambeili*

involved in medical matters and often remained lifelong members of various medical associations.

Understanding Otago Medical School, and the experience of women students there, requires some historical context. Perhaps the most important element was the rapid development and expanded wealth of the school's home base, the city of Dunedin, after the Otago goldrush of the 1860s. Dunedin was already a progressive city, and its well-educated, predominantly Scottish residents had high aspirations, particularly for women's education.

Otago Girls' High School (OGHS) — the very first state secondary school for girls in the southern hemisphere — was founded there in 1871, and in 1878 the University of Otago became the first university in Australia and New Zealand to admit women students. This was largely due to the lobbying of Learmonth Dalrymple, an educationalist who campaigned for secondary education for girls in Otago and had written about women's admission to those planning to establish a university there.

Alexander Wilson, rector of OGHS from 1885 to 1895, was instrumental in ensuring that the young women in his school received a high school education in courses that were not traditionally taught at other girls' schools but that were required to enter professions such as law, science and medicine. Wilson also believed that women were naturally gentle, moral and caring, and that if women better understood subjects such as botany, higher mathematics and Latin, their 'modifying influence . . . on men's manners and language' could penetrate male institutions.[12]

Elsewhere, the wider New Zealand school curriculum in the late nineteenth century did not serve girls well.[13] Those in the larger cities of Auckland, Wellington, Christchurch and Dunedin had better access to higher education, but even there the schools were highly stratified. Schooling was compulsory only up to the age of 13. Largely because of the cost involved, girls who attended any type of secondary school tended to come from wealthier families, and almost all were Pākehā.[14] Higher education was not generally considered necessary; more important was to prepare girls for a future in the domestic sphere. People in the upper levels of society, in particular, believed that a successful family was one where the wife and daughters did not have to contribute to the family income. And because schooling for girls was not seen as a necessity, there was little pressure on schools to provide a curriculum that challenged them academically.

This was reinforced by a 1923 report from the consultative committee on 'Differentiation of the Curricula between the Sexes' in the United Kingdom, which stated that the intellectual capacity of girls slowed down after puberty due to lower blood counts and poorer oxygenation and thus they should be judged more leniently by examiners.[15] Schools also had a degree of flexibility in what subjects they could teach.[16] Schools in the larger cities, including girls' schools, could afford to introduce a range of topics such as maths, science and languages, whereas small-town and rural schools received less funding and struggled to attract suitable teachers.[17] In addition, rural schools tended to focus on practical skills such as agriculture (for boys) and hygiene (for girls) that were considered of greater use to their students.[18]

The earliest adopters of a well-rounded education for women were located in Dunedin and Auckland, though Christchurch and Wellington were not far behind. Otago Girls' High School included physics and chemistry in its curriculum from its inception, and Auckland Girls' Grammar, founded in 1878, became known for its well-equipped physics laboratory.[19] Other schools taught only botany, a subject that required little or no equipment.[20] Some, such as Christchurch Girls' High School, founded in 1877, taught physiology as an alternative to botany: the school argued that it was better for teachers to explain the human body in a scientific, 'morally proper' way than for parents to attempt it.[21]

Given that most secondary schools did not teach the subjects required for entrance to certain university degree courses, coupled with the general consensus that girls needed to be prepared for marriage and not careers, it is not surprising that it took so long for women to be accepted into professional degree courses such as medicine, law and engineering.[22]

The attitudes that shaped the education system at Otago Girls' High School are paralleled in the founding of New Zealand's first university. From its establishment in 1869, the University of Otago had been open to both sexes in all the degrees of arts, medicine, law and music.[23] When it was integrated into the University of New Zealand as one of four colleges, along with Canterbury, Victoria (Wellington) and Auckland, in 1874, this policy was also

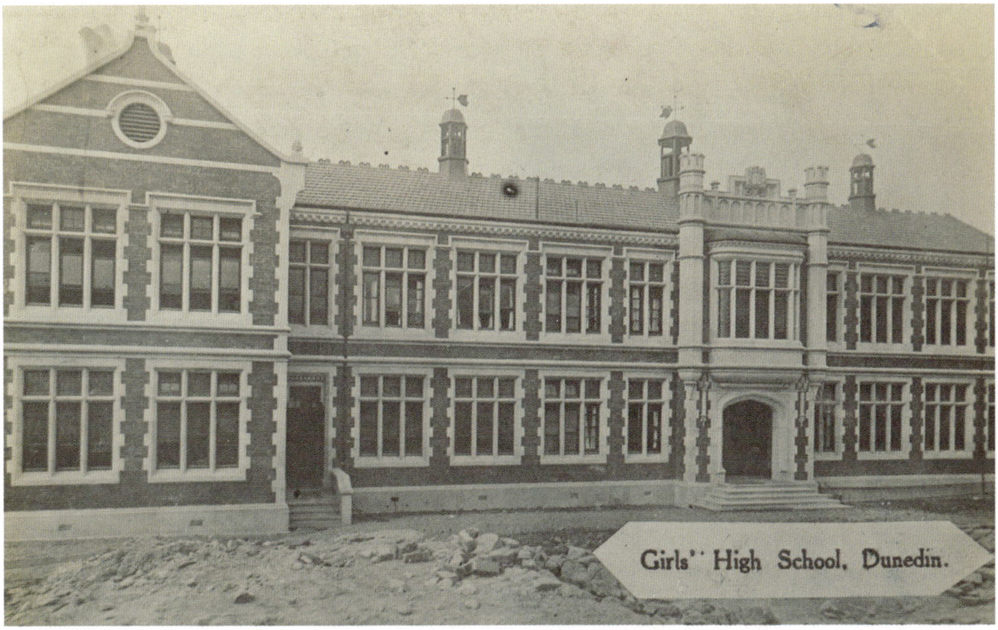

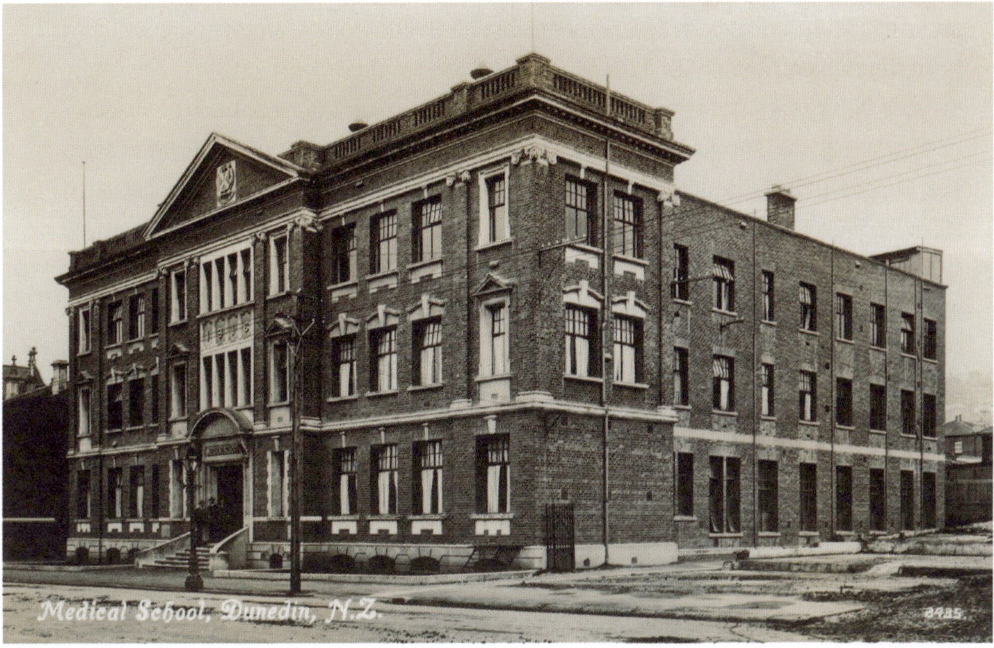

ABOVE: Otago Girls' High School, c.1911. *Hocken Collections Uare Taoka o Hākena, A.B.C. postcard, Box-307-012*

BELOW: Otago Medical School in the 1920s. This building on Great King Street is now known as the Scott Building. *Houghton family collection*

adopted (the University of New Zealand was dissolved in 1961 and the four colleges became independent universities).[24]

Initially, the medical school offered only a two-year course, and students completed their degrees at recognised universities in Britain. This was a barrier for women, since British universities did not admit women students until 1874, when the London School of Medicine for Women opened, and 1886, when what proved to be a more popular destination, the Edinburgh School of Medicine for Women, opened. These schools continued to attract New Zealand women who wanted a medical degree from a well-established university until 1914, when travel restrictions were put in place due to the First World War.

With the creation of a full five-year medical course in 1885, women in New Zealand could finally complete their medical education in their home country.[25] Yet it was another six years before the medical school accepted the first application from a woman student — Emily Siedeberg in 1891. In fact, until then, few women had completed any of the other degrees available at the university: the first to do so was Caroline Freeman, who graduated with a BA in 1885.[26] By the time Siedeberg made her request for entry to the medical school, only nine women had graduated from the university, all with a BA.[27]

Siedeberg was not the first woman to attempt to enrol as a medical student. In May 1882, the *Otago Daily Times* reported that Mary Tracey had obtained a score of 528 in her examinations and had thus won the Scott Scholarship, awarded by the University of Otago Council to outstanding students who wished to study at the medical school. She was one of two candidates advanced for the award; the other, a male, had a score of 368.[28] Although she completed many of the prerequisite courses for entrance to the medical school, possibly in time to join the first class of the five-year course, Tracey then disappeared from the records. The only other mention of her comes from William Goodlet, the laboratory assistant of one of the medical school professors, who later noted that Mary Tracey 'did not get any encouragement from Dr Scott at the time, and did not have any one to back her up. She was very much disappointed at not entering the Medical School.'[29]

Much had changed in Otago in the eight years between Mary Tracey's and Emily Siedeberg's applications to the medical school, and these societal and financial shifts may be the reason for Siedeberg's acceptance. Written accounts of Otago Medical School suggest that in the early 1890s, the University of Otago Council faced two important questions: 1) Should women be allowed to attend classes and

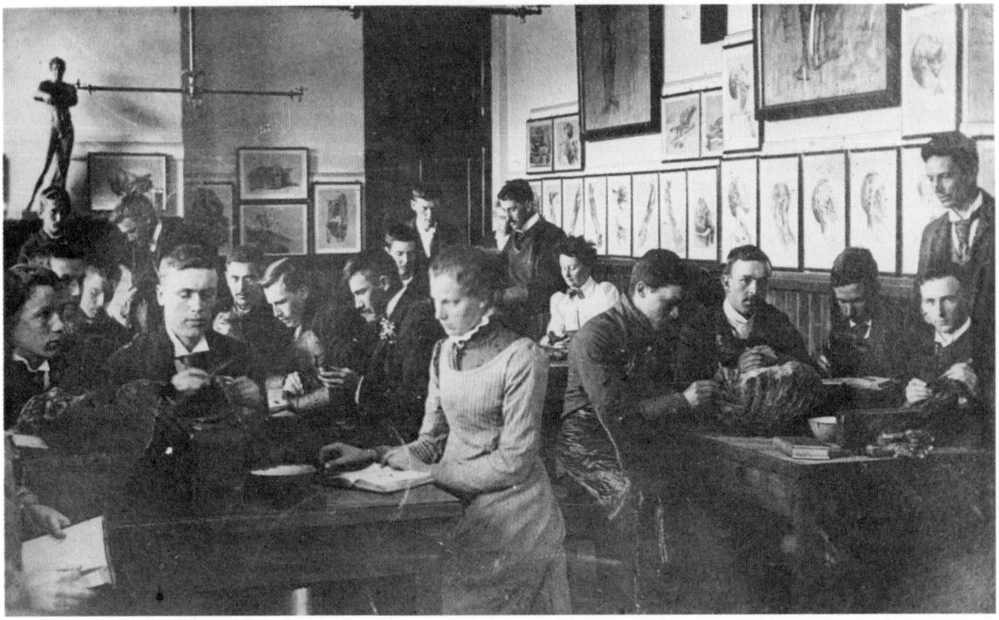

Margaret Cruickshank (centre front) and her fellow medical school students in the dissection room at Otago Medical School, c.1895. *W.D. Trotter Anatomy Museum, S05-517*

complete the degree? and 2) Should the medical school close?[30] The university had faced financial difficulties from its inception. There were never enough students across all its courses, and in the case of the medical school, many dropped out or transferred to overseas universities as a result of the rundown conditions of both the school and Dunedin Hospital.[31] The medical school was also understaffed, and many of the lecturers were either unpaid or worked for low salaries.[32]

The cause of the financial strife originated from poorly performing pastoral rents on farmland that had been gifted to the university. As wool prices fell during the slump of the 1890s, the university had to resort to borrowing money. As a result, each year the university fell further into debt. The year 1901 was the eighth in a row in which it had 'exceeded its income by £150 per annum'.[33] All of this occurred while the medical school's lecturers were pushing the council to hire more specialists, to properly equip the laboratories and classrooms, and to improve the state of the medical school buildings. The hospital, where the students did their practical work, was also described as employing poor-quality staff and having low standards of hygiene.

These extreme financial pressures coincided with a re-evaluation of the role of women in New Zealand society. When Mary Tracey enquired about admission into the medical school, discussions about female suffrage were under way but had not yet achieved traction. A request that women be allowed to vote had been presented to the New Zealand Parliament in 1878 but had been continually denied.[34] It was only with the establishment of various women's organisations and unions, most notably the Women's Christian Temperance Union, that the movement gained momentum. In 1891, the suffrage petition attracted 9000 signatures, in 1892 it doubled to 19,700, and in 1893 it stood at 31,871 — including the signature of Emily Siedeberg.[35]

The suffragists' demands were not especially radical. Women argued that they did not want to take over the public sphere by entering politics and the workforce; rather, once they had the vote they would use it to extend the role they already played — that of homemakers and 'guardians of moral health and welfare' — in order to better society.[36] Higher education, argued the feminist periodical *Daybreak*, 'tended to produce the highest form of womanhood' as it 'allowed women's "natural instincts" to be given free rein in the service of others'.[37]

Studies on the push for female suffrage in New Zealand have concluded that it was for this very reason — which could be seen as non-threatening to men —

that when New Zealand did achieve universal suffrage in 1893, women did not immediately enter politics: the first woman member of Parliament, Elizabeth Reid McCombs (née Henderson), was not elected until 1933.[38] Instead, women took up roles in education (teaching, administration and leadership) and in healthcare (medicine and nursing) — two fields in which they could continue their roles as carers in the public sphere.[39] Accepting women into higher education in these fields did not hurt their future positions in the family unit; rather, it better prepared them to carry out their roles.[40]

The changing opinions about women in the workplace during the 1890s meant that both the medical school and the hospital were more willing to accept women doctors and nurses. In the medical school women students meant more students paying the fees that the university desperately needed.[41] Furthermore, fully trained, professional female nurses cost Dunedin Hospital half the salaries paid to untrained male wardsmen.[42] Trained female nurses were welcomed because 'doctors needed to be sure that their instructions were being implicitly carried out night and day and only a thoroughly trained and disciplined staff of nurses could give them this assurance'.[43]

This book covers the period from 1896, when the first woman graduated from Otago Medical School, through to 1967, the year before New Zealand's second medical school opened in Auckland with the proportion of women in the new school's first intake immediately higher than any of the years at Otago.[44] During this period, over 400 women graduated from the Bachelor of Medicine and the Bachelor of Surgery degrees. Although it is difficult to determine the exact numbers, between one and four women students were admitted to the medical school each year from 1891 to 1916. From 1918 to 1967, there were usually no more than 12 women students (out of 120) entering the second-year class after their intermediate year.

Over these years, the numbers graduating in the sixth year ranged from as low as one in 1927 to as high as 16 in 1948 and 1960. In the final year of this cohort only 10 women graduated. The variation in graduate numbers compared to intake numbers can be explained by students needing to repeat a year or taking a year out to do a research degree (BMedSc), while others left altogether, often because they married or had children.

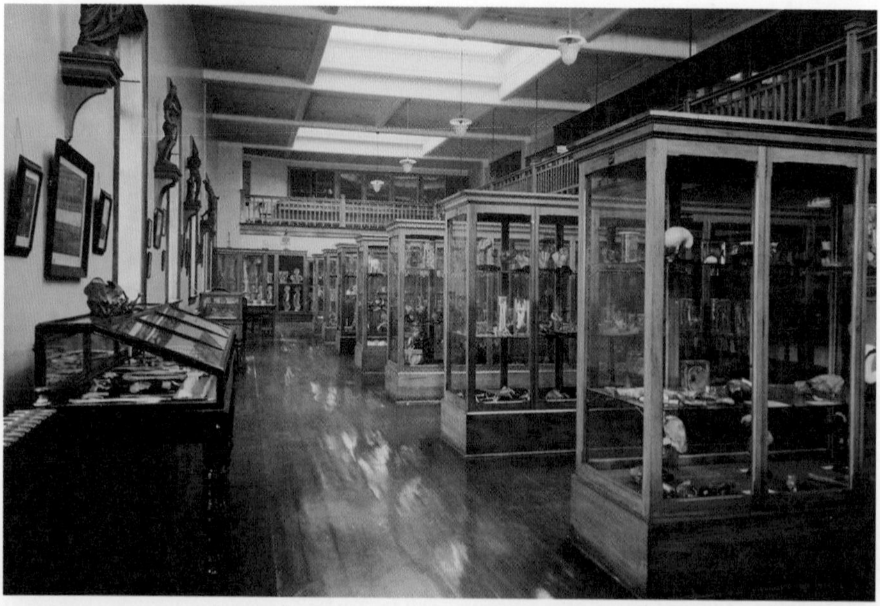

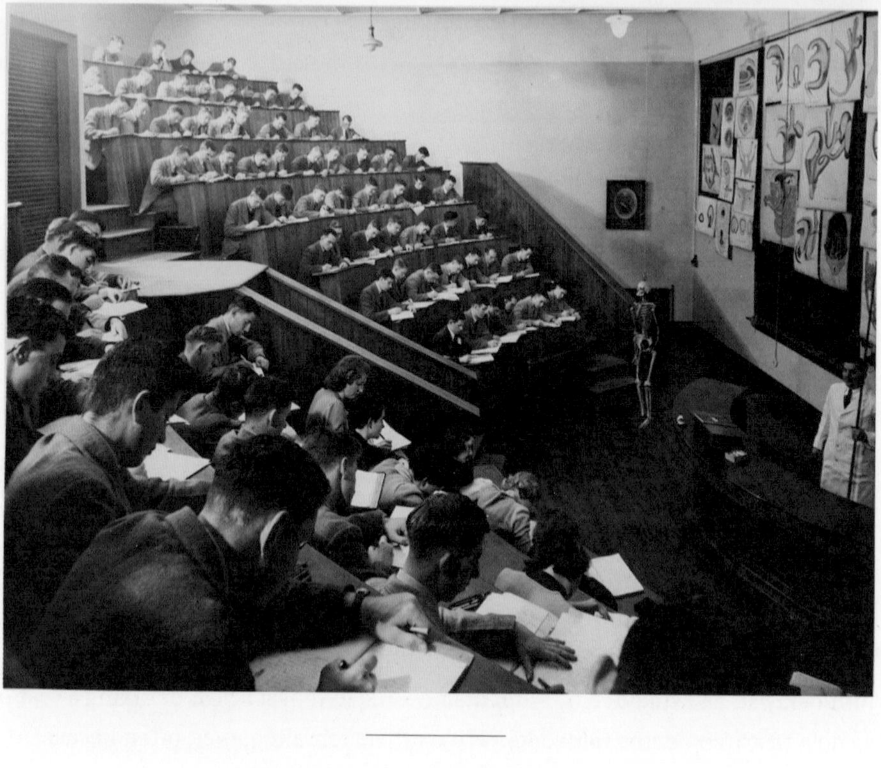

ABOVE: The Otago Medical School Anatomy Museum, 1949. *Hocken Collections Uare Taoka o Hākena, Prime Minister's Department photograph, Box-184-023*

BELOW: An anatomy lecture in progress at Otago Medical School, 1949. *Hocken Collections Uare Taoka o Hākena, Prime Minister's Department photograph, Box-184-024*

Despite over 400 women graduating during this time period, only 5 per cent of the 1995 obituaries published in the *New Zealand Medical Journal* between 1887 and 2017 are of women (and not all of them trained in New Zealand). The statistics do not get any better in the literature. From its inception through to the present day, Otago Medical School has produced six formal histories. The focus of all the histories is predominantly on the achievements of men, which is perhaps understandable considering that all the early lecturers and professors were medical men and that medical women were barred from most social events until the late 1960s.

But the attitudes of the authors towards topics such as the experience of women students are naïve at best. For example, in their history of the medical school, Charles Hercus and Gordon Bell opened their chapter on 'Women of the Otago Medical School' with the line: 'The women of the Otago Medical School merit a book to themselves, but that is beyond our competence.'[45] And in 1945 during his discussion of Siedeberg's experience of having flesh thrown at her during a laboratory session or being asked to leave the room for certain anatomy lectures, Dudley Jones, editor the annals of the medical school, wrote: 'Happily, the personal recollections of Miss Siedeberg . . . were of a less unpleasant nature.'[46] It is highly likely that Siedeberg felt constrained in what she could say at the time, since the future of women's acceptance to the medical school rested on her shoulders.

Outside of Otago Medical School histories, literature focusing specifically on women in New Zealand medicine has increased since the late 1980s, notably in writing by Michael Belgrave, Dorothy Page, Kathleen Anderson and John Armstrong.[47] In 1990 Margaret Maxwell published a book that featured short biographies of 14 prominent women doctors in New Zealand.[48] A larger publication followed in 1994 written by the New Zealand Women's Medical Association (NZWMA). In *The Goods' Train Doctors*, Jill McIlraith collated the oral accounts of more than 20 women who discussed their experiences of medical school, the difficulties of entering a male-dominated field, and the changes they brought to Aotearoa New Zealand's healthcare system.[49]

Four years later, the NZWMA initiated the Stories of Diversity and Success oral history project, which recorded interviews with seven prominent women doctors.[50] These interviews are stored at the Alexander Turnbull Library alongside other oral history interviews with women graduates from this period conducted by other groups.[51] At present, there are at least 25 interviews. In addition, several medical graduates have published autobiographies. In 2016 Cynthia (Cindy) Farquhar of the University of Auckland established the Early Medical Women of New Zealand (EMWoNZ) oral history project which, over the past nine years, has recorded over 70 interviews with medical graduates or their families and written over 150 detailed biographies, using recorded oral and written histories.

One of the contributors to this gap in Aotearoa New Zealand's history is the lack of adequate documentation. The graduation lists held by Otago Medical School do not include the full list of medical graduates, in part because graduates did not have to return to Dunedin to graduate in person. Also, it was common for students to take longer than the recommended time to complete the five- or six-year course. Many students repeated at least one year, particularly in the early days, meaning that entrance records do not always match graduation records. Unfortunately, many class and grade lists have been destroyed, and although identification photos were taken of each student from the 1950s, the remaining records are incomplete.

Gaps in the documentation can be filled by researching other archival sources. The PapersPast archive, for example, has digitised newspaper records nationwide from 1839 through to 1989.[52] For the entire period from 1896 to 1967, newspapers reported on births, deaths, marriages, school prizegivings and awards, university rankings, classes passed in universities, graduations, declarations of intent to apply for registration, locations of practices and attendees at social events. Nevertheless, documentation such as this tells only one side of the story.

This book aims to fill some of the gaps in the history of New Zealand's medical past by providing a comprehensive account of the experiences of women at Otago Medical School and in their subsequent careers. It draws together secondary literature, archival research and oral histories. Through interviews, graduates have presented their personal interpretation of the past, thus adding to the repository of knowledge.[53]

It is another step towards a more complete history of New Zealand's medical women. The research used is drawn primarily from the EMWoNZ oral history project whose research has relied on graduates who are still living and have been willing to record their oral history, or families of graduates who have contacted the project. Where the project has not been able to contact family members, the focus has generally been on women who have been mentioned most often in the archives or in published sources.

The project also focuses on the medical graduates who were 'firsts' — such as the first Māori, Samoan, Fijian-Indian, Jewish and Chinese graduates, or the first women to obtain a position or fellowship — in order to bring greater awareness to the achievements of medical women. Thus, while the project has highlighted the experiences of a greater number of medical women, it still only paints half of the picture, and there is still work to be done.

This book does not attempt to provide a 'factual' history of women students at the medical school or of women doctors during their varied careers. Every woman experienced her training and career differently and encountered different circumstances. This has sometimes led to conflicting accounts. Memory and hindsight play an important role in how events are recalled, and experiences recounted later in life may have a different narrative than those told as events unfolded. Importantly, the aim of the EMWoNZ project was to allow medical women to tell *their* stories, often for the first time.

Where an oral history could not be recorded, we used secondary and archival sources to establish the most accurate picture possible in order to write the biography. In instances where medical graduates were no longer alive, we interviewed their descendants, who told us what they knew of their relatives' experiences. Where oral histories have been recorded, they have been edited and supplemented with extra research.

These published biographies were given final approval by the participants themselves, or by their families, where possible. This means that there are certain gaps in the narrative where participants have decided to withhold information for reasons of privacy. In her history of refugees in New Zealand the historian Ann Beaglehole wrote:

> In presenting oral history, the writer's primary responsibility is to the people interviewed. The most important thing is to convey as accurately as possible the perspectives of the informants. Ideally, the informants' recollections should be presented in full, unedited and uninterrupted by comment, analysis or interpretation. The eloquence of the interviewees is also justification for keeping a writer's intrusion to the minimum. The role of the interviewer/researcher is merely to link together the

> interviewees' comments . . . However, in this book, it was decided to use the collected material differently . . . Informants have not been quoted in full, uninterrupted by comment or interpretation, but an attempt has been made to preserve the individuality of their personal statements while placing these within an analytic framework.[54]

A similar method has been used for this book. Biographies published on the EMWoNZ website comprise direct quotations from the interviews to maintain the authenticity of each woman's account. This book, however, places these same interviews in a more analytical framework to bring together the varied experiences into one coherent discussion and draw connections between experiences and broader contexts.

It is also important to note how this book refers to individual women. Most graduates who married did so after they completed their studies. Many then chose to practise under their married names, and it was by these names that they became well known in their communities. Some women married while at medical school, and a few who married chose to practise under their maiden names. For clarity, this book refers to the women by the names by which they became well known — even if it is different from their names as students.

For example, the first medical graduate, Emily Hancock Siedeberg, married late in life, and although she changed her surname to Siedeberg-McKinnon, she was mostly known as Siedeberg, and she is referred to by that name in this book. Susanna Williams (née Lemchen) married after completing her studies, and practised under her married name, Williams, for the rest of her career; this book thus refers to her as Susanna Williams. We have noted and celebrate the awarding of titles such as professors and damehoods, but we have chosen not to use honorifics throughout. Finally, we have given the graduation dates for each woman at her first mention in the text.

Chapters 1–4 deal with specific periods in the history of Otago Medical School, defined by wider societal events such as two world wars, a pandemic and the 1930s Depression that had an impact on student life and the clinical years (the last three years of study that were spent in a hospital rotation). Chapters 5 and 6 cover the decades 1948 to 1967; they include the postwar years, and the increasing role of women doctors in advocacy both at home and abroad. Chapter 7 analyses the complete time period of the book (1896–1967) with a focus on the achievements of women doctors in medical research.

In covering the period from 1896 to 1967 in this way, this book presents a new understanding of Otago Medical School and of the wider field of the study of medicine in New Zealand in the years before the second medical school opened, in Auckland. From its foundation, Otago Medical School was one of the most progressive medical schools in the Commonwealth. Nevertheless, New Zealand continued to be a relatively conservative society, and it was slow to accept women doctors. The women of this period paved the way for later women medical graduates and the establishment of a fairer health system for all New Zealanders.

Otago Medical School in 1901. The copy of this photograph in the medical school archives does not give names, but 10 women are pictured; some may have been members of staff. Agatha Monfries (née Adams; 1904) and Emily Nees (née Ridley; 1904) are in the second row, fifth and seventh from the right, respectively. The first Māori graduate, Peter Buck Te Rangi Hīroa, is in the third row from the front, fifth from the right. A male graduate is pictured holding a skeleton wearing a hat: in the early days this was not uncommon in class photos and perhaps indicates a way of coming to terms with learning about the basics of the human body by humanising a body skeleton. *Otago Medical School Archives*

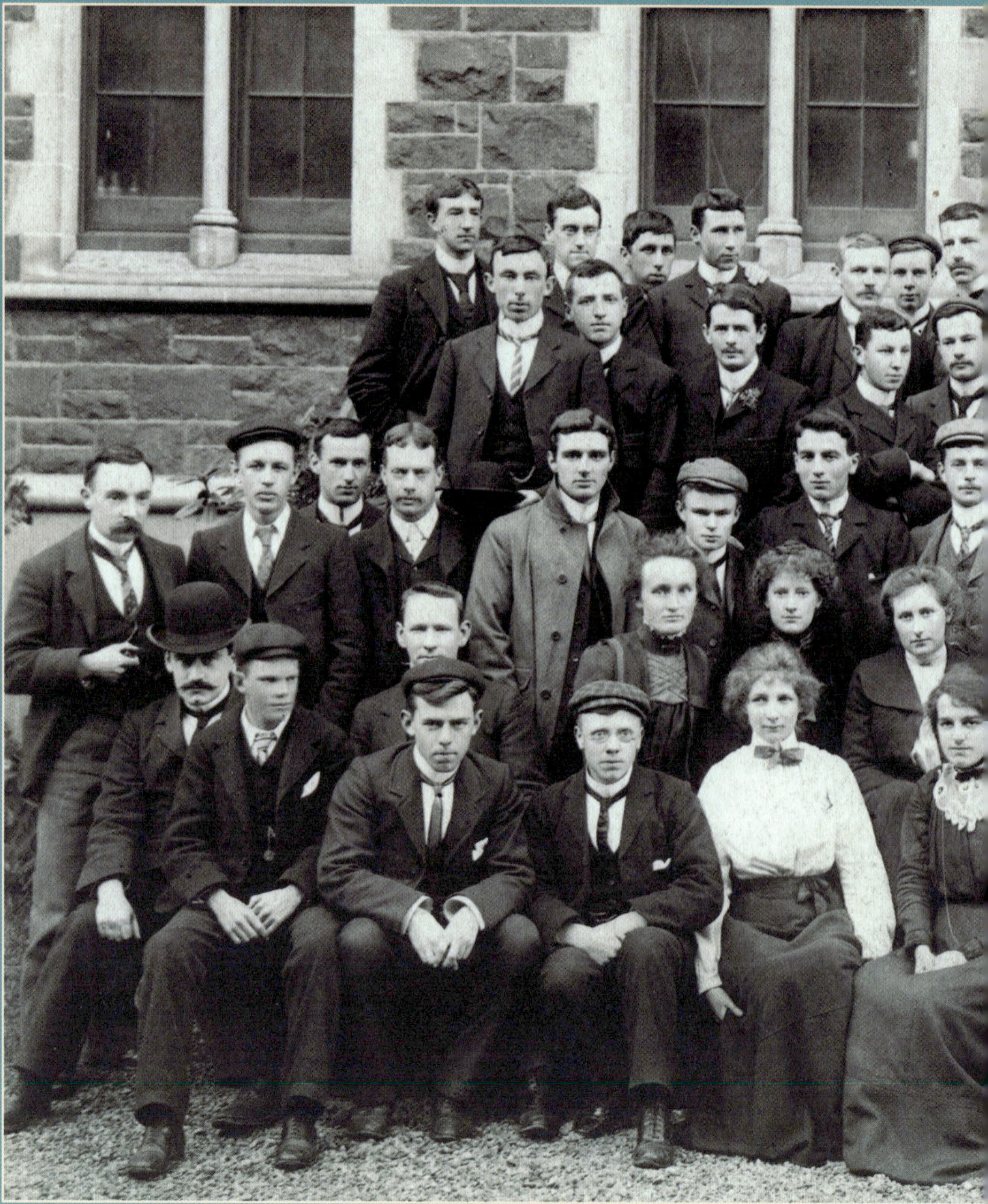

1. The pioneers 1891–1913

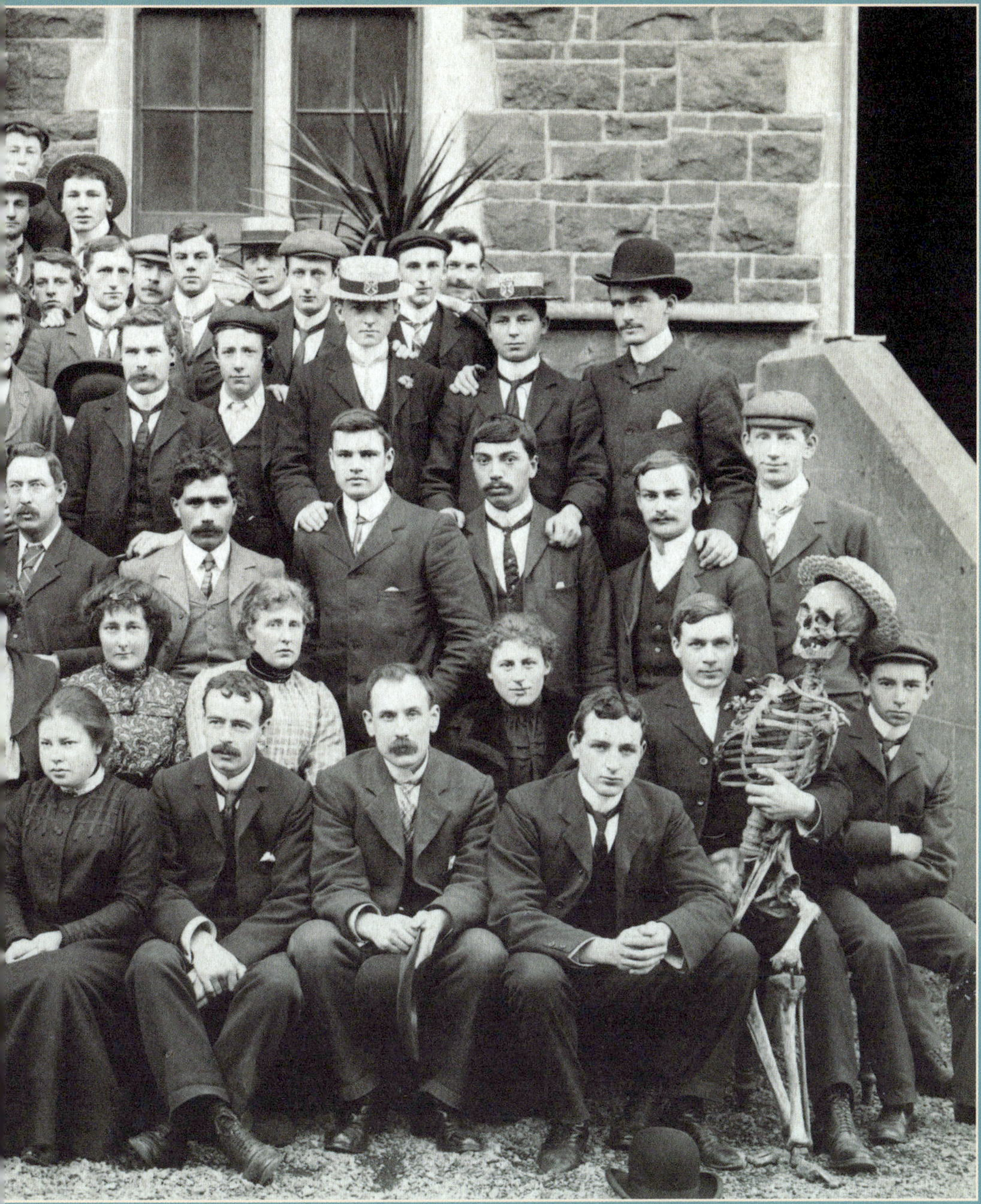

On 10 March 1891, 18-year-old Emily Hancock Siedeberg, a Dunedin-born graduate of Otago Girls' High School (OGHS), submitted a letter to the University of Otago expressing her desire to enrol in Otago Medical School. She explained that she had completed the necessary preliminary examinations and hoped now to proceed to a degree in medicine. She requested not only acceptance to attend the classes but also to receive the degree, should she successfully pass the examinations.[1]

This request was significant. Until 1885, because of inadequate resources, the medical school had offered only a two-year medical course, with the assumption that students would complete their studies at one of the approved universities 'back Home' in Britain. Yet most of these universities were not open to women, and of those that were, some only allowed women to attend classes but not to sit the final examinations and receive the degree.[2] Only the London School of Medicine for Women, established in 1874, admitted women for the full degree, and this remained the case until 1886, when the Edinburgh School of Medicine for Women was founded.[3]

Despite the relatively liberal attitudes circulating in Dunedin society in 1891, Siedeberg did not receive a resounding 'yes' from either of the bodies — the University of Otago Council and the Hospital Board — she applied to. All nine university staff members were willing to admit her, although two believed that women should be taught separately.[4] The problem lay with the hospital. Of the nine hospital staff members, six voted against Siedeberg's admission. Eventually, they decided to accept her, based on the fact that the university had accepted her.[5]

Emily Siedeberg truly paved the way for other women. She excelled at her

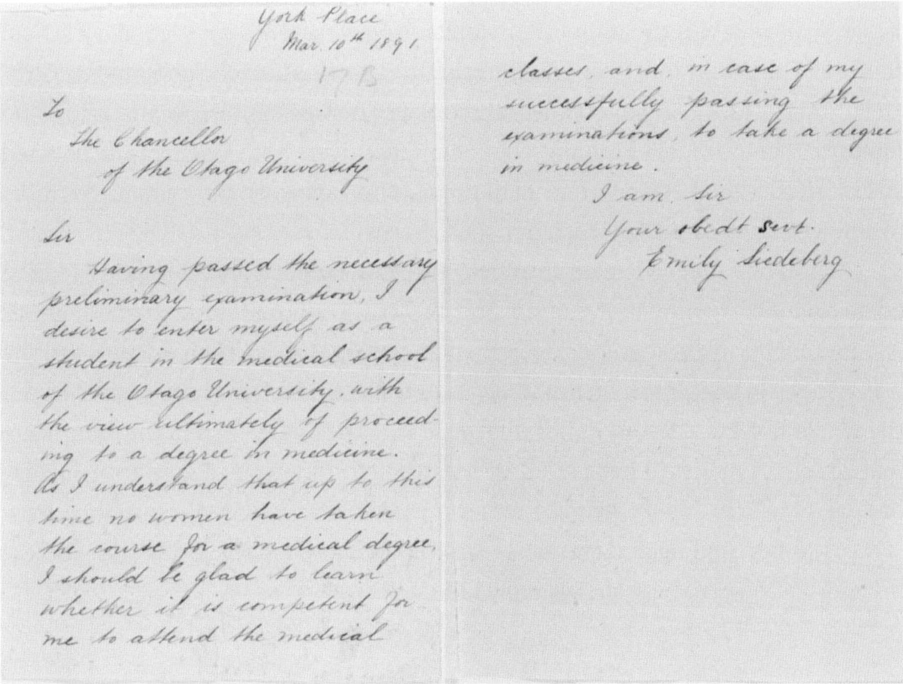

York Place
Mar. 10th 1891

17B

To
The Chancellor
of the Otago University

Sir

Having passed the necessary preliminary examination, I desire to enter myself as a student in the medical school of the Otago University, with the view ultimately of proceeding to a degree in medicine. As I understand that up to this time no women have taken the course for a medical degree, I should be glad to learn whether it is competent for me to attend the medical classes, and, in case of my successfully passing the examinations, to take a degree in medicine.

I am, Sir
Your obedt servt.
Emily Siedeberg

The letter written on 10 March 1891 by Emily Siedeberg to the chancellor of the University of Otago.
University of Otago Medical Library Historical Collection, MS-1689/001

---

studies and did not create waves, despite being targeted by some of her male peers.[6] She also encouraged Margaret Cruickshank (1897), a fellow OGHS graduate, to join her in the medical programme.[7]

The number of women graduates continued to fluctuate in the years before the First World War; most years there was only one. There were three in 1904; four in 1900; and none in 1898, 1899, 1901, 1905, 1907–09 and 1912–13. Each woman who entered the programme performed well and graduated within five to eight years,[8] an achievement that can be attributed in part to the educational background from which they came. Of the 14 who graduated before the First World War, nine had attended OGHS, and one had attended Braemar House, a private school in Moray Place, Dunedin, founded in 1894.[9]

The high percentage of Otago-raised graduates is also explained by their being able to continue living at home while studying, something many parents preferred over their daughters travelling overseas. Of the very early graduates,

Jessie Maddison was the only other woman to have attended a secondary school that was equipped to deliver an education to young women: Christchurch Girls' High.[10] Alice Horsley (née Woodward; 1900) was home-schooled so that she could look after her mother and siblings, but her parents were both teachers and ensured she received a good education in all of the required subjects; they employed tutors for subjects they could not teach her.[11]

Ina Moody (née Dugleby; 1910) was the only medical graduate in this era to come from a truly rural background. She was an exceptional student: not only was she in a higher class than her age group at Napier District High School, but she was also top of the class in many subjects, and she received the top overall score in the whole of New Zealand in her final year of schooling.[12] Despite this, her name had largely been lost to history, as all records before Dorothy Page's 2008 history of Otago Medical School referred to her mistakenly as Ingleby.[13] Constance Frost (1900) was born in England and arrived in New Zealand at the age of 17, and there is no information on where she was educated.[14]

We know little about why these young women chose to study medicine, or about their experiences at medical school. Emily Siedeberg was encouraged by her parents, and she, in turn, encouraged Margaret Cruickshank. Eleanor McLaglan (née Baker; 1903) was astonished when her parents first told her that they intended for her to study medicine.[15] Agatha Monfries (née Adams; 1904) was most likely encouraged by her brother, who had enrolled at the medical school two years before she did. Jane Kinder and Daisy Platts-Mills (née Platts), both graduates of 1900, worked for five and six years, respectively, before enrolling: Kinder taught at a secondary school and Platts-Mills worked as a governess. Was this a change of career direction, or did they work in order to build up a nest egg to cover the course fees and living costs of the five-year programme?

The only other detailed accounts of very early medical school experiences come from Eleanor McLaglan, who wrote a memoir; Catharine Brookfield (née Will; 1911), whose son wrote a family history; and Alice Horsley, who talked to her children about her studies and career. These women's experiences corroborate some of the complaints of their male peers: the hours were long (classes started at 9 am and finished around 7 pm, after which students were expected to study), and some of the lectures were dull and not well taught.[16]

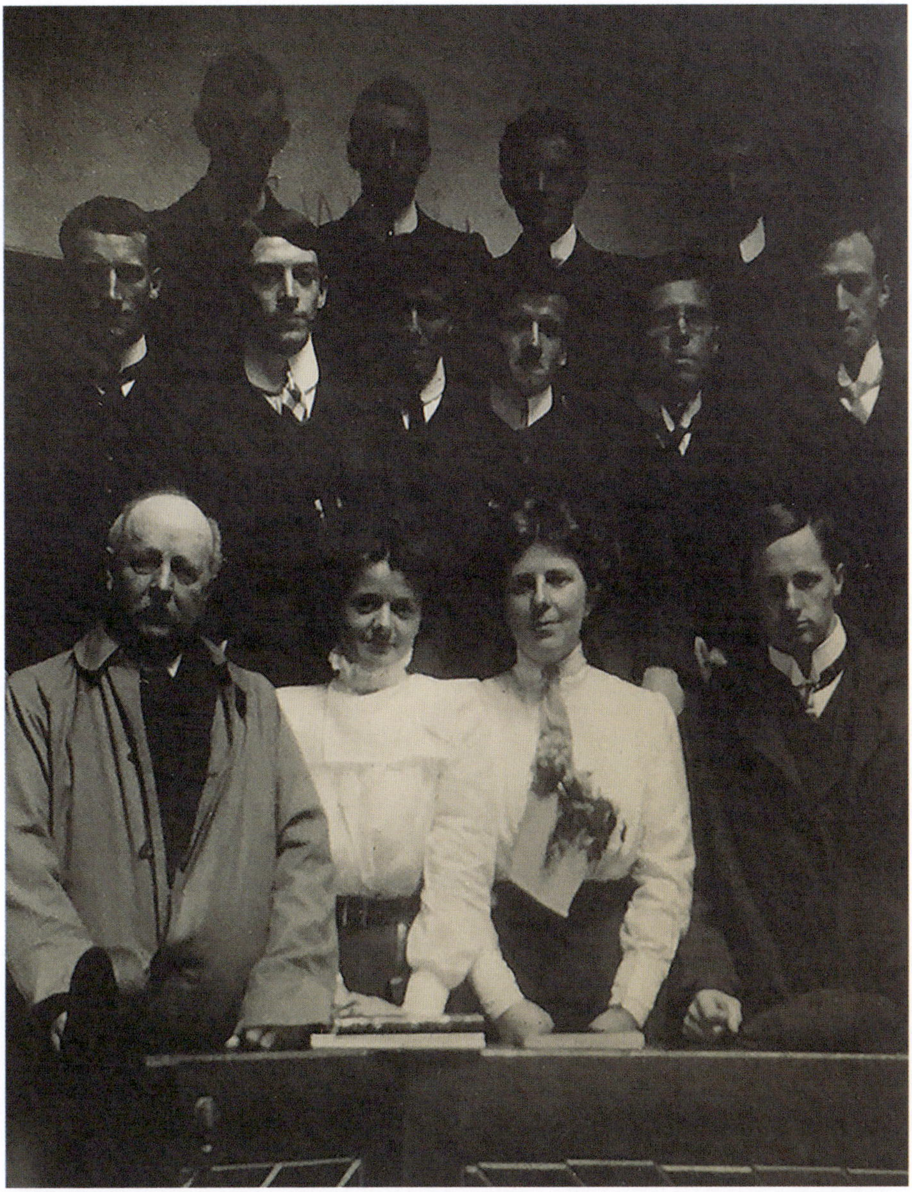

Medical students in a lecture theatre, c.1910. Front from left: Professor Daniel Colquhoun, Violet Field (Edinburgh graduate), Catharine Brookfield (née Will), R. B. P. Monson. Middle: H. O'Callaghan, P. Ardagh, W. P. Johnston, W. B. Wishart, H. D. Robertson, R. W. Edgar. Back: D. R. Fenwick, H. L. Widdowson, A. O. Evans, J. E. Brown. *McMillan family collection*

The major differences for the women were that many felt behind on topics such as physics that had not been offered at their schools; and that they were asked to leave the room for some topics the male professors felt uncomfortable explaining to mixed classes. As mentioned in the Introduction, Alice Horsley recounted one of the lecturers announcing, '"I now come to the part of my lectures I refuse to give before women. Therefore the women must leave the room or I will leave," and they were forced to retreat to "hoots, jeers and stamping".'[17]

Eleanor McLaglan recorded the strict rules about uniforms — something many of the women graduates mentioned right through to 1967.[18] Women were expected to wear 'a black or navy full-flared serge skirt which swept the ground . . . a cotton shirt blouse, white or striped, a high starched collar and a straw boater hat . . . Corsets were tight and designed to produce the hourglass shaped figure.'[19] McLaglan also mentioned an occasion on which a lecturer mistook her for the only other woman in the class and told her that she had not done well enough to sit finals; she had actually come top of the class.[20]

McLaglan recalled that the women students generally sat together at the front of the classroom. Some claimed this was for 'protection' from the men; others that the lecturers required it. Historian Kathleen Anderson, however, has explained that since there were only ever between one and four women in any given class in the early years, it would have been unusual if they had not sat together.[21] McLaglan remembered when the women students started arriving early to lectures to claim seats at the back and avoid being the victims of the occasional peashooter attack.[22]

The degree was five years long (it became a six-year course in 1920), including the medical intermediate examination. Completing the medical intermediate year was a requirement before being accepted to the medical degree course, but it could be undertaken at any of the four university colleges, located in Dunedin, Christchurch, Wellington and Auckland. Information on where they completed their medical intermediate year was available for only seven of the 14 women: four in Dunedin, two in Auckland and one in Christchurch.[23] Presumably the other seven had completed the course in Dunedin, as they had attended OGHS and were already in the area.

Newspaper reports of examinations show that Emily Siedeberg, Margaret Cruickshank, Daisy Platts-Mills and Agatha Monfries took the expected five years to complete the course. Alice Horsley, Eleanor McLaglan, Emily Nees (née Ridley; 1904), Ada Paterson (1906), Ina Moody and Catharine Brookfield took five or six

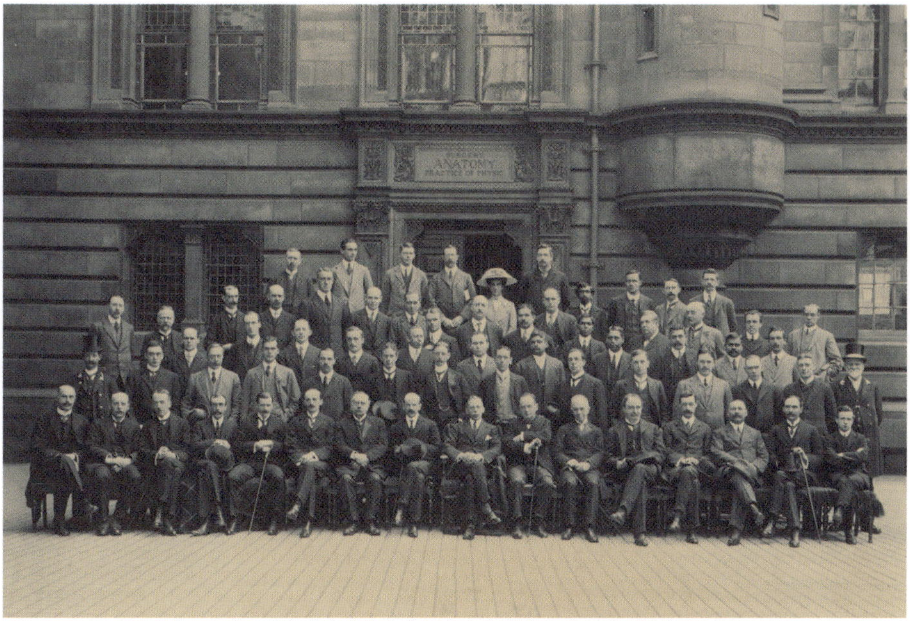

Emily Siedeberg, wearing a broad-brimmed hat, with her fellow University of Edinburgh medical students in 1912. *Hocken Collections Uare Taoka o Hākena, Andrew Swan Watson photograph, P2018-013-163*

---

years — it is unclear whether this was because they had to repeat courses in the medical intermediate or the medical degree itself. Jane Kinder took six years, Jessie Maddison seven and Constance Frost eight, but this was not unduly long. William Christie, the first male to graduate from Otago Medical School in 1887, took six years. The woman who took the least time — a mere four years — was Winifrede Bathgate (1904). She had already completed a BSc and presumably did not have to do the intermediate year.

In general, we know more about the lives and careers of these women after graduation. At some point in their careers (either directly after graduation, such as Siedeberg, or many years later, such as Cruickshank), six travelled overseas for postgraduate education, which at this point was not available in New Zealand. Popular destinations were the Rotunda or Coombe hospitals in Dublin, the School of Medicine for Women at the University of Edinburgh, a hospital in Berlin (possibly the Charité), or any of the teaching hospitals in London. Cruickshank was the only woman graduate from Otago Medical School in this era to obtain a Doctor of Medicine (MD).

All 14 of these early women went on to practise medicine, and many were successful. Six opened their own general practices, and one bought an already established practice from a retiring doctor.[24] These early practices were based in their homes, making it easier to combine having a career and a family.[25] Eleanor McLaglan began a career in the School Medical Service in 1914. She was seconded there to do research on goitre, which she had identified as a problem in certain geographical areas. She was hired by Charles Hercus, who later became a worldwide authority on public health, to travel around New Zealand examining the thyroid glands of school students. Hercus created a map of the incidence of goitre and low iodine levels in the soil based on her figures, and this data eventually led to the introduction of iodine as a supplement in table salt in New Zealand.[26]

Many of these women held more than one job. Emily Siedeberg, Alice Horsley and Daisy Platts-Mills, for example, spent most of their working lives in their private practices, but they also all had adjunct positions — in anaesthetics at the hospital, clinic consultations for a few hours a week or vaccination services at local pharmacies — in order to make a living. Siedeberg and Horsley had at least three additional appointments, not including their volunteer positions, and Platts-Mills had at least four.

In these cases, some may have chosen to do the extra work, perhaps wanting to help their communities, but other women worked several jobs because they struggled to find a permanent or stable role. Eleanor McLaglan had at least 16 appointments throughout her career, none of which lasted long. Constance Frost was forced to reapply for her job at Auckland Hospital every year for 17 years because the hospital was determined to find a male doctor to replace her. She had to supplement her work at the hospital with other jobs in the community because, at first, the post was unpaid. The board finally employed her full-time in 1918, only two years before her premature death in 1920 from influenza.

The fact that these women managed to at least find a position in New Zealand, whether permanent or not, stands in contrast to those who studied overseas and then came home. Historian Michael Belgrave has argued that many New Zealand-born women who trained in Britain and then returned after their studies were unsuccessful in establishing their own practices, and some even went so far as to warn prospective medical students away from the career because of the difficulties in making a living.[27] The problem seemed to lie in 'breaking in' to the market.

The successful women, such as Siedeberg and Horsley, often had the financial backing of their families as they established themselves; McLaglan, whose parents had died before her graduation, attributed her struggle to find a footing in the New Zealand market to her lack of financial backing. This pushed her into what she considered an 'undesirable job' at the School Medical Service, a job she believed was regarded as not practising 'proper medicine'.[28]

Studying in New Zealand also allowed the women graduates to make professional connections that seemed to make a difference in establishing their careers. Emily Siedeberg obtained her first job — as locum tenens — from one of her lecturers, Truby King, who was the medical superintendent at Seacliff Lunatic Asylum (as it was then known). King also gave Eleanor McLaglan a job as a medical officer at Seacliff when he took a leave of absence, though as this was a psychiatric hospital there may not have been a lot of competition. When ophthalmology surgeon Lindo Ferguson employed Winifrede Bathgate as his assistant at Dunedin Hospital in 1907, she became the first woman on the clinical staff there.[29] Agatha Monfries obtained a locum at Siedeberg's practice. Other women were successful in establishing a practice or a reputation in their local areas: Platts-Mills in Kurow and Duntroon, McLaglan in Te Kōpuru, Monfries in Taumarunui, Paterson in Picton, Cruickshank in Waimate and Moody in Clinton. They all showed remarkable determination: even those who struggled to find a permanent position managed to keep on working rather than give up their careers.

Five of the 14 women who graduated between 1896 and 1913 died young. Jane Kinder died at the age of 33 of tuberculosis contracted while managing the Torrens Island bubonic plague quarantine station at the mouth of the Port River in Adelaide, Australia, in 1902. Margaret Cruickshank died of influenza in 1918, aged 45, while she was dealing with the epidemic in her South Canterbury community of Waimate. Constance Frost died in her fifties in January 1920 after contracting influenza from her work in the pathology laboratory during the epidemic. Agatha Monfries died of peritonitis in 1911 at the age of 31, two days after she gave birth to her stillborn son. Ina Moody died in 1930, aged 44, after struggling for at least 15 years with unspecified 'health complications'. Her illness had forced her to stop practising after she married.

In 1909 and again in 1913, Ferdinand Campion Batchelor, a lecturer in midwifery at Otago Medical School, stated that admitting women to medicine had been a failed experiment: although he had been 'won over' by women students, he still believed that they were not 'shaping up to the demands of professional medicine'.[30] 'While any fool of a man could succeed in practice, the brightest and most intelligent of women were failing to become established as medical practitioners . . . it was one thing to emerge with a medical degree and quite another to earn a living.'[31] Why spend the time and money training women if they were not going to use the knowledge, critics asked. There were some who thought that medical women only had two options — either 'marry' their career or give it up entirely.[32]

But Batchelor spoke too soon: all of these 14 early women graduates worked after graduating. Only Catharine Brookfield and Ina Moody stopped practising once they married. The other six graduates who married continued to practise. In fact, Daisy Platts-Mills' son said that it was because his mother continued to work that the family did not fall into financial ruin. Alice Horsley's husband's successful pharmacy business enabled her to provide her services free of charge to those in need. We cannot know what would have happened if Margaret Cruickshank, Constance Frost and Jane Kinder had not died prematurely, but it can be agreed that the careers of at least six women in this era were not affected by societal pressure to cease practice once they married, a pressure that diminished in the coming decades.[33]

Although some women experienced difficulties finding permanent employment in a system that was not open and receptive to women achieving a higher education, most succeeded in some degree in their ambition to have a medical career. In doing so they were paving the way for later generations. They were able to establish practices and developed reputations for being kind, caring, vital members of society. Indeed Cruickshank, Horsley, Frost and Kinder put themselves in harm's way — sometimes with disastrous consequences — and they all left a legacy of research and advocacy that opened doors for later graduates.

EMILY HANCOCK SIEDEBERG-MCKINNON (NÉE SIEDEBERG)

1896 graduate — first woman medical graduate in New Zealand, first woman to establish a private practice in Dunedin

When she was 10 years old, Emily Siedeberg overheard her parents in discussion: 'I think we will make a doctor of Emily,' her father said.[34] Her first thought was, 'Only men are doctors', but she later decided that 'it would be a grand life'.[35] Siedeberg, born on 17 February 1873 to Anna Thompson, a Northern Irish Quaker, and Franz David Siedeberg, a Jewish architect from Prussia, grew up in a family that was relatively liberal in the context of late nineteenth-century New Zealand.[36] Franz Siedeberg had high expectations for his daughter from a young age. His opinions about education were progressive, and when the family moved to Dunedin for his work, they also found the best city in New Zealand for girls' education. The booming city was a hub of activism in education as well as suffrage.

Franz Siedeberg had bought his daughter the book *Our Famous Women*, which covered the struggles of the Blackwell sisters and other eminent women 'who have won their way from poverty and obscurity to fame and glory'. According to Siedeberg's niece, this book 'opened up vistas of what life meant, the struggles ahead, the difficulties to overcome. She had been shown a purpose in life and so grew up with the sure knowledge that it was her destiny to be a doctor.'[37]

Siedeberg attended the Normal School on Moray Place, where she did so well that she received a National Board scholarship to attend Otago Girls' High School. These scholarships, which could be life-changing for families who could not otherwise afford to send their daughters to secondary school, were offered annually to 'the most deserving pupils of the primary schools. The winner of such a scholarship is entitled to free tuition at one of the secondary schools established in the principal towns of the district.'[38] According to an 1890s' report on women's education, the scholarships could also provide a pathway to university: 'It thus frequently happens that a clever child of poor parents gains a District Scholarship after free attendance for a few years at a primary school, and so passes without expense to a secondary school, where in due time, a University Junior Scholarship is won, and presently, the highest honours which the University can give.'[39]

Siedeberg attended OGHS until age 17, when she began the process of enrolling

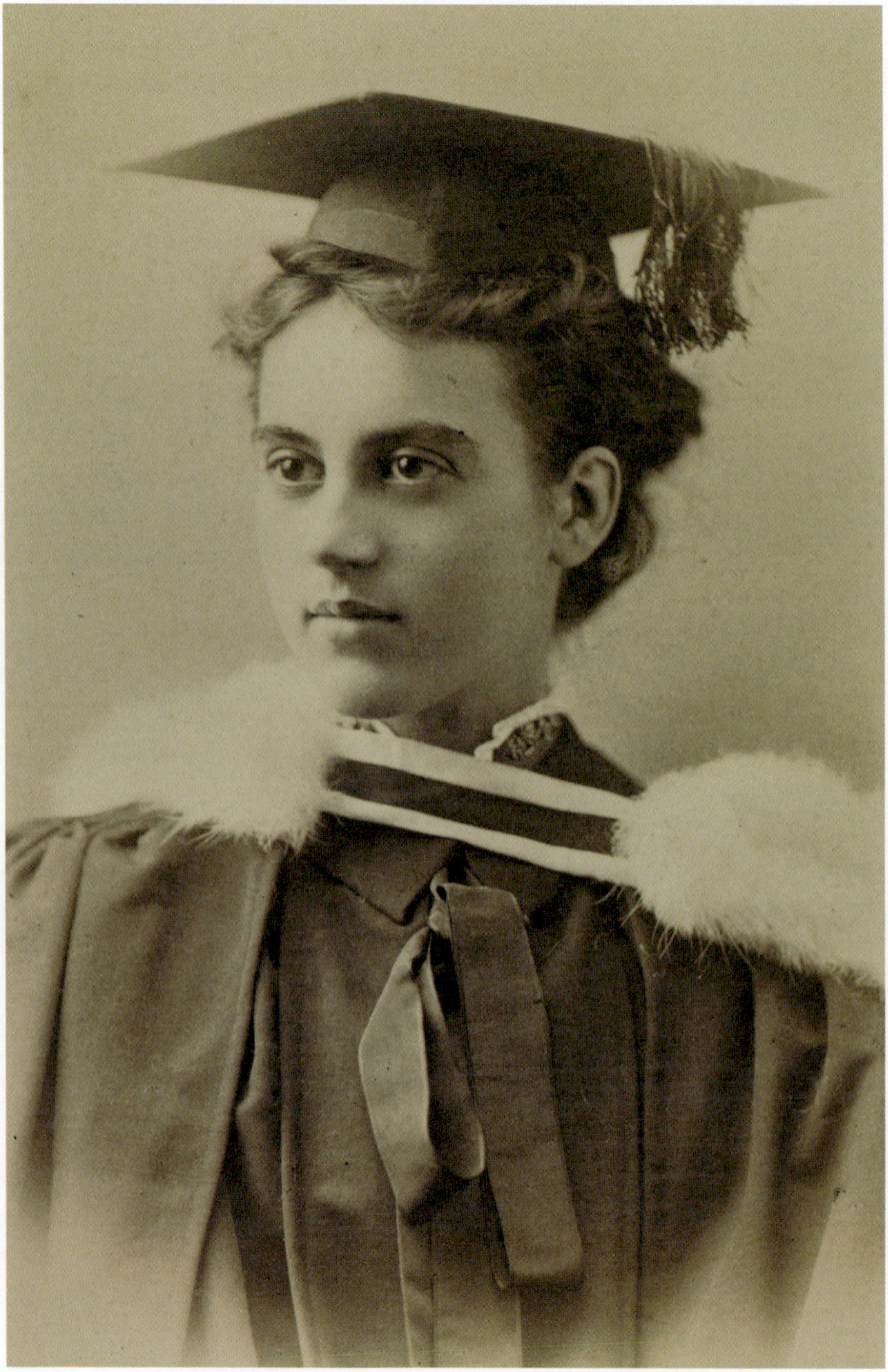

Emily Siedeberg at her graduation in 1896. *Hocken Collections Uare Taoka o Hākena, F. L. Jones photograph, Box-148-002*

in Otago Medical School.[40] The process for admission was gruelling, and no woman had yet been successful.[41] Despite initial hesitation from the university and hospital staff, her application was accepted,[42] and on 29 April 1891 her name was added to the register of medical students at the University of Otago.[43]

The dean, John Halliday Scott, was quite upfront with Siedeberg about how she would need to conduct herself in order to be accepted by the men in her classes:

> He led me to understand that the attitude of the students towards me would depend entirely on how I conducted myself. The good old Victorian mothers had trained their daughters in self-respect — 'keep men at a distance, don't allow them to touch you or take liberties, never show your feelings or look invitingly at them'. So I behaved accordingly and no frivolities or incidents of much importance occurred in the dissecting room or elsewhere.[44]

Scott told her that if she could hold her own in a class of students who were prone to doing pranks, then she would be just fine.[45] Her mother had also advised her to 'keep men at a distance and never to show her feelings'.[46]

+ + +

Siedeberg completed her studies within the standard five years and graduated in 1896 with an MB ChB (Bachelor of Medicine, Bachelor of Surgery), making her the first woman medical graduate in New Zealand.[47] She then left for Ireland, where she studied at Rotunda Hospital in Dublin and gained a postgraduate Diploma in Obstetrics,[48] followed by postgraduate courses in gynaecology and children's health and skin diseases at a university in Berlin.[49] She returned to Dunedin at the end of 1897 and set up her own practice, which she maintained for 30 years.[50]

For the first two decades, she was the only woman medical practitioner in Dunedin.[51] Business was initially slow but she was able to continue with help from her father, who gave her a house in York Place with consulting and waiting rooms and a horse and gig for making house calls. Her first patients were women and children, and she slowly built up her practice with her reputation for never saying no when someone needed help, no matter the conditions: 'day or night, hail, snow or storm, in good health or off-colour'.[52]

In 1900, Siedeberg was appointed as the honorary medical officer for the Dunedin branch of the Society for the Protection of Women and Children, and in 1905 she was appointed the first medical officer (and later superintendent) of St Helens maternity hospital in Dunedin, where she established the first antenatal clinic in New Zealand in 1918.[53] From 1907 to 1930 she was the medical officer at the Caversham Industrial School (later the Girls' Receiving Home).[54] She became renowned for her midwifery work and in 1920, 'she recorded proudly that she had not a case of eclampsia (toxaemia) for 11 years, at a time when this disease was a major killer of women in childbirth'.[55]

Although Siedeberg disapproved of prostitution, she was committed to helping prostitutes and other women in need. She took pregnant women into her home and tended to them, delivering and helping to find a home for their babies. When her male colleagues heard what she was doing, they condemned her for it: they believed that she was disgracing the medical profession by helping 'loose' women.[56]

She actively spoke out in favour of women's rights within marriage. She argued that there should be strong measures in place to control venereal disease and that the existence or transmission of these diseases should be a legitimate reason for divorce.[57] In 1899, she had been a founding member of the Dunedin branch of the Society for the Protection of Women and Children, which sought to protect women and children from neglect and abuse.[58] In 1921, she founded the New Zealand Medical Women's Association and was elected as the first president.[59]

Emily Siedeberg was awarded the King's Jubilee Medal in 1935 and was appointed Commander of the Order of the British Empire (CBE) in the King's List of New Zealand Honours in 1949. She was awarded a life membership of the New Zealand branch of the British Medical Association in 1929 and a life membership of the New Zealand Registered Nurses' Association in 1939.[60]

After Siedeberg married a retired banker, James Alexander McKinnon, late in life she stopped working at her practice and concentrated solely on her work at St Helens. In 1941 she was instrumental in building the Otago Pioneer Women's Room, in Moray Place, where Otago women could meet and hold social activities.[61] Siedeberg finally retired in 1938. She died at the age of 95 on 13 June 1968. In her memory, the University of Otago established the Dr Emily Hancock Siedeberg Scholarship, awarded annually to the top woman student across the three clinical schools in the sixth-year graduating class. The city named a street after her in 1993 as part of the Suffrage Centennial Year.

MARGARET BARNETT CRUICKSHANK

1897 graduate — second woman medical graduate in New Zealand, first registered woman medical practitioner in New Zealand, first New Zealand-trained woman to gain a Doctor of Medicine in New Zealand

Margaret Barnett Cruickshank and her twin Christina were born on 1 January 1873 in Palmerston, Otago, to George Cruickshank, a Scottish engineer, and Margaret Taggart.[62] They were the first of seven children, and by the time the last child was born their mother's health was failing. Margaret and Christina helped with caring for the younger children and looking after the house, and after their mother died, they assumed her role and responsibilities.[63]

From the age of 10, they decided to alternate attending school so that one was always home to help the family while the other was learning.[64] The twin who attended school would come home and teach the other in the evening and they would switch every six months.[65] Despite these constraints, they were ahead of their peers by the end of primary school.

The girls went on to Palmerston District High School, where they both did well and were awarded National Board scholarships to attend Otago Girls' High School in Dunedin. The scholarship paid their fees, and their father paid for their board.[66] In 1891, they were joint dux at OGHS and were awarded university junior scholarships to the University of Otago.[67] Christina followed the path of education, but Margaret was unsure what course to enrol in. She discussed her options with a trusted teacher, who encouraged her to speak to fellow OGHS graduate Emily Siedeberg, who encouraged her to pursue medicine.

At first she was hesitant, but later she enrolled in the medical school. She enjoyed the course and graduated with an MB ChB in 1897. Because Emily Siedeberg had travelled to Britain for postgraduate studies before registering, Margaret Cruickshank became the first New Zealand-trained woman medical graduate to register in New Zealand.

Through a former teacher Cruickshank heard that there was a job opening in Waimate for a medical assistant. She travelled there for an interview, was offered the position on the spot, and accepted straight away. The head of the practice was Herbert Clifford Barclay, and she initially boarded with him and his wife, Ruth.

Her first recorded case at the practice was on 3 March 1897, when she acted as anaesthetist for a surgery performed by Barclay. She continued in this role, as well as seeing patients, until 20 March 1898, when she performed her first surgery and Barclay administered the anaesthetics.

+++

Cruickshank became a partner in the clinic in 1900, and by 1908 she was performing the majority of the surgeries. She spent most of her time at Barclay's private practice but she also obtained a position at the local school, and later at the public hospital.[68] Meanwhile, she continued her studies. In 1903 she graduated MD from the University of Otago — the first of three postgraduate qualifications she would obtain throughout her career.

Cruickshank did not report any hostility from her male colleagues during her career in Waimate; indeed, after her arrival in 1897 the *Waimate Times* wished her well: 'The day of the lady doctor, like the women's franchise and the labour legislation, seems to be upon us . . . We cannot do less than wish this clever pioneer much happiness and success in the profession she has selected.'[69]

Some of her success in Waimate has been attributed to her knowledge of the difficulties of rural life. She was happy to walk the many miles between clients and, while at their homes, often helped with the housework. Like many doctors of this era, she asked her patients to pay for her services only if they were able to. This trait of going above and beyond was typical of many of the early women doctors but it was exacerbated when the number of doctors increased and many struggled to find paid work.

Cruickshank was a firm believer in educating the public about medical and other matters. After a railway accident in Waimate, the town established a St John Ambulance and medical course, and she was chosen as the lecturer for first-aid classes. The community responded positively to these courses and her colleagues at Waimate Hospital thanked her for her work.

Between 1909 and 1912, a woman doctor writing under the pseudonym of 'Margaret Faithful' contributed articles to the *White Ribbon*, the magazine of the Women's Christian Temperance Movement, that covered a range of topics from the promotion of healthy living and nutritional information on certain foods and diets to an explanation of common illnesses.[70] It has never been confirmed, but

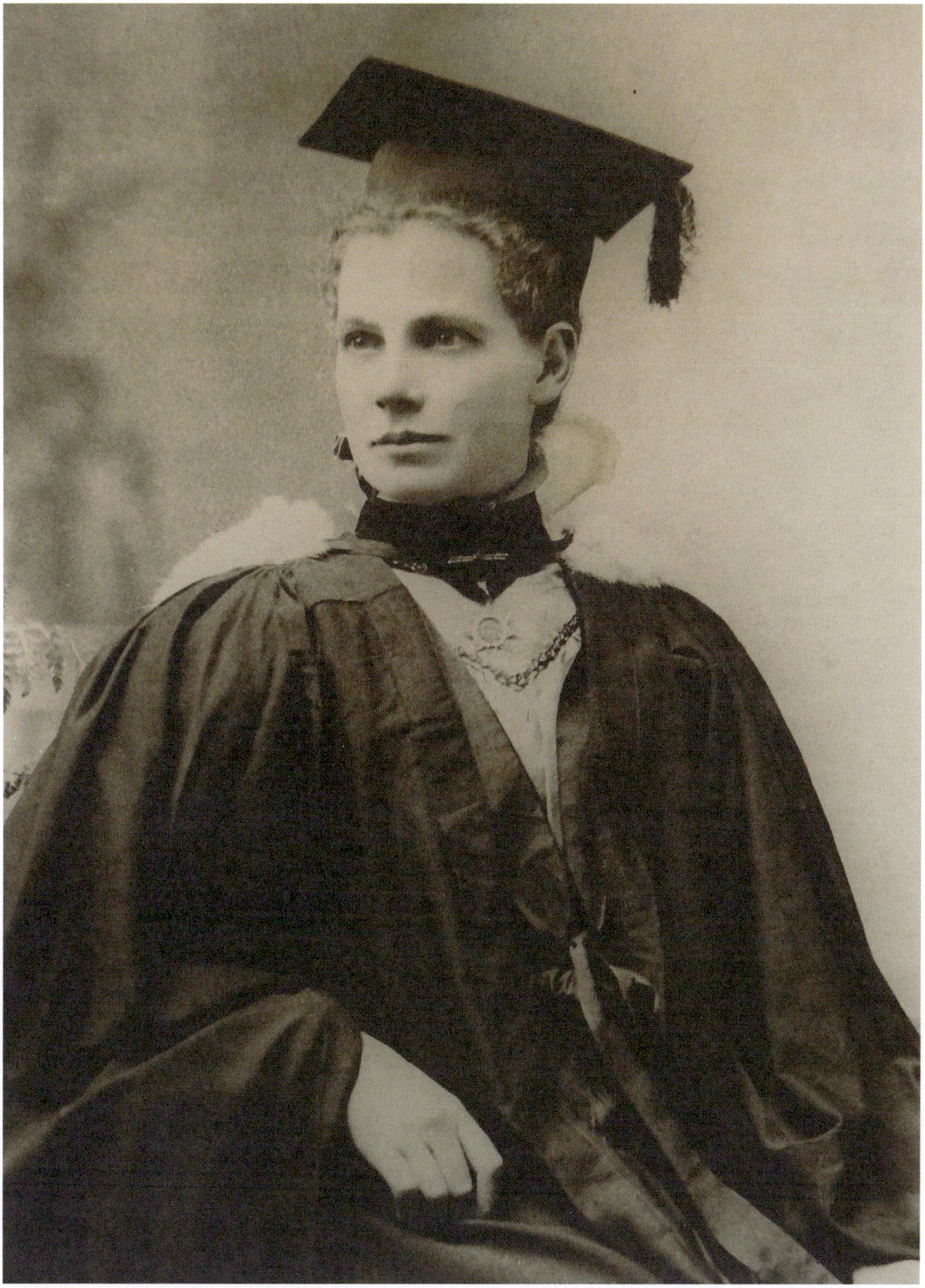

Margaret Cruickshank photographed following
her graduation ceremony in 1897. *Waimate Museum*

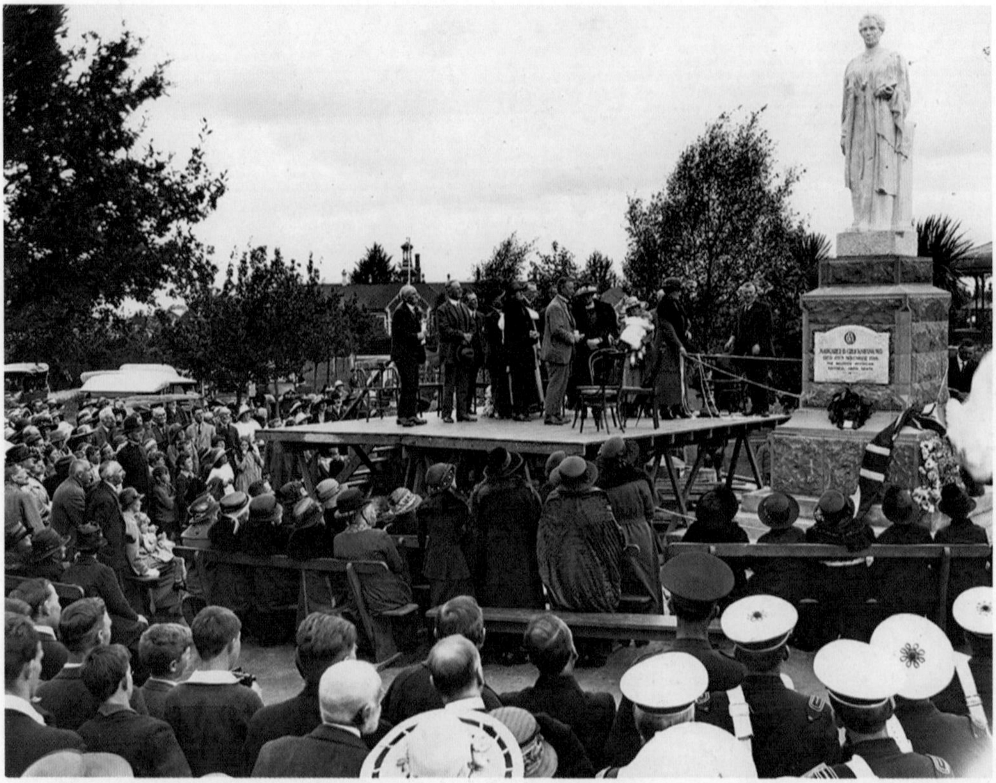

The unveiling of the statue erected in memory of Margaret Cruickshank in 1922 in Waimate. *Waimate Museum*

Criuckshank is assumed to have been the author — partly because of the nature of the content but also because the articles stopped appearing the year she left Waimate for a year-long overseas holiday.

On her trip abroad in 1913, Cruickshank visited America and Italy and then went to Britain, where she completed postgraduate courses in Edinburgh and Dublin.[71] She also visited the St John Ambulance headquarters in London to find out how she might adapt their courses for a New Zealand audience.

In 1914 Barclay left Waimate on an 18-month sabbatical and Cruickshank returned to manage both the clinic and two patient loads.[72] When war broke out, Barclay informed her that he had joined the Royal Army Medical Corps and would not be returning; he was leaving her in sole charge of the clinic.[73] Cruickshank took on these increased responsibilities for the next four years, alongside her volunteer work for the Red Cross. In addition, she was appointed superintendent at Waimate Hospital, which included lecturing.

+++

In 1918, the influenza pandemic reached New Zealand, and Cruickshank reported that the local situation was quickly getting out of control. She urged the Waimate District Council to raise hygiene standards at hotels and to close public bars to prevent the spread. Her driver fell ill during the epidemic, so she ended up cycling to visit her patients and continued to attend to as many people as possible, working most days and nights. She eventually became ill with influenza and pneumonia, and on 18 November she was admitted to hospital, where she died 10 days later.[74] On 25 January 1922, five years after her death, the town erected a marble statue in her name. In memory of her service, E. Morrison wrote in 1923:

> We wish that, in years to be, the story should be told of a woman who was brave, and strong, and kind, and true as steel, who had a heart with room for others' sorrows, and hands swift and sure in deeds of loving service; who gave her life as truly for duty's sake as any soldier on the 'gallant, glorious' field. She is dead, but her influence on others is a living thing that cannot die.[75]

ALICE HORSLEY (NÉE WOODWARD)

1900 graduate — first woman doctor employed at Auckland Hospital, first woman doctor to open a private practice in Auckland[76]

Alice Horsley was born on 3 February 1871, the first child of William and Laura Woodward, both originally from England.[77] Her parents' love affair was a whirlwind romance of which neither of their families approved. They eloped to London, where they married, and then boarded a ship bound for South Africa.[78] When the ship docked in Dunedin, Laura was pregnant and the couple disembarked and made their way to Auckland.

The Woodwards bought a 154-acre property in what is now East Auckland. They were one of the first 10 Pākehā families in the area, and they were not good farmers. At a young age, Alice was expected to help out on the farm, including slaughtering animals and grooming visitors' horses.[79] When depression hit in the 1870s, many Auckland farmers struggled to survive. Her father took a teaching job at Pigeon Mountain School (the forerunner to Pakuranga School) and six months later Laura joined him on the staff as an assistant teacher.[80]

Alice started school at the age of eight; she was most likely home-schooled until this point. She was considered the 'smart one' in the family, always with her head in a book,[81] but her schooling was interrupted by childminding and farm work. When she was a teenager her father had to stop teaching because of poor health, and she stayed home to look after him and her younger siblings so their mother could continue working. Her desire to become a doctor may well have stemmed from this time spent caring for her ailing father.

She was determined to be a doctor, and many people helped to fill the gaps in her education: the inspector of schools encouraged her, the parson whose cows she milked taught her Latin and the family doctor taught her chemistry. In 1893 Horsley achieved the two general examinations required to enter university and by the age of 22 she had also passed the additional requirements of either Greek, French or German, as well as the elementary mechanics of solids and fluids. She entered medical intermediate at Auckland University College to complete chemistry, biology and physics.[82]

Horsley travelled to Dunedin some time in the mid-1890s. She is recorded as attending anatomy and physiology classes at the medical school in 1895, although her family believes she may have begun her studies in 1894. She talked about enjoying her time in Dunedin, while noting that the women were treated differently to the men. One lecturer refused to teach them about anatomy below the waist, so they had to leave the classroom: 'Mixed classes were segregated, with the young ladies in front, target for pea-shooters and guffaws, vulnerable to verbal attacks by the lecturers.'[83] She also mentioned that she was always the last to be assigned to a cadaver, which she believed was because she was a woman: 'A student to whom she was assigned as a partner for anatomy classes exclaimed that he had to do his dissection with "a blessed damozel".'[84] She completed her final exams at the end of 1899 and qualified early in 1900 alongside three other women. She registered in June 1900, making her the fourth New Zealand graduate.

+ + +

At the end of 1899, Horsley was offered a house surgeon position at Auckland Hospital, where she was 'welcomed with little enthusiasm by most of her male colleagues in that conservative profession'.[85] The male doctors were vocal in their disapproval of the board hiring a woman doctor but all of this changed early in 1900, when there was an outbreak of a suspected bubonic plague. News of the outbreak spread like wildfire and many shops and services closed. The hospital proposed setting up a plague hospital in the Auckland Domain, but none of the male doctors was keen to take on the 'dangerous' position:

> Who was going to put their lives at risk from this fearful disease for which there was then no known cure? Young Doctor Woodward, registered only that month, offered to supervise the hospital, going into isolation for the duration of the trouble if necessary. The feared epidemic never eventuated, though sporadic cases of plague cropped up for the next eleven years. But the heroic offer by a very new doctor was not forgotten, and did her no harm in the eyes of Aucklanders.[86]

In 1902 Horsley's position at Auckland Hospital was finally formalised with an offer to become the honorary anaesthetist — this is believed to have been a part-time position.[87] She remained in this role until 1947.

After her house surgeon years at Auckland Hospital, she decided to go into private practice on Queen Street — the first woman in Auckland to do so. When a man turned up and asked to see 'the doctor' she responded with, 'I'm the doctor', to which he replied, 'You can't be the doctor, you're a woman.' 'Well, come in and let's see what I can do,' she replied. He ended up being her patient for the next 50 years.[88]

She met her husband, Arthur John Horsley, while he was serving his apprenticeship at the chemist shop beneath her practice. They were married on 9 December 1903 at St James Anglican Church in Māngere. Both of their practices flourished. His chemist shop became one of the most important and busiest shops on Queen Street, and his income allowed him to support the household so that she could run her private practice. According to family historian Patricia Whitford, 'She soon had no need to rely on family connections for her busy practice. She was also able to supplement fees from her patients by taking an appointment as honorary anaesthetist at Auckland Hospital. Anaesthesia was a field where women faced somewhat less fierce opposition than in other specialties, as it was comparatively poorly paid.'[89]

In 1917 the family moved to a slightly larger house on lower Symonds Street in the city (known as Doctor's Row), where she set up a private practice. She did not keep regular hours, and her nephew Hughlings Jackson remembers that every time he visited, there were at least four people in the house.[90] The patients would always wait: 'You turned up and you'd turn up at any hour, 24 hours, 7 days a week. And she never turned a patient away.'[91] She never asked any of her patients for payment; often she treated people free of charge or accepted payment in kind, and on some occasions she even gave money to needy patients.

Although her private practice and anaesthetics work at the hospital were enough to keep her busy, she also worked outside of her practice: she provided aid during the 1918 influenza epidemic, joined the 1931 medical relief party after the Napier earthquake, and in the 1930s joined the Dock Street Mission clinic as a physician.

Alice Horsley was still working in her eighties. Her husband had died in 1950, and she was afraid she would start losing her memory so she bought some books and taught herself Greek. She was nursed by her daughter Molly in Papatoetoe until her death on 7 November 1957.

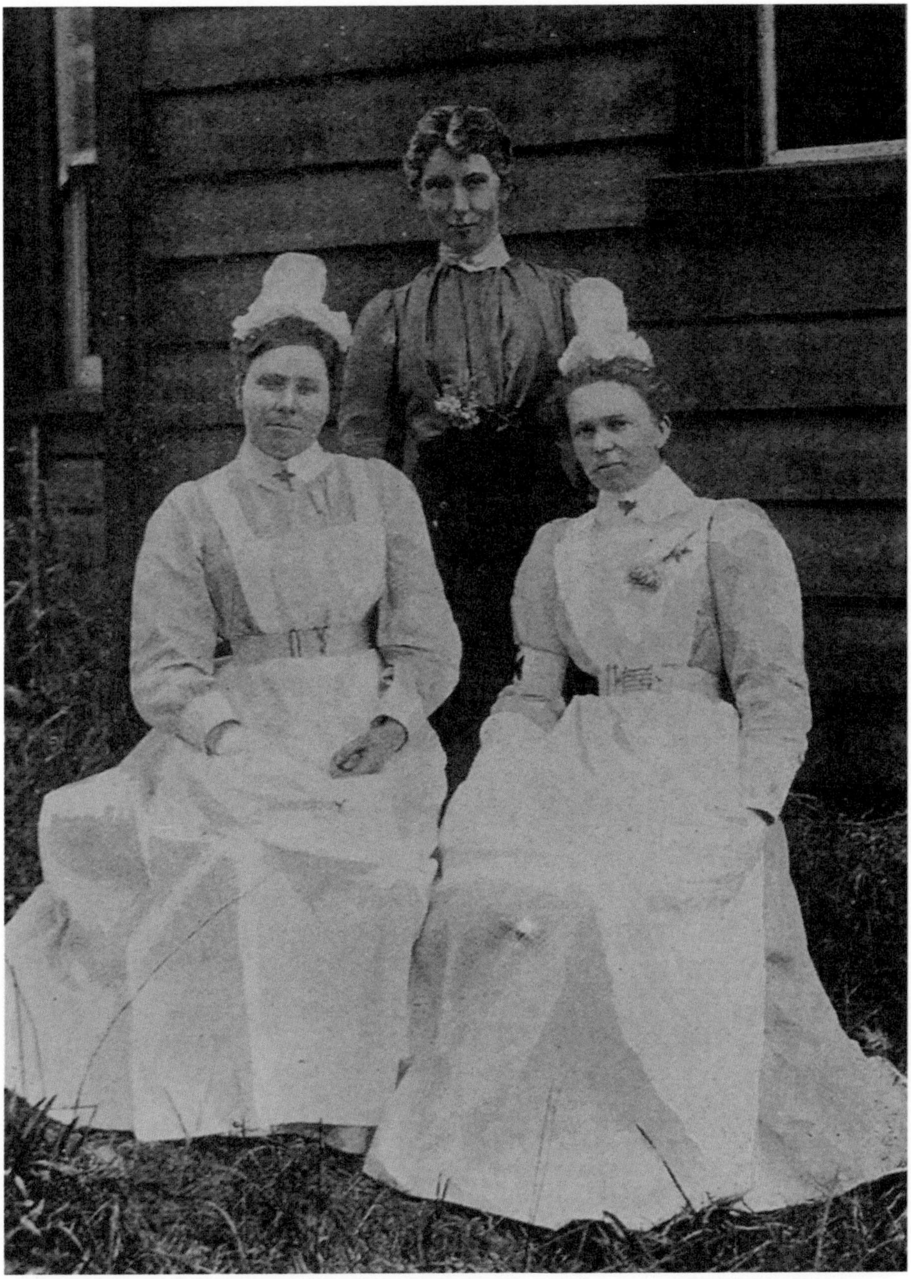

Alice Horsley, centre, with two nurses who assisted her during the 1900 bubonic plague outbreak in Auckland. *Courtesy Anne Morris*

CONSTANCE HELEN FROST

1900 graduate — second woman doctor to obtain a position at Auckland Hospital

Constance Frost was born in London around 1862 to Thomas Frost and Mary Ann Antwis. The family moved to New Zealand around 1879, when she was 17, and settled in Onehunga, Auckland. The first recorded mention of her was in the *Auckland Star* in January 1884, when she announced her intention to study medicine.[92] She studied at Auckland Training College and completed a BA at Auckland University College in 1892. Frost then travelled directly to Dunedin at the conclusion of her BA to pursue medical studies.

She took eight years to complete the five-year course and graduated from Otago Medical School in 1900 at the age of 33, one of four women graduates, the largest group yet.[93] Early in 1900, the *Observer* reported that Frost would be taking up a position as house surgeon at Auckland Hospital after her graduation. Hospital positions for women medical graduates were 'almost non-existent in New Zealand', so this appointment was quite an accomplishment.[94] However, the role never eventuated. Instead, Frost accepted a position as resident medical physician at Adelaide Hospital, in Australia, alongside fellow graduate Jane Kinder: they were the only women doctors at Adelaide Hospital at this time.[95]

The medical programme in Adelaide had recently closed, which meant that male doctors were in short supply and the hospital was willing to broaden its horizons. The positions were temporary, though Frost and Kinder were both reappointed the following year. In 1902, Frost became assistant bacteriologist at Adelaide Hospital, a position she held for 18 months. In this role, she focused on the study of bacteriology and was in charge of the entire laboratory.[96]

Frost returned to New Zealand in 1903 and settled in Auckland, where she remained for the rest of her career. At first, she established a practice in her home on Dominion Road in Mount Eden: the opening hours were 9 to 10 am and 5 to 7 pm.[97] She also held daily clinics at two pharmacies: from 11 am to 12 pm she saw patients at Fenton's Pharmacy on Karangahape Road, and from 2 to 4 pm at Edson's Pharmacy on Queen Street.[98]

Alongside her practice, she worked as a pathologist and bacteriologist at Auckland Hospital: the two positions were combined because there had been no other applications for either appointment. In 1913, this expanded to include the role of public vaccinator.[99] Frost's appointment was temporary for the entire time she was employed there. The board only ever intended for her to hold the position for one year while they continued to advertise for a male doctor.[100]

+++

When Frost first began working at the hospital there was no laboratory. She acquired all the necessary items and equipment and, over time, developed her reputation as a 'skilled bacteriologist'. She was also actively involved in hospital matters, advocating for better working conditions, including increasing the quality of work in the laboratory to improve its functionality. Her position initially came with many benefits, though these gradually dropped away over the years at the board's instruction, highlighting the problematic nature of her unpaid position at the hospital. Kathleen Anderson has noted that there is no known reason why she remained in this continually temporary position other than that she must have enjoyed the work.[101]

In 1908 Frost attempted to permanently move away from her highly demanding pathology job by applying for the advertised role of honorary physician. Her application was denied; she once again accepted the temporary position of honorary pathologist. In 1911, the hospital committee finally recognised the demands being placed on her and recommended that the position be a salaried one. But they continued to look outside for an employee, even expanding their search to the whole of New Zealand, 'England and elsewhere at a salary of £400 per annum'.[102]

Once again, there was no interest, most likely because the salary was considered too low. In 1913, Frost was again elected to her honorary post. Though the hospital committee suggested a small annuity of £100, the board was more generous and approved a payment of £250 per year. In May 1918, when she requested to be granted the full-time position of pathologist, the request was finally granted. The role came with a pay rise to £500 per annum but it remained temporary and continued to be advertised throughout the colonies and in England.[103]

Interestingly, it appears that the members of both the hospital committee and the board kept their low opinion of Frost within the walls of the hospital. In April 1906 the committee spoke publicly to the *New Zealand Herald* about her appointment as pathologist and bacteriologist: they complimented her work and said that it was 'quite equal to anything of the kind in the colony. The work carried out was really of a most searching character, and most valuable.'[104] It is both tragic and difficult to fathom today that this opinion was not reflected in their behaviour towards her as employers.

In 1918, the influenza epidemic reached New Zealand and quickly spread throughout the country, and in January 1920, it finally caught up with Constance Frost. She contracted influenza in the laboratory and on 29 January died at her home on Dominion Road. The hospital finally managed to hire a male doctor — Walter Gilmore — to fill her position after her death. By the end of his first year he was earning £1000 per annum, making him the second-highest paid doctor at the hospital. Kathleen Anderson has surmised that Frost has been 'ignored historically' because she did not conform to the traditional role expected of women doctors: to care for women and children by focusing on paediatrics, obstetrics, gynaecology or general practice.[105] Despite the fact that Constance Frost was the second woman doctor to obtain a position at Auckland Hospital and worked there for 17 years, the official history of the hospital makes no mention of her.[106]

AGATHA HELEN JANE MONFRIES (NÉE ADAMS)

1904 graduate — first woman doctor to practise in Taumarunui

Very little is known about Agatha Helen Jane Monfries' early life. She was born in 1880 to Robert Noble Adams and Jane Ellen Aitchison, attended Otago Girls' High School, where she did well academically, and in 1896, qualified for matriculation on the junior scholarship papers.[107] She missed being head girl by only one mark. By the time she was contemplating going to university, her brother Robert was in his second year at Otago Medical School; he graduated in 1902 and began practising in Tākaka that year. It was most likely his influence, as well as that of her teachers at Otago Girls', that encouraged her to apply to medical school.

In 1897, she passed the medical preliminary on the junior scholarship papers. In 1898, the *Otago Daily Times* reported her exam results: third class in junior physics, second class in practical physics, first class for chemistry lectures, and second class for chemistry practical. During her student years she was a member of

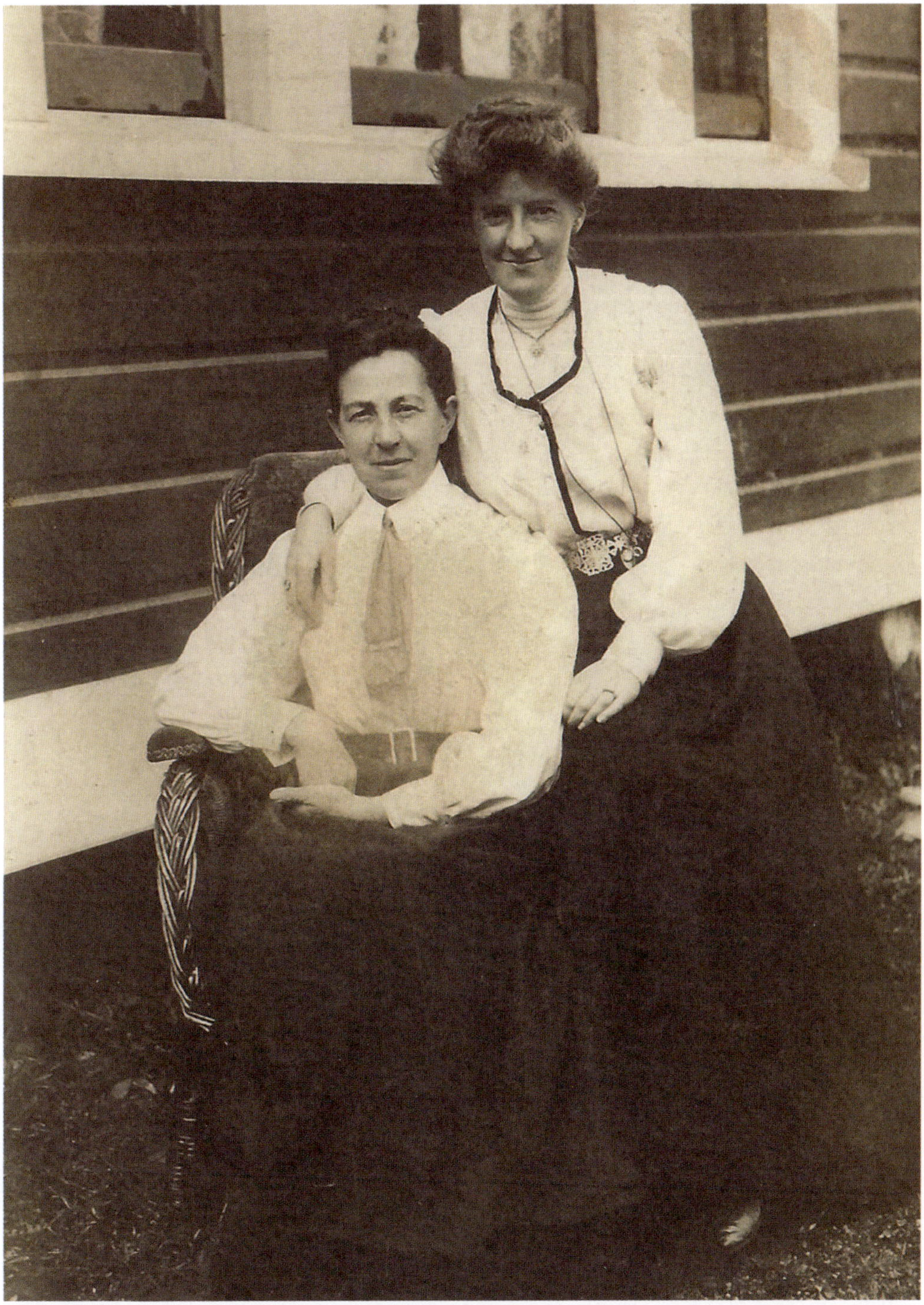

Agatha Monfries (right), c.1908, during her time as locum for E. H. Howard at Murchison. Seated next to her is Howard's wife, Georgina. *Muir family collection*

the University Debating Society, and she occasionally performed piano solos. She graduated with an MB ChB in 1904 at the age of 23, along with two other women graduates.

In October 1904, Monfries placed an advertisement in the *Otago Daily Times* advising that she was open for consultations at her rooms on George Street on 'the diseases of women and children'.[108] She became involved in the local community: she attended meetings of the Society for Promoting the Health of Women and Children; offered her services as honorary medical advisor to the orphanage of the Presbyterian Social Service Association; and she acted as locum for the Rock and Pillar Sanatorium for Consumptives at Waipiata in the Maniototo.

She also assisted her brother at Tākaka for a short time, and was a locum for Rosa Collier at Middlemarch, Fergus Paterson at Geraldine, and Emily Siedeberg in Dunedin. She did an extended locum in 1908 for E. H. Howard (father of Nina Muir; 1925) at Murchison while he was doing postgraduate study in England; she lived with his wife, Georgina, and their daughters while she was there. In 1907, she was appointed medical superintendent at the Plunket-run Home for Babies in Dunedin by special recommendation of the society's founder, Truby King.

On 20 March 1909, aged 28, she married James Inch Monfries (34) at St John's Church, Wellington. After their marriage, she became the first female doctor in Taumarunui. She bought William Cairns' practice and was appointed medical officer to the Taumarunui Hospital for a year but found the district too large and the workload too heavy. In 1910 she practised in Manunui and the surrounding area. Monfries also held the position of native health officer for the district and officiated as Māori health doctor. Monfries worked for two years in the Taumarunui and Manunui districts before giving birth to a son, who was stillborn. Three days later, she developed peritonitis and died on 22 February 1911, aged 30.[109]

ADA GERTRUDE PATERSON

1906 graduate

Ada Gertrude Paterson was born in Caversham, Dunedin, on 6 June 1880, to James Paterson and Margaret Smith Ayton. She attended Otago Girls' High School, excelled in her studies and graduated as dux in 1898.[110] Little is known of her time at Otago Medical School, but she presumably sat medical intermediate there and completed it in one to two years. She must have performed well throughout her time at medical school, as she completed the five-year course without any repeats or delays and graduated early in 1906. She then went straight to Ireland, where she undertook postgraduate studies at Rotunda University in Dublin and graduated in 1908 with a licentiate in midwifery.

Paterson returned to New Zealand and started her first job in general practice in Picton, where she worked for four years. She became a valuable member of the community during this time, and her farewell party was described as 'one of the most largely attended and enthusiastic gatherings ever held in Picton'. Those present called her a '"people's doctor", kindly, supportive, and ever available to help'.[111]

In 1912 she was appointed medical inspector of schools. Her first assignment was in Dunedin, where she was employed as one of the first four women doctors working in the School Medical Service: her job entailed conducting physical examinations of thousands of schoolchildren each year. In 1916 she was transferred to Wellington. Across these two positions, she developed a concern for girls' health and the mental and physical health of children.[112] She came to believe that girls were not raised in equal circumstances to their male counterparts, something she argued was pertinent, especially in childhood. In 1921 Paterson decided to pursue this concept further, and she took a year-long sabbatical to investigate work in the field of children's health in Australia, Britain and North America. When she returned, she promoted classes and schools designed to help children who were displaying behavioural issues.

The Education Department had merged into the Department of Health in 1921, and in 1923, after the retirement of E. H. Wilkins, Paterson was appointed as director of the Division of School Hygiene.[113] Her role involved efforts to raise the public perception of the School Medical Service by talking to school boards, service clubs and women's organisations. Her desire to establish school medical inspections beyond primary schools was set back by the Depression of the 1930s. Instead, she put her energy into promoting children's health camps, a programme initiated by Elizabeth Gunn (a New Zealand-born medical graduate of the Edinburgh School of Medicine for Women) in 1919.[114] Paterson founded the Wellington Children's Health Camp Association, which went on to establish the Raukawa Children's Health

Camp, New Zealand's first permanent camp, and the model for further health camps in Ōtaki in 1932. She was pivotal to its establishment, working with banks to arrange overdraft allowances and managing the recruitment of volunteers.

Outside of her work for the Department of Health, Paterson was also an advocate for women and juveniles, and she often appeared as an official representative at the courts. She was one of the first members of the New Zealand Federation of University Women. In 1936 she was diagnosed with cancer. She had a mastectomy but died on 26 August 1937 in Wellington.

INA BURNMAN MOODY (NÉE DUGLEBY)

1910 graduate — first woman to graduate who did not come from one of the four main city centres

Ina Moody was born in Auckland in 1886 to Walter Alfred Dugleby and Annie Neale. She was one of five children, and at some point in her childhood, the family moved to Napier, where she excelled academically at Napier District School. At the end of 1898 she achieved a National Board scholarship with a score of 584 and in 1899 she was dux of the school.

She was unable to attend the prizegiving ceremony because of illness and so the minister for education visited the school the following year to present it to her along with a gold medal. The local newspaper reported that 'Mr Walker highly complimented Miss Dugleby . . . upon her attainments, stating that not only had her honest work borne fruit but it had also set a wholesome example to her fellow workers.'[115]

Illness had prevented her from sitting the scholarship examination that would cover her fees for secondary school and the minister declared that 'he would give his moral and official support towards securing her a scholarship rendered vacant by one of the winners not taking it up'.[116] At the end of 1900, she was finally able to sit the examination, and placed first in the whole district with a score of 757. She also again received the senior scholar prize and won the Caledonian Society medal for achieving dux in the district.[117]

Following this success, Moody moved to Napier Girls' High School, where she passed her matriculation examination in 1902 and was made dux. In 1903, aged 17 and having been at high school for only three years, Moody completed the preliminary medical examination for the junior scholarship. When she obtained only a 'credit' result she decided to repeat the year and attempt the examination once more. At the end of 1904 she again sat the junior civil service examination, in which she came first in the country, and the junior university scholarship, in which she came second. With the scholarship, Moody was able to attend university with all fees paid; she would only need to pay for her board and living costs.[118]

It is not known why Moody decided to pursue a career in medicine, but she must have made the decision early on, as she enrolled in Otago Medical School as soon as she received notice of the scholarship. She travelled to Dunedin in March 1905, where she was enrolled to study the medical intermediate and then the medical degree. She graduated as the only woman medical student in her class at the beginning of 1910: the *Poverty Bay Herald* reported that she was the first girl from Napier to gain this distinction.[119]

+ + +

After completing her studies, Moody obtained a position at the clinic of Rosa Collier, a 'lady doctor' who had trained outside of New Zealand, in Balclutha.[120] She and Collier listed their hours for Balclutha, Clinton, Waiwera, Waipahi and Clydevale in the *Clutha Leader*. Patients could also phone them at Balclutha and Clinton. Moody attended house calls in her horse and gig. One particularly foggy evening one of the horses missed a turn and drove straight into a barbed-wire fence. The newspaper reported: 'The doctor sprang out over the wheel, and the groom managed to lift the buggy over the fence, when the pair took fright, and one came over the fence again. The mare that did so was badly cut about the legs. The other horse, which stood quietly on the paddock side of the fence, escaped with a slight injury. Dr Dugleby escaped with a shaking.'[121]

The position was only short-term, and by July 1910 she was working as a locum in the north of New Zealand. After this, she was appointed public vaccinator for the district of Waikouaiti, Otago, a position she held for two years. She was well liked in the area, and when her position ended the residents of Waikouaiti threw her 'an enjoyable social and dance'.

> A presentation was made in the form of a solid silver tea service and tray, a cake basket, and fruit dish. Eulogistic speeches were made by the Mayor and others, who referred to the high esteem in which the guest of the evening was held and the regret felt at her leaving Waikouaiti. Dr Fowden, with whom Dr Dugleby has been practising, suitably responded on her behalf. Mrs Backett and other ladies also arranged a pleasant kitchen evening, when Dr Dugleby was asked to accept numerous useful articles.[122]

It is not clear why she left this position, but she was now engaged to be married to Arthur Stanley Moody, a Dunedin doctor; they married on 17 March 1913 at St Mary's Church, Dunedin. The newspaper announced: 'Dr and Mrs Moody, who are well known in the south, were the recipients of numerous valuable and handsome wedding gifts.'[123] After her marriage, there were no further reports about her life or work until her death in February 1930, although Arthur Moody continued to practise. Her obituary in the *Auckland Star* noted that Dr Ina Moody had stopped practising due to health complications, which led to her death.[124]

CATHARINE LOUISA BROOKFIELD (NÉE WILL)

1911 graduate — first woman junior house surgeon appointed to Dunedin Hospital

Catharine Louisa Brookfield was born on 25 April 1886 and attended Green Island School, outside Dunedin, with her younger sister and brother.[125] Their father, Bill, was a New Zealand-born Edinburgh medical graduate who had returned home to set up a general practice late in 1884. The family lived on a farm and had their own cow and at least one horse, which Bill used to conduct house calls.

After primary school, Brookfield attended Braemar House, a private girls' school founded in 1895 in Dunedin. It was run by two sisters, the Misses Miller, who impressed on their students a reverence for life, a sense of civic responsibility and service, and the need to contribute to the good of humanity while gaining a liberal education. Brookfield took the course for matriculation; her subjects included mathematics, English, French, Latin and natural science, which included

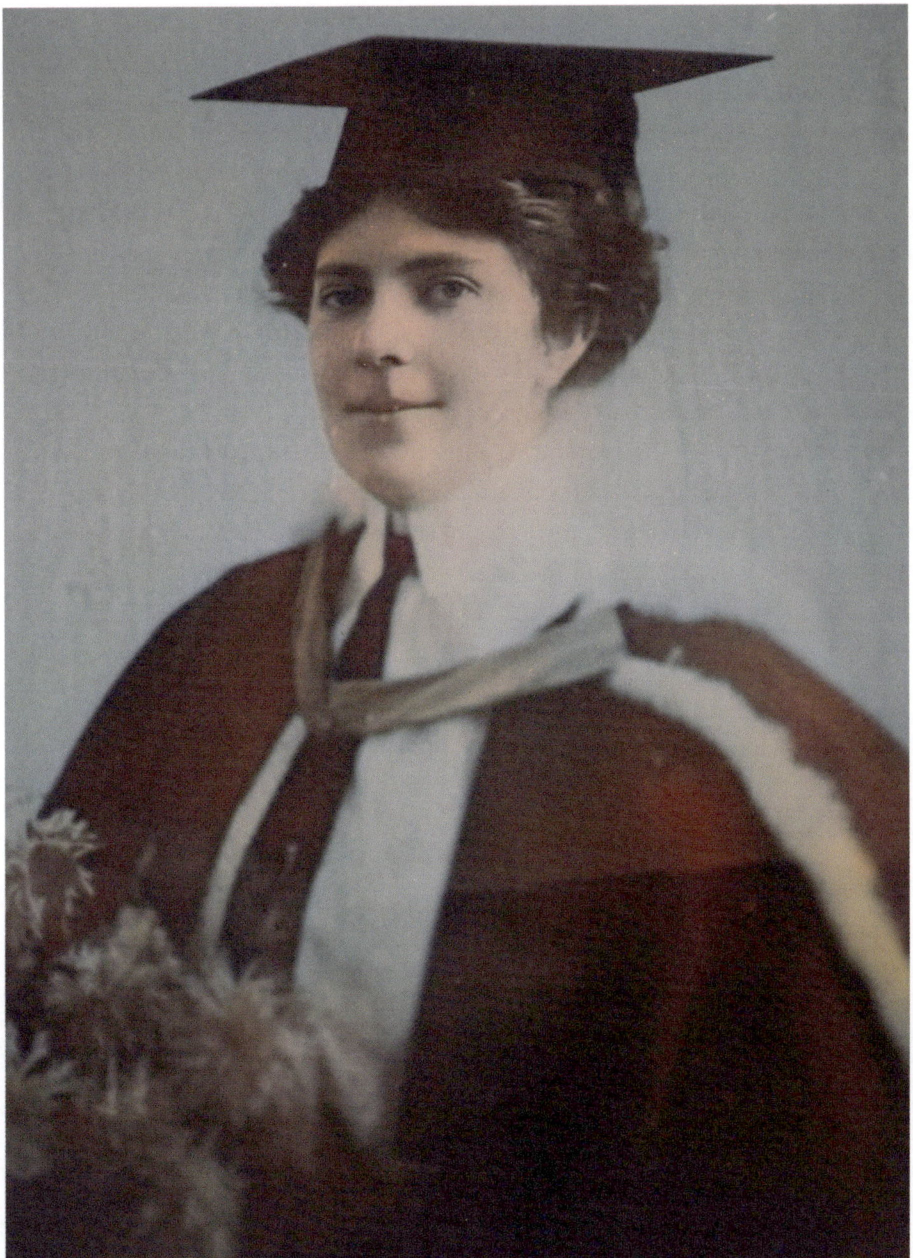

Catharine Louisa Brookfield (née Will) on her graduation day in 1911. *Family collection*

physiology. She did well at school and her name was prominent on the Braemar honours board.

Her father encouraged her to pursue medicine as a career at Otago Medical School — something that had not been possible in New Zealand during his university years. She enrolled in early April 1904, when she was almost 18. At first she commuted from Green Island but she found the workload challenging and after a few weeks she switched to boarding in Dunedin. She had done no physics and possibly also no chemistry at high school, and failed these subjects in the finals. She spent 1905 at home, but with strong encouragement from her father she returned in 1906, repeated her medical intermediate and passed.

She began her medical training in April 1907 in a class of 14 students; there was another female student in the first year, but on graduation she was the only woman listed — the other student had transferred to Edinburgh to finish her studies. Brookfield successfully passed her exams year by year, and in 1911 she graduated MB ChB.

+++

Catharine Brookfield applied for a position as junior house surgeon at Dunedin Hospital and, to her surprise, was appointed as one of the four house surgeons — the first woman to be appointed to this role — on an annual salary of £100. In the spring of 1911, she was appointed acting medical officer at the tuberculosis sanatorium at Pleasant Valley, a few kilometres south of Palmerston. She was reappointed as medical officer in March 1912 at double the salary (£200 per annum). She was the sole resident doctor for 12 months — the last position she ever had.[126]

Her future husband, Athol William Purchas Brookfield, was in the same year of medical training. They became engaged on 17 June 1911, but he failed his final examinations in 1911, and had to repeat them the following year. He eventually passed in 1912, and later that year began working as a general practitioner and surgeon in Papakura, Auckland. When they married in Auckland on 12 September 1913, Catharine moved from Palmerston to Auckland to join him. They had no honeymoon and started married life in a rented house on Clark Road, Papakura, where they lived until they moved back to Dunedin in 1921 because of Athol's ill health. He died during surgery for asthma at the age of 36.

The Brookfields had three children: one son and two daughters. Their son,

Melville, followed in his parents' footsteps and went to medical school; Evelyn studied for a BSc, and Daphne trained as a nurse. After her marriage and having children, Catharine Brookfield's focus turned from medicine to her family. She was very attentive to them and, for many years during the 1950s and 1960s, she would spend two months in Auckland visiting her sister and her daughters' families. In Dunedin, she had many old school friends, and she made new ones among her fellow Presbyterian worshippers at First Church. She was a regular attendee at the Otago Classical Association and at Greek play readings and was a member of the Victoria League, which connected people from Commonwealth countries. From 1959 onwards, she suffered from failing health. She died on 16 January 1967.

Otago Medical School students at Dunedin Hospital in February 1908. Ina Moody (née Dugleby; 1910) is fifth from the right in the second row; Catharine Brookfield (née Will; 1911) is seventh from the right. The other two women, J. G. Gow (née Collie) and Mrs Land (née Williams), did not graduate from Otago. *Otago Medical School Archives*

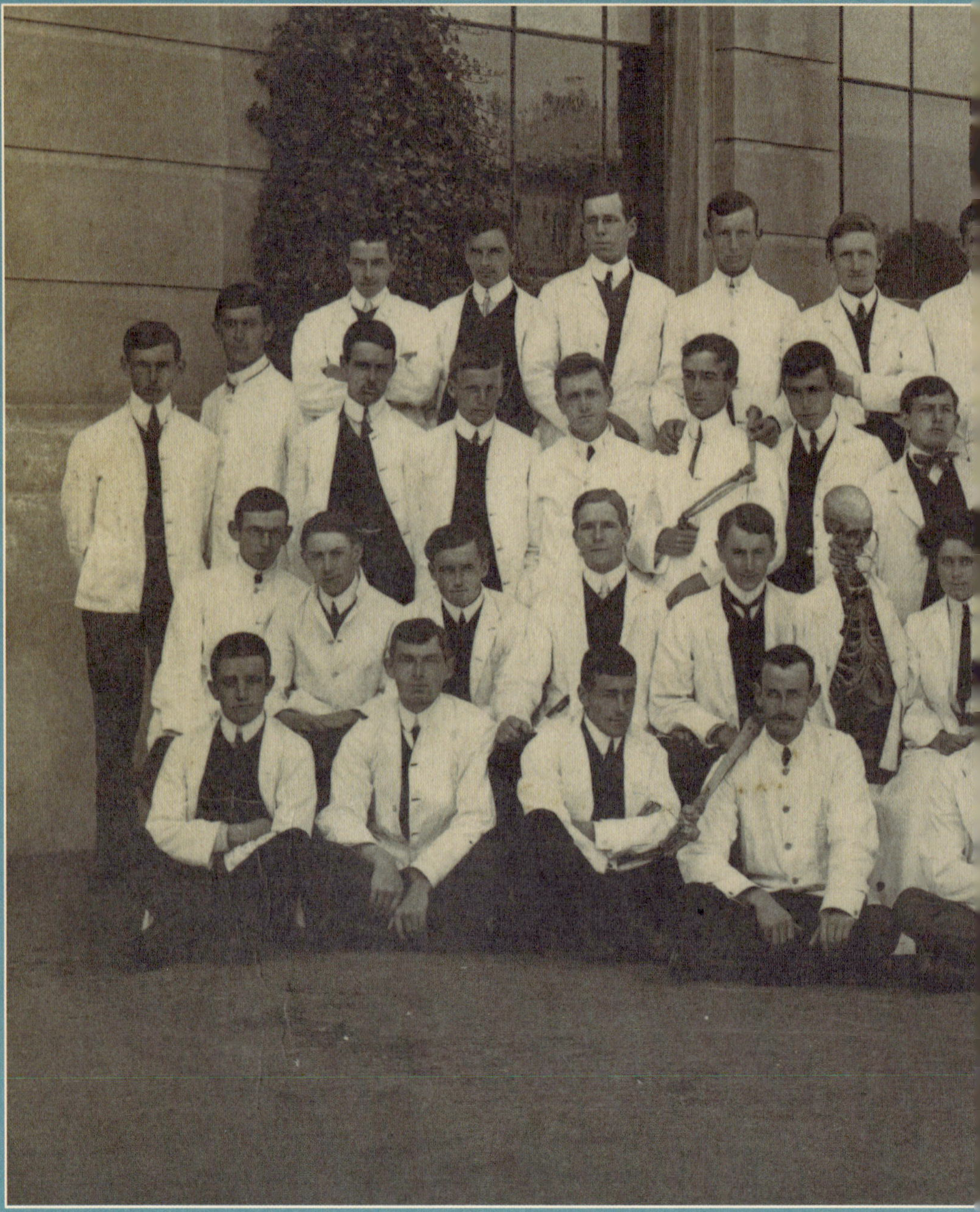

2. The war years 1914–1919

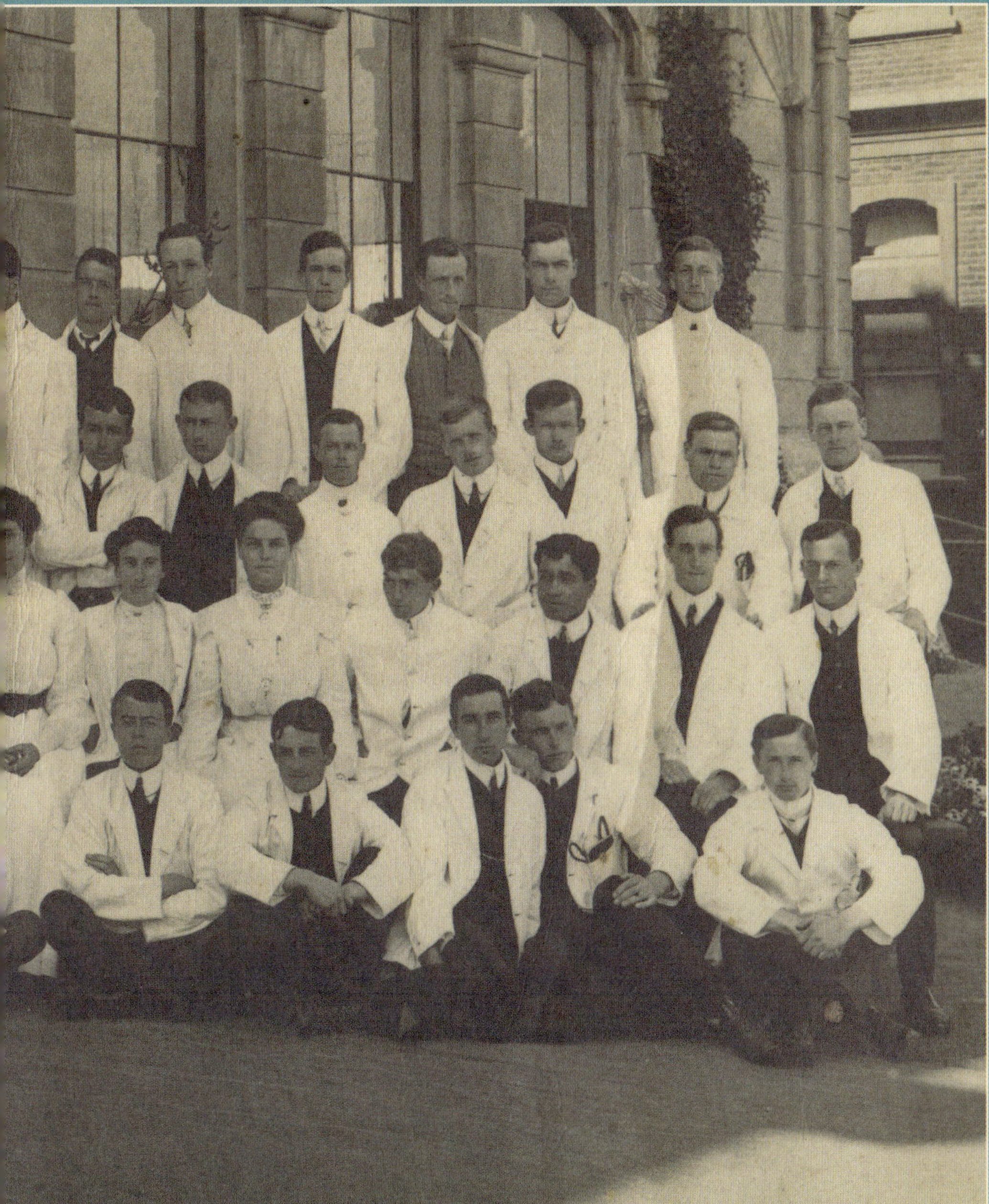

The prevailing atmosphere in New Zealand in 1914–19 is best described as one of crisis and catastrophe. On 4 August 1914, Britain declared war on Germany, and New Zealand, as a loyal dominion of the empire, had no choice but to join.

The outbreak of war caused a huge upheaval in New Zealand society, including a reassessment of the role of women: large numbers of men had left the country to serve in the forces and their roles needed to be filled. New Zealand was unique in this regard compared to other countries at the time. Elsewhere, there was a large increase in women in employment as a result of the gaps left by men who had enlisted, but in New Zealand the change was not so marked, possibly because the number of women in the workforce had already doubled in the preceding decades.[1]

Women's labour statistics may also have been under-reported in the decades leading up to the war. With a low population and over 50 per cent of the population living rurally, women had worked on farms and supported family businesses out of necessity, forms of unpaid work that were not included in the census. According to historian Melanie Nolan, the war merely accelerated a process that was already under way.[2]

Of course, this does not mean that women were readily accepted everywhere. In 1913, changes in regulations for female employees gave employers the right to make working conditions unfavourable for their female workers: 'Lower rates of maximum pay were introduced; women were barred from sitting the public service entrance examinations; and upon marriage women were forced to resign their positions.'[3] Nolan reported that some women were receiving only 25 shillings (£1 5s) a week for the same jobs that men had been doing for £3.[4]

This pay gap had a considerable impact on women during the war, especially those entering commercial or professional jobs. Most were placed on temporary contracts and were paid considerably less than men in the same positions. There was no room for vertical mobility or job stability, a sign that most employers viewed having female employees as a temporary solution until the men returned home.

In 1915 the Women's National Reserve was established to help women find employment in order to free up men for overseas service. In some industries, this proved successful. In August 1915, for example, positions were advertised for 'general' employment, such as letter carriers or tram conductors. These jobs that did not require much training were aimed at women who had never worked before.[5] However, when the Women's National Reserve approached the efficiency commissioner for Canterbury in 1917 with a list of 500 women ready to engage in work, he said he was 'appreciative of the women's offer' but was unwilling to offer them positions until all qualified men had been 'absorbed in essential industries'.[6]

At first there were limited opportunities for women to contribute directly to the war effort. For example, 400 trained nurses were initially denied permission to serve overseas; it was not until April 1915, when the New Zealand Army Nursing Service was established, that they were approved to leave. In the end, they served on several fronts, from France and Britain to Greece and Egypt.[7] One New Zealander, Esther Allen, who had the finances to support herself, paid for her own travel overseas and volunteered her nursing services in Britain.[8] When Agnes Bennett, an Edinburgh medical graduate who was practising in New Zealand, offered her services to the New Zealand Army but was rejected, she and her sister, a trained nurse, funded their own way overseas and served in hospitals in Cairo and Scotland.[9]

Although women were denied the opportunity to serve in the war, they were asked to contribute to the war effort through assembling care packages and fundraising. In 1914, Waimate GP Margaret Cruickshank participated in one of the largest fundraising campaigns in New Zealand — the Queen Carnival. Each town put forward a candidate, and the public cast 'votes' in the form of monetary donations that would go towards relief for the poor in war-torn countries.

Cruickshank was elected for Waimate, and for most of the competition she was the leading contender. The final day of the carnival was held in Tīmaru, and many travelled from Waimate to support her. Witnesses described her as 'tall and gracious, in her beautiful court dress of satin and lace, her fair hair with its tints of gold, arranged in a coronal'.[10] Although Cruickshank did not win, her participation raised £10,000 for the war effort. In 1920, the Red Cross calculated that the funds raised across the country from the Queen Carnivals totalled £1,348,876; 'the equivalent of one pound seven shillings for every man, woman and child at a time when women textile workers earned between two shillings and one pound seven shillings per week'.[11]

Women doctors made a valuable and necessary contribution to the war effort. Many of the medical men had been enlisted overseas, leaving gaps in hospitals and general practices that were filled by the ever-increasing number of medical women graduates.

Two graduates, Doris Gordon (née Jolly; 1915) and Francesca Dowling (1915), along with two male classmates, were offered the coveted position of house surgeon at Dunedin Hospital when all the male staff left for war. Gordon described these years as high-pressure. Surgery was just beginning to move away from the 'cut-and-slash get-it-over-quickly technique' that had been necessary in the pre-anaesthetic days.[12] By later standards, their seniors worked 'roughly', causing shock to the patient, anxiety for the anaesthetist, tension for the nursing sister, frayed nerves for the surgeon, and frequent rude words for the house surgeon. Seventy per cent of the anaesthetics were administered by interns, who were still in training. Gordon was grateful that the doctor in charge of the house surgeons, John Tait Bowie, stood by each of them for the first dozen or so surgeries and only let them go solo when he was sure they knew what they were doing.

The sharp drop in the number of male students was also felt at Otago Medical School. Men who were training in medicine were technically exempt from conscription, but many chose to enlist and this opened up more opportunities for women wishing to enrol in the programme. Kathleen Todd (1923), Frances Preston (née McAllister; 1922) and Augusta Klippel (née Manoy; 1922) were in the 'unusual' 1917 intake, in which eight women were accepted in a class of only 48 students, twice the number that had previously been accepted and entirely attributable to the lack of male applicants.[13]

The increased allowance for women medical students conveniently coincided with the opening of St Margaret's College, a Presbyterian-run hall of residence for women, in 1911. It initially housed 15 women students in a vacant Presbyterian manse at 333 Leith Street — a temporary solution until a purpose-built premises,

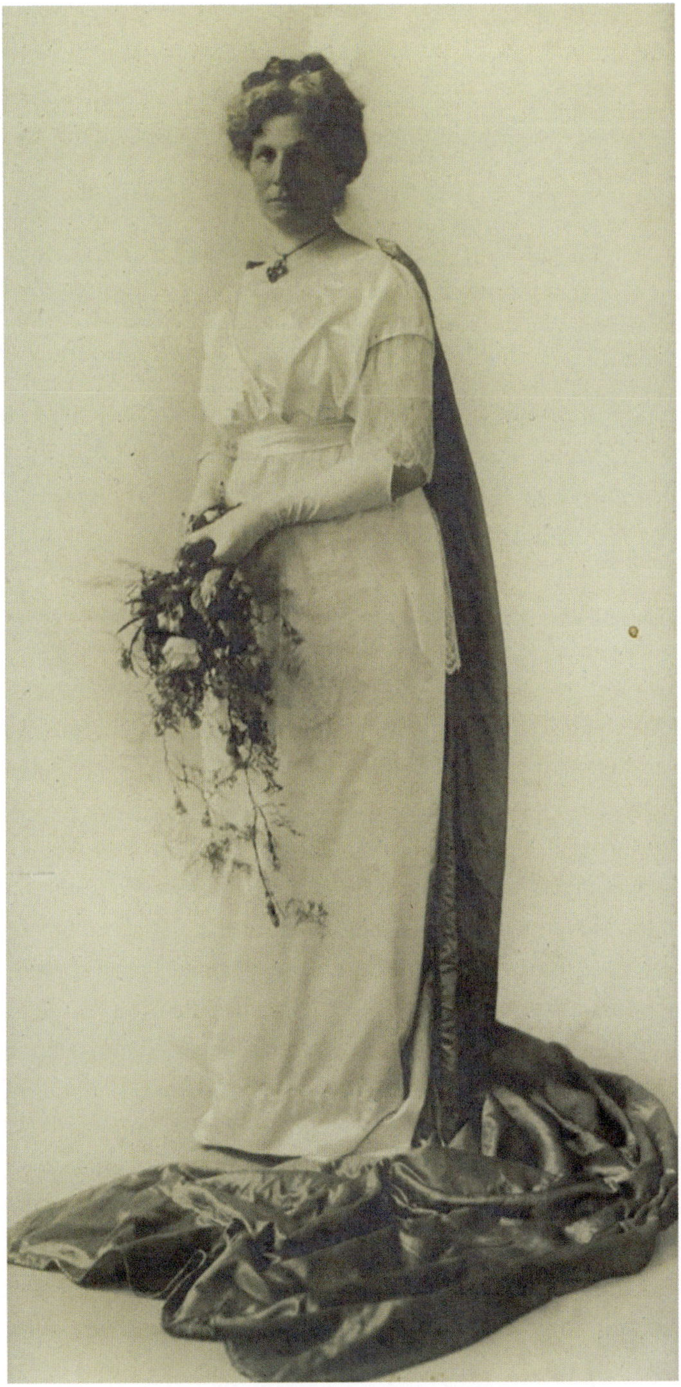

Margaret Cruickshank dressed as a First World War Carnival Queen, Waimate, 1915. *Waimate Museum*

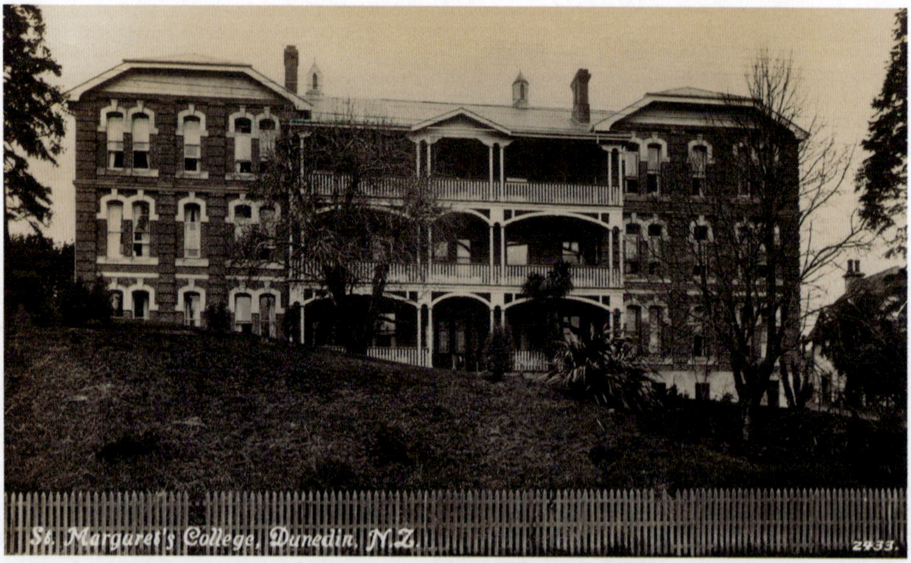

St Margaret's College photographed by 1928 graduate Nellie Houghton. *Houghton family collection*

located opposite the main university buildings, was completed in 1914. Although St Margaret's was founded and managed by the Presbyterians, it had an ecumenical admission policy.

Doris Gordon and Francesca Dowling were the first two women medical students to stay at St Margaret's, but it quickly became the preferred option over private board for students whose families were not from Otago. The promise of a safe hall of residence for their daughters gave these families reassurance.

The centennial history of St Margaret's describes life there in the early years. The matron, Miss Jean Callender, 'managed every aspect of daily life in the College and held the girls accountable to a strong work ethic and high standards of personal behaviour. She organised meals, laundry, and cleaning, enforced House rules, looked after girls who were ill or homesick and led daily Bible readings and religious devotions. In many regards Miss Callender operated as a surrogate maternal figure for young women transplanted from home life to university.'[14]

There were other changes to the medical school during this period. After many petitions calling for upgrades to the school, the university finally began making improvements to its programme and the buildings. In his history of the medical school, Gordon Parry argued that this was possible because the high demand for medical officers meant the government 'suddenly began to take heed of the School and its needs. Money became more readily available.'[15]

In 1913 the university introduced a Diploma in Public Health, and the medical school built relationships with hospitals other than Dunedin where students could complete their clinical experience. In 1916 the medical school opened two new buildings — pathology and bacteriology (which incorporated a public health laboratory). The buildings came with new teachers, and some subjects were separated: bacteriology from pathology, and public health from medical jurisprudence.[16] By 1918, the Faculty of Medicine was the largest in the university.

By 1917, New Zealanders were tiring of the war and its effects. The list of casualties continued to rise — a staggering one in four New Zealand men between the ages of 20 and 45 had been killed or wounded while on service. Food prices were mounting, too: families were struggling to make ends meet, and women often took in boarders or looked after other people's children, while their own children left school and went out to work to help support the family.

The signing of the Armistice on 11 November 1918 was welcome news and a day to celebrate. Augusta Klippel, at this point a third-year student, remembered it clearly: 'We were celebrating it in the Octagon and I who am absolutely tuneless who can't sing God Save the King stood up. There is a fountain in the Octagon . . . in Princes Street near to the Stock Exchange. I clambered up on that thing and conducted the "Marseillaise".'[17]

But the joy was short-lived. With the returning servicemen came what was known as the 'Spanish flu' — the influenza pandemic of 1918. It is thought to have arrived in mid-October in Auckland, possibly on the troopship RMS *Niagara*, which had left Vancouver for Auckland on 21 September, although this has never been conclusively established. By the time medical authorities realised how serious the illness was, the soldiers who had been on board the ship had returned to their homes across New Zealand.

The timing was tragic. Doctors returning from overseas and those who had remained were dealing with a disease that was rabid and deadly. Many Health Department officials succumbed early, leaving the department inadequately staffed and the country in a critical condition.[18] At a public meeting in November 1918, Margaret Cruickshank cited Christchurch as an example of what could go

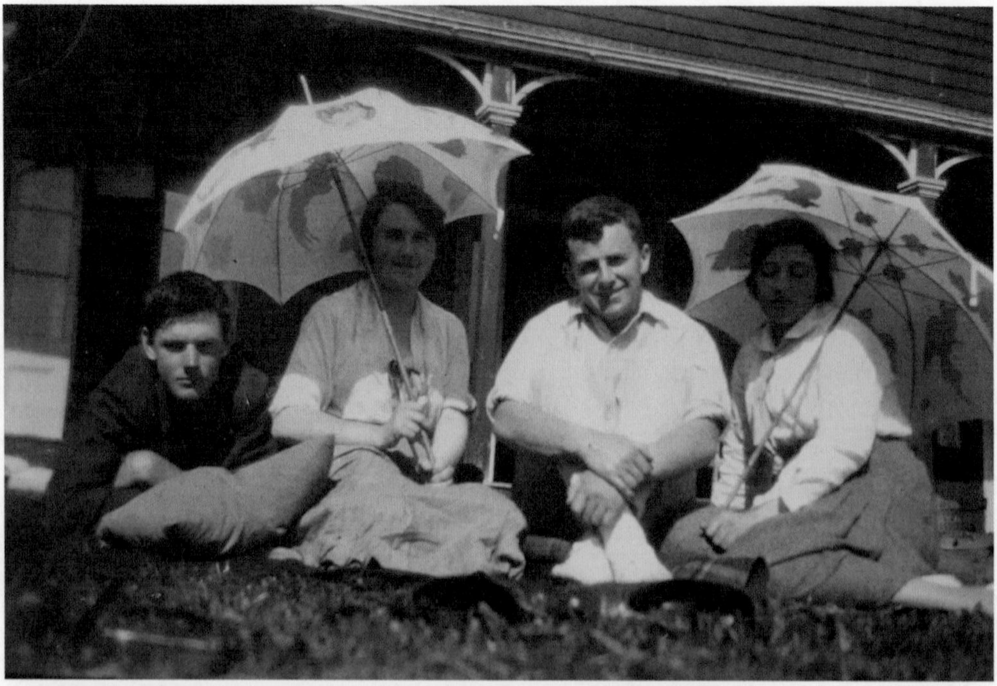

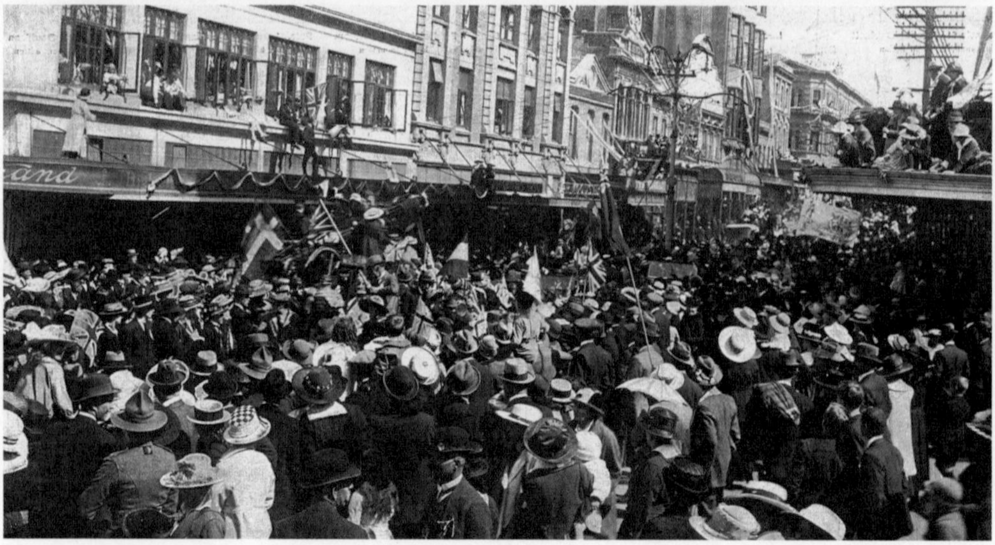

ABOVE: Medical school friends, 1915. Elspeth Fitzgerald (née Cameron) is second from left and Beatrix ('Tui') Bakewell at right — both graduated from Otago Medical School in 1920. Elspeth's future husband, Robert Fitzgerald, is third from left. *Courtesy Susan Cambridge*

BELOW: Armistice Day celebrations in Dunedin's Octagon, 20 November 1918. *Hocken Collections Uare Taoka o Hākena, Guy photograph, Otago Witness*

wrong if precautions were not taken early. The city council had decided to go ahead with a People's Day show on 8 November to celebrate the end of the war, but the celebrations likely caused the flu to spread through the city and neighbouring towns: approximately 462 people died in Christchurch alone.[19]

Spurred into action by Cruickshank's speech, the Waimate District Council placed regulations on public spaces, and it decided that only the most serious cases were to be admitted to the hospital; minor cases were expected to self-isolate at home.[20] This placed the burden of care on families. St John Ambulance and the Red Cross sent workers to families and into communities to assist with care, exposing thousands to the virus in the process.[21] Jean Smith (née Cockerell) recalled the care her mother administered at home: 'Quinine was the best thing to cure the plague, but they ran short of it, they just couldn't get enough. I know mother used to come home and give it to us; it was terrible stuff to take, but it did save us.'[22] Those left to self-isolate were often found dead the following morning.[23]

Alice Horsley became renowned for her work in Auckland during the pandemic. After administering anaesthetics to soldiers in the military hospital, she would then visit the influenza hospitals.[24] When a quarantine facility was set up in the Auckland Domain, she volunteered to isolate with the flu patients. Her whole family contracted the illness, but they all survived after nursing each other back to health.[25]

The situation became so dire that even second-year medical students were enlisted to help, and the Department of Health gave final-year students full medical authority, apart from signing death certificates. Frances Preston recalled working from 2 pm to 10 pm or later: 'Practical nursing was not on our curriculum and the knowledge we gained of handling patients, sponging, giving enemas, even laying out the dead was invaluable for later country practice.'[26] But the medical school staff were not always in support. When Kathleen Todd offered her services, anatomy professor Percy Gowland told her, 'You'll all get it . . . and you must get on with your anatomy; this material can't be wasted; we can't give you another chance.'[27] In the end, he agreed that they could volunteer as long as they agreed to do three hours of dissection every morning.

Moana Gow (née Anderson; 1921), who was in her third year, was sent out on placement early. At a farm in an isolated valley she found both parents of the family had died of influenza, and she had to ride to the next farm to get temporary care for the orphaned children.[28] Eva Hill (née Day; 1921) recalled that the influenza epidemic, which occurred during her third year, was the most instructive event of her student years.

> Doctors and nurses at the hospital went down with it, so we students took over as general nursing staff. We were very green but we just got on with it; we had to. I learnt to do everything from changing soiled bed linen without disturbing a sick patient to laying out the dead . . . Dunedin came almost to a standstill. The trams stopped running. Fourth and Fifth Year students were given a crash course in minor anaesthetics, hypodermic techniques, and drug prescriptions, so that they could take over from those town GPs who'd been laid low. It was like a dead town. Young people went down like flies. We had all the jobs to do including bedpan drill . . . I nursed right through the epidemic, the whole six weeks, usually twelve hours a day, and didn't even catch a cold, but you'd never know from one day to the next whom you'd find had died.[29]

Since the very nature of their jobs required them to attend to sick patients, it is no wonder that many women doctors themselves fell victim to the flu. Doris Gordon, who was working in Stratford, caught it very early on and called on her colleague, T. L. Paget, to return from the military camp where he was stationed to assist her.

> While we were asking him, I got the first shiver. Both gentlemen noted it and T. L. Paget said in his forceful way: 'Home to bed for you. That's the quickest cure. I'll carry on alone . . . Away you go.' He was correct in his theory that the cure would be quicker in ratio to how promptly the victim gave in and went to bed. I was at work again in six days, very sorry for myself.[30]

Kathleen Todd recalled that the majority of her class, herself included, came down with the flu as Gowland had predicted, but thankfully they recovered.[31] Not everyone was so lucky. Francesca Dowling died on 22 November 1918; as noted in the previous chapter, Margaret Cruickshank died on 28 November 1918; and Constance Frost died in January 1920, making a total of three New Zealand women doctors who died during the epidemic.[32] Doris Gordon later wrote:

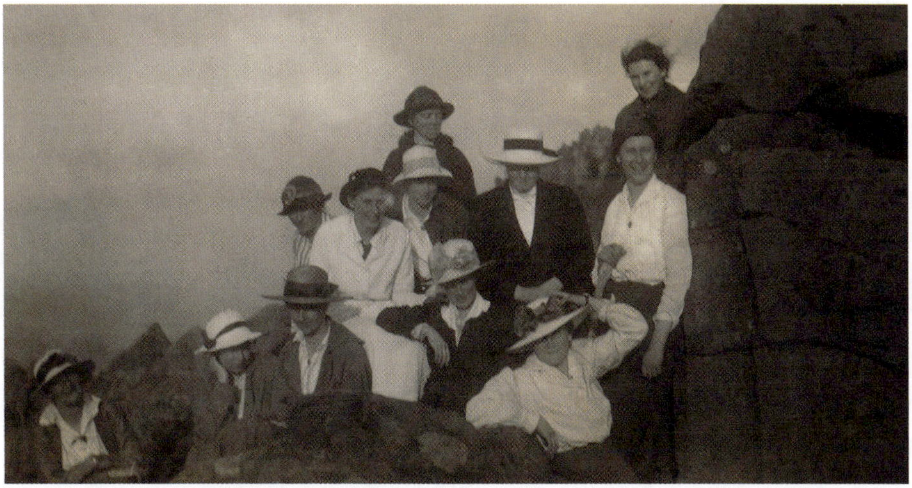

Medical school students on a trip up Dunedin's Mount Cargill in 1917, photographed by 1928 graduate Nellie Houghton. *Houghton family collection*

> Never in all my medical training had I ever expected to be responsible for lives in a Black Death Plague . . . I spent most of my time verifying that the victims of Armistice Day celebrations were pulseless and signing their death certificates. Someone in the capital had taken action and closed hotels, schools, churches, places of amusement and all non-essential industry. Authority had ordered funerals to take back streets and to hurry. Funeral processions were banned and often relatives had to help the overworked gravediggers.[33]

And Frances Preston noted:

> When it was all over, everyone who survived was exhausted; catching up for lost time made continued hard work for both teachers and students. It was a sudden and tragic introduction to life and death. No one could live through such an experience and remain quite the same; in short, we began to grow up.[34]

The pandemic that raged through New Zealand claimed around 9000 lives in the first six weeks, and it continued to spread for another one and a half years.

Ever since it established the full medical degree in 1885, Otago Medical School had struggled to attract and retain students. The prevailing belief that the better programme was to be found 'back Home' in Britain endured, and some students started their degrees at Otago then transferred to Britain to complete them.

That all changed during the war years. The travel restrictions that came with a world war meant that staying in their own country to pursue a medical degree was the only option for many students, and this led to more enrolments at Otago Medical School. In the first two decades that women were admitted to the programme (1896–1919), only 23 women had graduated; in the 1920s alone, there were 62 graduates.

The increase in student numbers, along with the challenges of treating injured soldiers and the pandemic, finally persuaded the government that it should support the medical school by funding facilities, hiring more staff and subsidising more fees. Unfortunately, although women were being accepted by the medical school in increasing numbers, the country as a whole remained slow to offer them jobs after they graduated. This, coupled with the high number of returned servicemen with medical training, led to a shortage of jobs for women doctors. As a result, many medical women turned to better opportunities overseas.

DORIS CLIFTON GORDON (NÉE JOLLY)

1915 graduate — first woman in New Zealand and Australia to secure a Fellowship of the Royal College of Surgeons, first Honorary Fellowship for the Royal College of Obstetricians and Gynaecologists

Doris Gordon was born on 10 July 1890 in Coburg, Australia.[35] She and her older brother, Frank, enjoyed a comfortable life with their parents, Lucy Clifton Crouch and Alfred Jolly, in Victoria until the 1893 financial crash. In 1894 their father moved to New Zealand in search of better prospects, and secured a job at the National Bank in Wellington. The family joined him there later in the year, and they lived in various rental homes before settling in their own house at Karaka Bay. The family later moved to Tapanui in West Otago, where they lived from 1905 until 1910.

The family's German-manufactured Thurmer piano, which they brought from Australia, played an important role in their lives. Lucy Jolly gave piano lessons to local children, as well as to Doris. Initially home-schooled, Doris Gordon was an indifferent student compared to her enthusiastic brother. She briefly attended Miss Shepherd's Academy for Young Women at age nine and Worser Bay School at 12, where she received her only year of uninterrupted formal education, earning a standard 5 certificate. From 1903 to 1905, she attended St Francis Xavier's Academy in Seatoun but often missed school to care for her mother, who suffered from heart problems.[36] She excelled in various subjects and received numerous prizes.

When the family moved to Tapanui, Gordon refused to attend the local high school. Her family recognised her unique talents and decided to focus on her music. She became proficient in music and passed the Royal Academy of Music senior exam in Gore in 1909. She also taught Sunday school to a class of 40 children. She felt a calling to become a medical missionary and announced this to her parents:

> Do you know what I'd like to do next? I'd like to study, pass the matriculation, and go to university and become a doctor. 'You study!' they exclaimed together. 'Yes,' I said meekly. 'And what do you want to do if you are a doctor?' asked mother. 'She probably wants to be a missionary,' said my father, who was observant. He rose quickly to his feet and in a manner that was both a challenge and a promise said, 'If you can pass matriculation, I'll pay for you to study medicine.'[37]

With the help of a family friend at the Teacher's Training College in Dunedin, Gordon studied the necessary subjects, passed the exams and began high school at Tapanui. She graduated from there in 1910 and went straight to Otago Medical School, where she passed three out of four medical intermediate subjects, allowing her to start first-year medicine in 1912, boarding at St Margaret's College. She excelled in her studies, and despite a disappointing anatomy exam in 1912 and a bout of appendicitis in 1913, she achieved top marks in her first professional examination in anatomy. In order to complete the MB ChB, students were required to pass the first professional examination at the end of their third year, the second professional at the end of their fourth year, and the third professional at the end of their fifth year.

During her training, Gordon developed a passion for improving the conditions

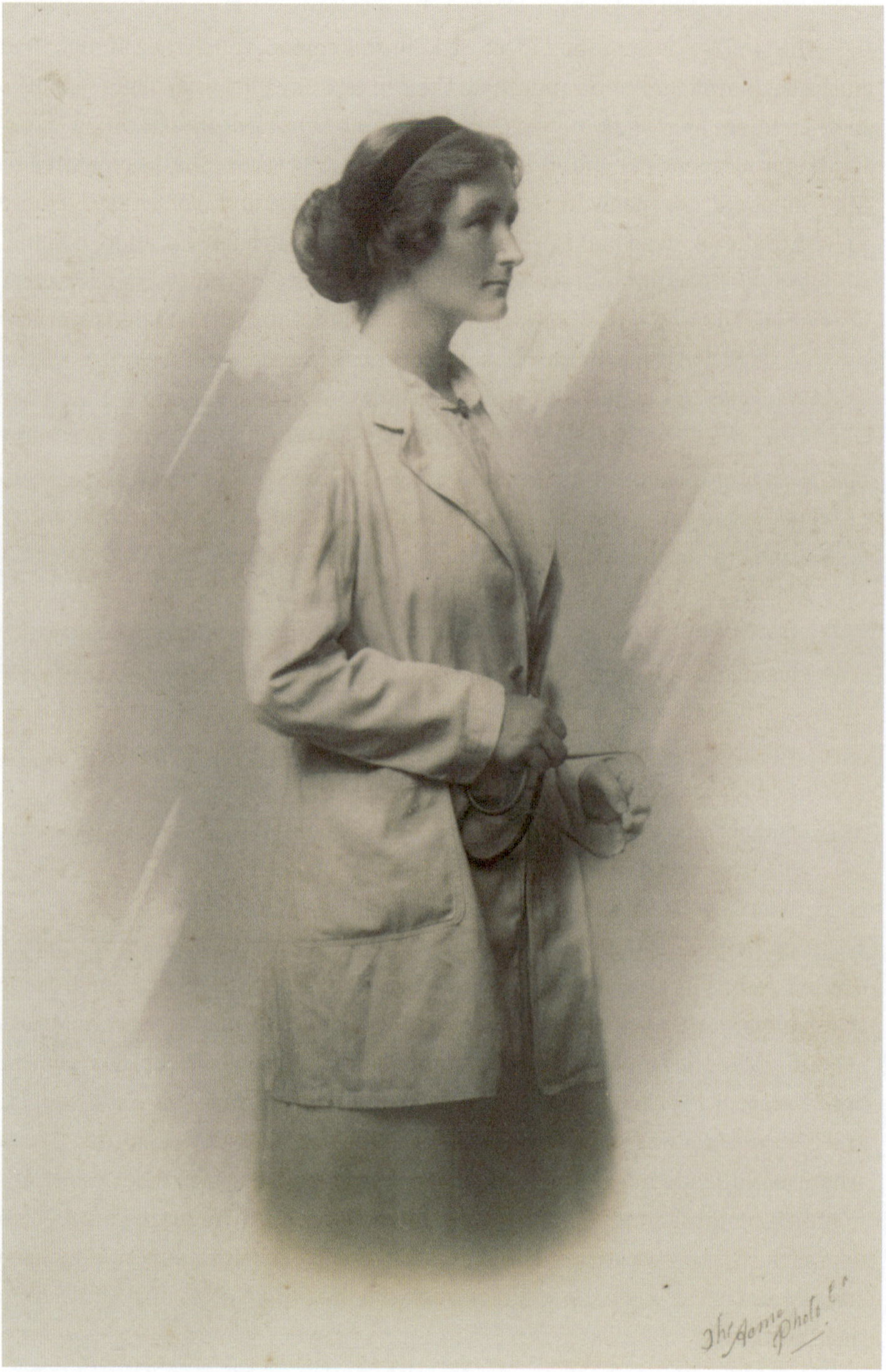

Doris Gordon as a young doctor (date unknown). *Courtesy T. Gordon*

of childbirth, particularly for underprivileged women. In 1914 she and her friend Francesca Dowling attended births at night at the Forth Street maternity hospital (founded by the Dunedin Hospital Board for the joint purpose of caring for 'fallen women' and providing instruction in midwifery for medical students), and at the Salvation Army refuge home for single girls, which allowed only women medical students to attend births. The conditions at these homes fuelled her determination to find a safe, universal method of pain relief for women in childbirth.[38]

In her final year of medicine in 1915, the military and civil authorities were competing for young doctors and the medical school was suddenly having to supply junior medical officers to the armed forces. This resulted in the final-year class of 1915 having their vacations cancelled and sitting the final exams in August 1915, rather than the usual February of the following year. Gordon had the good fortune to work at Dunedin Hospital with John Tait Bowie, who taught her to use her own powers of diagnosis rather than depending on 'modern machinery' such as X-ray machines. She believed her clinical work with Bowie eventually led to her gaining top marks in the medical and surgical final examinations.

On the Tuesday after she found out she had passed her final exams, Gordon received a telegram telling her she was required urgently and was to report for duty at Dunedin Hospital the following day with three other graduates. Within a week all the house-surgeon staff had gone to war, and the new staff were left to sink or swim.[39]

+ + +

Doris married fellow medical student William (Bill) Gordon in Palmerston North on 6 April 1917; they returned to Dunedin six days later and moved into a small flat on Pitt Street. Bill, along with the other male medical students, volunteered for the war effort as soon as he qualified, and he left for overseas on 26 April. He rose to the rank of captain and returned to New Zealand in mid-1919 as medical officer of the transport ship SS *Pakeha*.[40]

In addition to her hospital responsibilities, Doris Gordon took up a full-time position as university lecturer in bacteriology and public health under Sydney Champtaloup. She also began working towards a Diploma in Public Health. In late June she began studying abattoirs, food shops, dairy supplies and food factories as part of her research towards her diploma. She turned down a position at the

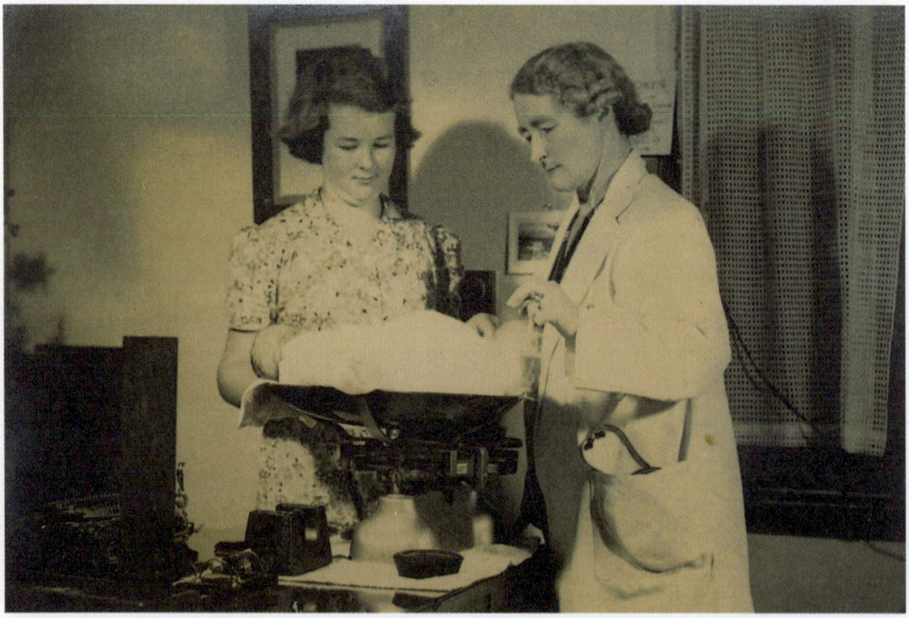

Doris Gordon and her daughter Alison weighing a baby
at Marire Hospital, Stratford. *Courtesy N. Gordon*

Department of Health — her instinct warned her to 'avoid state service, take the rougher, harder way of general practice'.[41]

The director of the Wellington office of the Department of Health introduced her to T. L. Paget from Stratford, who reportedly hated lady doctors. However, he must have been impressed because in mid-1918 he offered her a position as his long-term locum, along with his nine-bed private hospital, Marire, to mind while he was overseas on military service. Theoretically, the practice she had taken over from him was considered a 'light one' — until November 1918, when the influenza pandemic arrived.

When Bill came home and returned to civilian life in August 1919, he was able to take over Doris's locum duties. In 1919 they bought Paget's Stratford practice and private hospital, and set up a joint general practice which was their base for the rest of their working lives.[42] As she had planned, they developed the fine art of anaesthesia using pure chloroform inhalation, and later they gradually switched over to open ether. During their combined 74 years of using chloroform, they never had one mishap.

In addition, some of their maternity patients were offered 'twilight sleep', a combination of morphine and scopolamine, if the patient wanted partial or total oblivion while in labour; but they withheld this combination of drugs if the birth involved twins, toxaemia or premature labour as there was a risk of having 'puny' infants. Gordon sat up at night monitoring her patients while they were under anaesthesia.[43] Her own experiences with childbirth and raising four children enriched her medical practice.

In 1924, Gordon sent her thesis, 'Scopolamine–Morphine Narcosis in Childbirth', to the London examiners for the New Zealand MD degree. Later that year Lindo Ferguson, dean of Otago Medical School, sent her a telegram: 'Thesis accepted with commendation, my personal congratulations on the work you do for midwifery.'[44] She was successful in the clinical test but failed in the written section. She never retook the exam.

In 1922 Gordon became aware of the first 'rumblings' of state control of medicine, and she told her father she could not get the Edinburgh Fellowship of Surgeons quickly enough. Her opinion was founded on worry about the government interfering with the interests of doctors. Later, in 1927, her concerns led her to found the New Zealand Obstetrical Society (NZOS), partly 'to refute allegations that obstetricians were a forcep-interfering pest-bearing coterie'.[45] It is not clear how obtaining a fellowship would change her personal circumstances: perhaps being better qualified would give her more influence over the situation in New Zealand.

Her father offered a loan to enable her and Bill to go overseas as soon as a locum could be booked. Her mother agreed to look after their children, Peter and Ross. In December 1924 the couple boarded a freighter for England, with Bill acting as the ship's doctor. Each day they did 50 pages of revision in preparation for Edinburgh. They planned to sit their exam six weeks after landing, as they hoped to fit in a study trip to Vienna. They both passed, and Gordon became the first woman in New Zealand and Australia to be made a Fellow of the Royal College of Surgeons.[46]

In 1926 Gordon voiced a need for 'an association of midwifery practising doctors, similar to the British Obstetrical Societies, to better their work, correlate effort and to speak with a united voice on obstetrical platforms'.[47] The *New Zealand Medical Journal* reported that an obstetrical society would commence in the spring of 1926, and that the British Medical Association would be asked to recognise it.[48] Correspondence, including the aims and objectives, went out to every doctor in New Zealand. Fed up with the 'shalts and shalt-nots' from the Department of Health, 180 doctors signed as foundation members. At the inaugural meeting of the NZOS (later the NZOGS, when gynaecology was added in 1975), held at Otago Medical School on 5 February 1927, Doris and Bill Gordon were elected to the joint office of secretary–treasurer.[49]

In the late 1920s, on behalf of the NZOS, Gordon spearheaded fundraising efforts for a midwifery lecturer at Otago Medical School: they successfully raised £25,000, with the promise of about £6000 more to come. The NZOS was to be consulted on the appointment, and on the make-up of the advisory committee. Gordon's fundraising efforts only added to the accolades she received from the British College of Obstetricians and Gynaecologists in 1933: she was one of their foundation members, and she was made an Officer of the Order of the British Empire (OBE) in the 1935 Queen's Birthday Honours.[50]

+++

The Medical Council finally saw that a postgraduate obstetrical and gynaecological unit based in Auckland was essential for medical graduates to gain residential midwifery experience without depending on Britain. Dunedin was committed to training the medical undergraduates. The NZOGS, no doubt encouraged by Gordon's networking and background work in England on a 1939 visit, carried on the momentum in the war years. On 11 December 1940, the NZOGS held a conference in the British Medical Association Chambers in Wellington to discuss the proposed unit. Gordon instigated a public appeal to finance the postgraduate chair of obstetrics and gynaecology: they raised £101,203 by 1947.[51] In 1946, health minister Arnold Nordmeyer appointed Doris Gordon as director of maternal and infant welfare in the Department of Health.

Auckland eventually got its women's hospital and its postgraduate professor. In 1943, the US Army built a temporary military hospital in Cornwall Park to accommodate casualties from the war in the Pacific. The Auckland Hospital Board acquired the hospital and, after the war, established an obstetrical unit: the first baby was born there in June 1946.[52] In 1953 Harvey Carey was appointed the inaugural chair of the Postgraduate School of Obstetrics and Gynaecology. Douglas Robb, campaigner for improved medical education in New Zealand and later chancellor of the University of Auckland, saw this as the start of medical

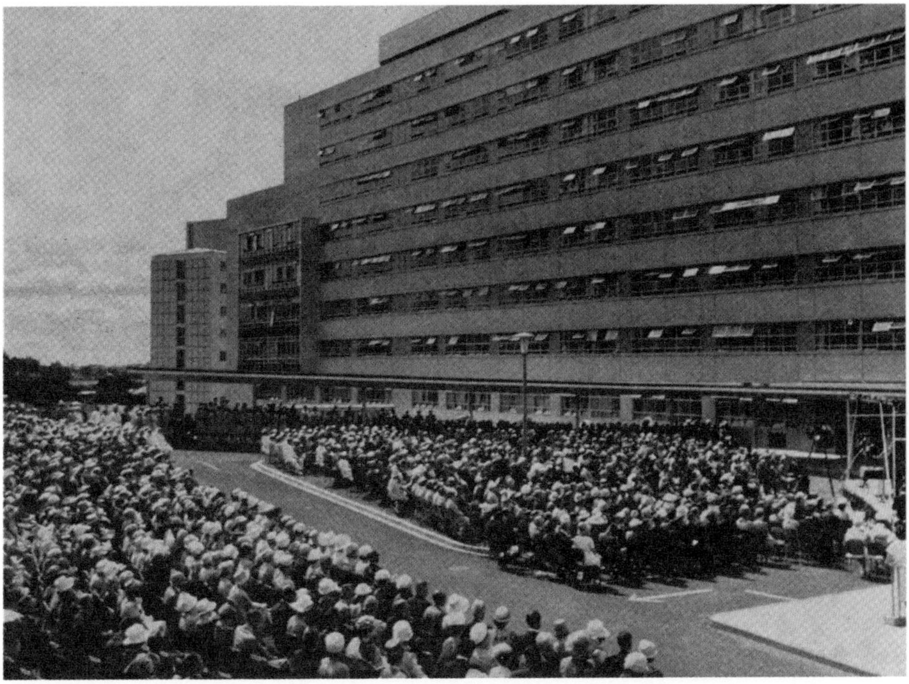

The opening of the National Women's Hospital in Auckland on 14 February 1964. *Auckland Libraries*

education in Auckland. National Women's Hospital (NWH) was officially opened on 14 February 1964.[53]

In December 1953, the Royal College of Obstetricians and Gynaecologists in London informed Gordon that, as part of their Silver Jubilee celebrations, they planned to make her an honorary fellow of the college in recognition of her services to obstetrics and gynaecology; the only condition was that she must be present to be admitted. She told her family over afternoon tea that she was going to England and that, at the age of 64, she would serve as the ship's doctor.[54] She decided it would also be a good opportunity to visit the publishers with the manuscript for her autobiography, *Backblocks Baby-Doctor*, on which she had been working for the past three years. Her son Peter and his wife were in England and accompanied her to the ceremonies, where she was presented to the Queen Mother and, a few days later, to the Queen and Duke at a royal garden party.[55]

In the second volume of her autobiography, Gordon described the open family home that she and Bill maintained at Stratford. After the Second World War they sponsored (and hosted) 32 immigrants from war-torn European countries such as Belarus, Hungary, Serbia, East Germany, Switzerland, Denmark and Holland. Their son Ross and his family lived beside his parents, and Gordon was able to enjoy her grandchildren for a few years. She died from a heart attack on 9 July 1956 at the age of 66.

After her death, the NZOGS and the National Council of Women raised £4793 to establish the Doris Gordon Trust to 'promote, sponsor, cooperate in, and otherwise further the study and/or practices of Gynaecology and Obstetrics'. After the OGS wound up in the 1990s the trust became inactive, but a new Doris Gordon Memorial Trust was established in 2016 between the New Zealand branch of the Royal Australian and New Zealand College of Obstetrics and Gynaecology and the National Council of Women to promote education in women's health, including an annual Doris Gordon Memorial Lecture.[56]

MARY FRANCESCA COMPERE DOWLING

1915 graduate — first woman to be awarded the New Zealand Medical Travelling Scholarship

Little is known of Mary Francesca Compere Dowling's early life. She was born in 1892, the second of the three children of Mary Bary and Richard Egbert Dowling. Her mother had been mistress of West End School in New Plymouth for many years. Francesca (as she was known) attended Central School and West End School, where she did well. She then attended New Plymouth High School, where she was named dux in 1908.[57] She received a senior national scholarship at the end of 1909 with the top score (2867) for the Taranaki Board area, which entitled her to a university scholarship. She was also awarded the Taranaki Scholarship, which she held for at least four years.

Dowling studied for the medical intermediate at Victoria University, Wellington, then enrolled at Otago Medical School in 1912. She lived at St Margaret's College while she was at medical school. Her friend Doris Gordon described 'Francie' in her memoir: 'Francie had big brown eyes which she could use to look roguish, intelligent, or pathetic as the occasion warranted. Before exams she was wont to lament that she knew nothing. She would then cram like a lunatic, stagger out of the exam rooms looking a wreck, and gather much sympathy. Finally, we at St Margaret's learned that more often than not she came top of everything.'[58]

As described earlier, because of the shortage of medical personnel the final MB ChB examinations were brought forward to August 1915, and the results were announced on 11 September.[59] Dowling graduated top of her class at Otago Medical School and was the first woman to be awarded the New Zealand Medical Travelling Scholarship, which included free tuition for one year in England or Europe, along with £150 in expenses. She had to defer her travel plans, however, as the scarcity of doctors in New Zealand meant that her services were needed there. Instead, Dowling, Gordon and two male students stayed on in Dunedin for their two years as house surgeons.

In October 1915, the *Christchurch Sun* announced the engagement of Francesca Dowling and fellow student Arthur Kidd.[60] Kidd had served in the New Zealand No. 1 Stationary Hospital at Amiens, France, and then with the 1st Field Ambulance, until he was wounded at Messines, Belgium; he returned to New Zealand after his convalescence. But soon after the announcement, one of them called off the engagement. It is not clear why, but in her autobiography Doris Gordon mentions that Dowling felt attracted to one of the house surgeons. Her behaviour as a young woman engaged to be married was no doubt frowned on, and at the end of 1916, neither she nor the young man was offered a second-year house surgeon position at the hospital.[61]

Dowling did a locum in early 2017 at Mangaweka, where she was called on to judge the baby show at the St Patrick's Day sports.[62] By August 1918 she had established her own practice as a GP in Hāwera (where her brother was the pharmacist).

On 20 November 1918, Dowling was reported to be seriously ill with influenza; she died two days later, at the age of 26. Her obituary in the local paper suggested that 'the strain of the hard and unceasing work she was called upon to do in the week or two preceding her illness' may have contributed to her early death.[63]

MABEL AILEEN CHRISTIE (NÉE HANRON)

1917 graduate

Mabel Christie was born in Peshawar (formerly India, now in Pakistan) in 1885, the sixth of the 11 children of Michael and Alice Hanron. Her father, who was orphaned in the aftermath of the Irish Potato Famine, had travelled from Ireland to India in early adulthood to train as an engineer with the British Army. The changing fortunes of colonial India eventually unsettled the family, prompting their immigration to Nelson, New Zealand, in 1888.

Christie spent her school years on the struggling family farm in Stanley Brook, Nelson, where her mother quietly pursued a revolutionary plan to ensure that 'no daughter of hers was to slave over a hot stove, day in day out, nor was she to soil her hands and grow old before her time'.[64] She was determined that 'the boys were to work on the farm to provide money for the girls to obtain a good education', despite the impecunious position of the family and occasional criticism from within the local community.[65] After her matriculation from Nelson Girls' College in 1904, Christie taught at primary school until the family could finally afford the medical training her mother had planned for her.

Christie studied first at Victoria University College in 1911, then continued her medical degree at the University of Otago from 1914. Life in Dunedin was harsh. There was little family money available for food and board for her or her sister, Nora, who was studying dentistry, and their health suffered. She graduated MB ChB in 1917, the nineteenth medical woman to graduate from the University of Otago. Her first appointment was as a house surgeon and physician at Dunedin Hospital, followed by a year as medical officer at Mangōnui Hospital in the Far North. Her daughter later recalled stories of weighty responsibility and isolation, including a late night spent refreshing her anatomy knowledge before operating alone to remove a gangrenous upper limb; the patient survived.

+++

Mabel married her classmate, Robert Lyall Christie, in 1919 and almost immediately moved with him to Sāmoa, where he took up an appointment as medical officer at

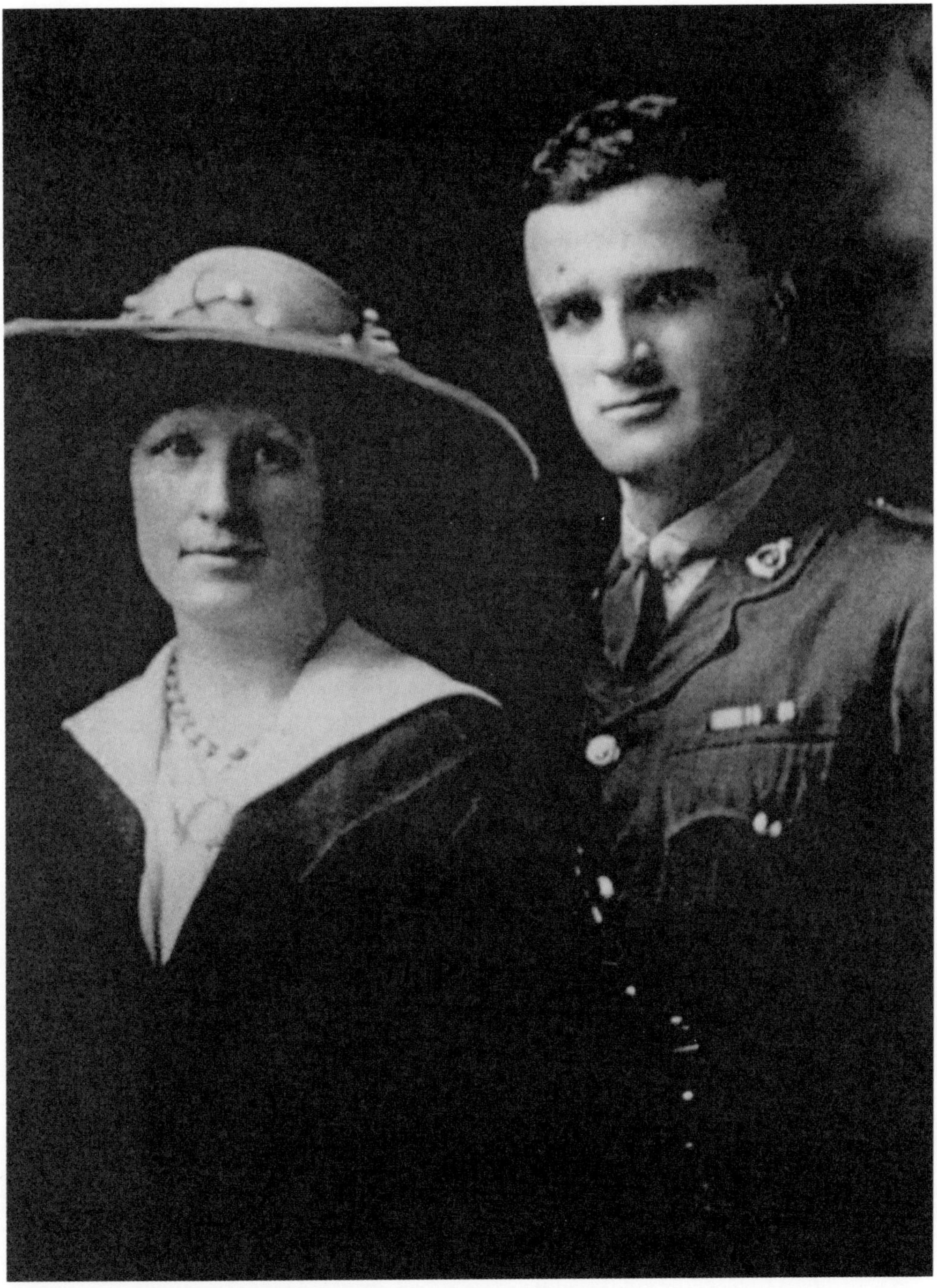

Mabel Christie (née Hanron) with her husband, Robert, in 1919. *Courtesy Nora Lynch*

Apia Hospital. She was 35 years old when she gave birth to a daughter the following year. This was to be her only living child; a subsequent son was stillborn.

Christie resumed her medical career in Sāmoa, where she worked to improve health services to mothers and children alongside Regina Keyes Roberts, wife of the American vice-consul, and local nurses. In 1925 she travelled to 85 villages 'on foot, horse and canoe for nine months . . . to explain and help establish the health committees and train the committee executive in basic first aid and sanitation'.[66]

An annual report of her work, presented to the New Zealand Department of Health in 1926 (reflecting the annexed status of Western Sāmoa at that time), makes interesting reading. Contemporary colonial patronage lies juxtaposed with authentic compassion, respect for Samoan women, and practical public health wisdom. Her assertion that 'the baby needs no other food than its mother's milk, and not only is other food unnecessary but is doing the baby a great deal of harm' is still relevant now, a century later.[67]

In 1927 the Christies moved to Rarotonga when Robert was appointed medical superintendent of the Cook Islands. It is unclear whether Mabel practised medicine during their four-year sojourn there. The family returned to live in New Zealand permanently in 1931, as their daughter approached secondary school age.

Robert Christie died in a motor vehicle accident in Wellington the following year. Mabel was just 47 years old: her daughter believed her mother never fully recovered. Thrust into the role of breadwinner, in 1933 she took a position as medical officer at the Waikouaiti Health Camp, a role commonly filled by medical women at the time. She subsequently worked in Auckland in her own private practice between 1935 and 1936, advertising her services as a physician and dietitian and sharing rooms in Civic House, Queen Street, with her dentist sister. Her daughter understood that the practice failed because, in the midst of a global Depression, 'everyone paid the doctor last'.[68] It appears Christie never worked again. She bought land, moved to West Auckland in her early fifties and lived there until her death in 1955 at the age of 70.

Her granddaughter, Nora Lynch, wrote in 2020:

> As I reflect on the life of a grandmother who I never knew, I am struck by the tenacity of her family who defied financial constraint and social mores to facilitate education for her and her sisters. As for the woman herself, it is difficult to really know her character but her pioneering child

health work in Samoa suggests abundant energy, sharp intellect and a social conscience. It is not difficult to believe the family narrative that the sadness of early widowhood extinguished a light which was never properly reignited.[69]

MARION KING BENNIE CAMERON (NÉE WHYTE)

1918 graduate — first lecturer of anaesthesia at Dunedin Hospital

Marion King Bennie Whyte was born in Glasgow, Scotland, in 1895. Her family moved to New Zealand in 1898, where her father, Alexander, a Presbyterian minister, helped found Iona College in Havelock North and later Columba College and John McGlashan College in Dunedin in 1918.[70] Whyte probably attended Havelock North Primary School on Te Mata Road. In 1906, she won a national scholarship with a score of 551, which gave her a junior scholarship to study at Napier High School. She also obtained a national scholarship at the end of 1907 with a score of 686, the third highest in New Zealand.[71]

After the family moved to Port Chalmers, Whyte attended Otago Girls' High School, where she was dux in 1912.[72] At the end of 1910, she received the second highest ranking in the Otago Education Board senior scholarships, and at the end of 1912, she was one of 10 New Zealand scholars to be awarded a junior university scholarship. Whyte began her studies at Otago Medical School in 1913. She was a resident of St Margaret's College and, in later years, became the official college doctor and had to deal with serious outbreaks of measles and polio among the young women residents.[73] By mid-June 1917, she had passed her third professional examination in applied anatomy, public health and medical jurisprudence, and she attained her MB ChB in 1918. She was a house surgeon at Dunedin Hospital for one year, followed by one year in the pathology department at the medical school.

Whyte started her Dunedin general practice combined with obstetrics and anaesthesia in 1920. According to the electoral role, she lived and had her practice at 267 High Street until 1957. In April 1927 she became one of the three members on the anaesthetic staff of Dunedin Hospital, and in 1928 she was appointed the first lecturer in anaesthesia, a role she continued to hold for the next 20 years. Her

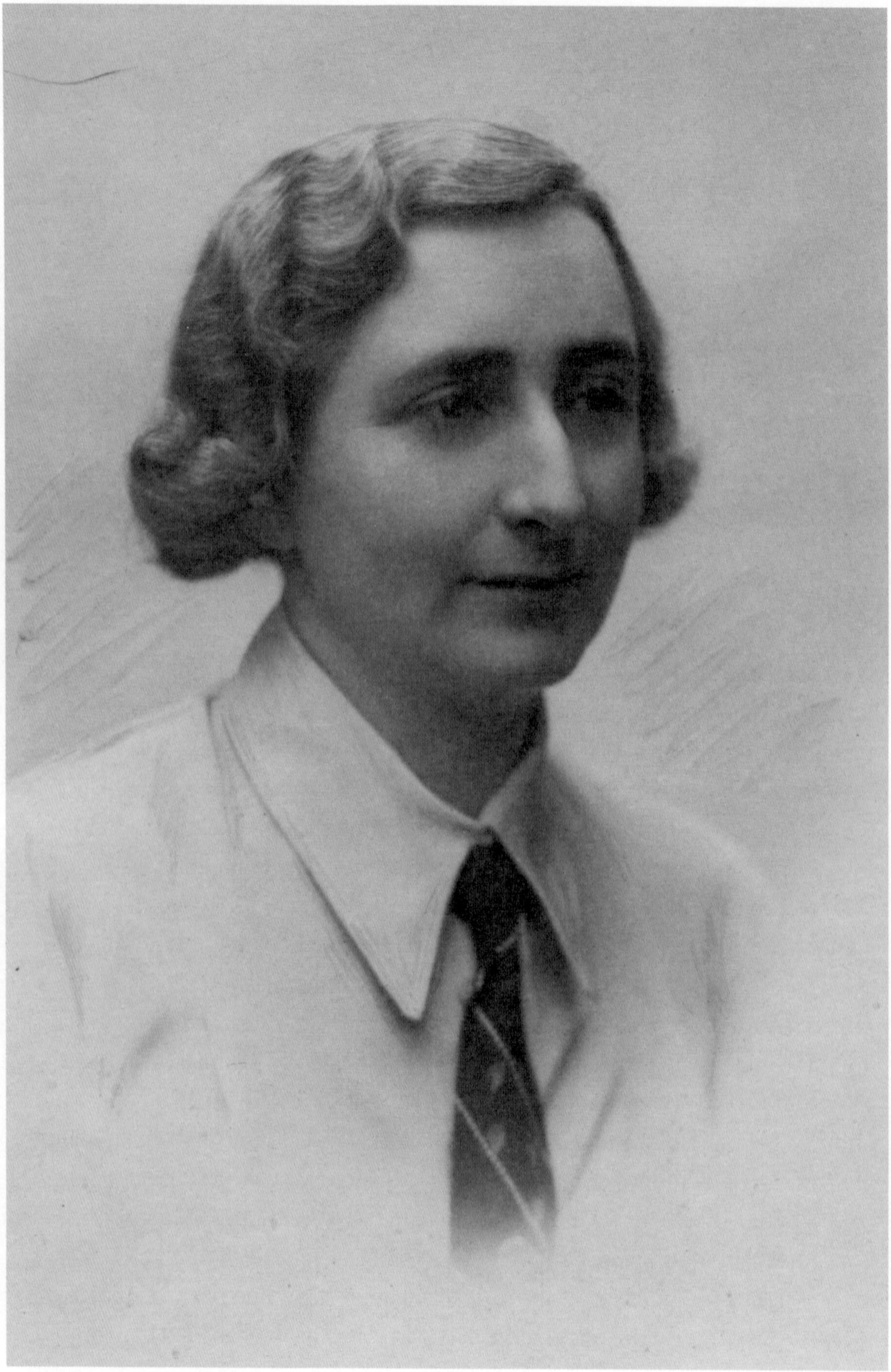

Marion King Bennie Cameron (née Whyte), c.1927. *Courtesy J. I. Clayton*

appointment indicated that the specialty was receiving some recognition after concerns in 1925 about 'deaths and anaesthesia'.

Before taking up the position, Whyte travelled to the United States and Britain from March to November 1927 to learn about the modern anaesthesia practices in these countries, which included time spent with the world-famous anaesthetist Elmer Isaac McKesson, who had developed the McKesson Nargraff gas machine. After this trip, she was regarded as a New Zealand pioneer in the use of endotracheal intubation, the use of the gas machine, intravenous fluids and spinal anaesthesia. She took over the teaching of the fifth-year anaesthetic course, which included both lectures and practical instruction, and was affectionately known as 'Maid Marion'.

In 1936 she was paid £66 per annum, with one guinea (about £1.05) for out-of-hours emergencies. She retired from her hospital and university lectureship work in 1948. Over these two decades, her time as an anaesthetist stretched from the chloroform on the kitchen table era to the complexity of modern anaesthetics for neuro and thoracic surgery.

In 1954 Whyte was elected Fellow of the Faculty of Anaesthetists of the Royal Australasian College of Surgeons (FFARACS) and was a regular attendee at college meetings. Whyte was a founding member of the New Zealand Women's Medical Association in 1921, and was appointed secretary–treasurer in 1924. In 1974 she was conferred Golden Jubilee membership of the Medical Women's International Association.

From 1958 until 1965, Whyte had her practice at Stuart Chambers, 83 Moray Place, and lived at 210 Highgate in Roslyn, Dunedin. After her marriage in 1963 at age 68, she changed her medical registration surname to Cameron, but she was always called by her maiden name. She maintained her registration until she was 86 and continued to live at her home in Highgate until her final weeks at Mater Hospital; she died on 17 September 1983. She was remembered for her devoted and loving service to her patients.

EMMA GERTRUDE ATMORE (NÉE APPLEGATE)

1919 graduate

Emma Gertrude Atmore was born in Coromandel township in 1894.[74] Her parents, Eliza Turvey and George Hubert Applegate, both originally from England, had immigrated to New Zealand when they were quite young. They met and married in Christchurch in 1887 and went on to have five daughters; Gertrude (as she was known) was the fourth. She showed academic ability early on and won a junior national scholarship to attend Auckland Girls' Grammar School, where she was a boarder.[75] In fifth and sixth forms, she won first prize for mathematics and science.

She was determined to go to Otago Medical School. As a prerequisite for admission a candidate had to have proficiency in a foreign language, so in her final year, in addition to Latin, she took German, squeezing a three-year curriculum into one year. According to the family history, she topped the whole of New Zealand in German that year, and was subsequently admitted to medical school. The family was not well off, and her father told her that if she failed a subject, then 'home she would come'.

Atmore was the only woman in her class. One of her fellow undergraduates remarked on how the quality of life for women students altered with the arrival of the beautiful, fair-haired girl from Coromandel — they called her 'the golden girl'.[76] It was a very male-dominated environment, and there were certain lectures she was not able to attend because 'they dealt with subjects unseemly for a lady', but she was still expected to be able to answer any exam questions on that topic. She graduated in 1919 and spent that year and the next as a house surgeon at Invercargill Hospital.

Atmore's first job was at Thames Hospital. She was based at Coromandel township and was medical superintendent for Coromandel. She used to travel on the *Lady Jocelyn* to Mercury Bay Hospital in Whitianga (approximately 65 nautical miles — 8 hours' travel at 8 knots). Local farmers would be waiting to take her to any patients needing attention. She would then travel back, probably overnight, often running to catch the boat before it left for Coromandel township.[77] In 1921 she became superintendent of the Otaki Sanatorium for tuberculosis patients, in the Manawatū. From 1919, the sanatorium accepted only female patients; this is

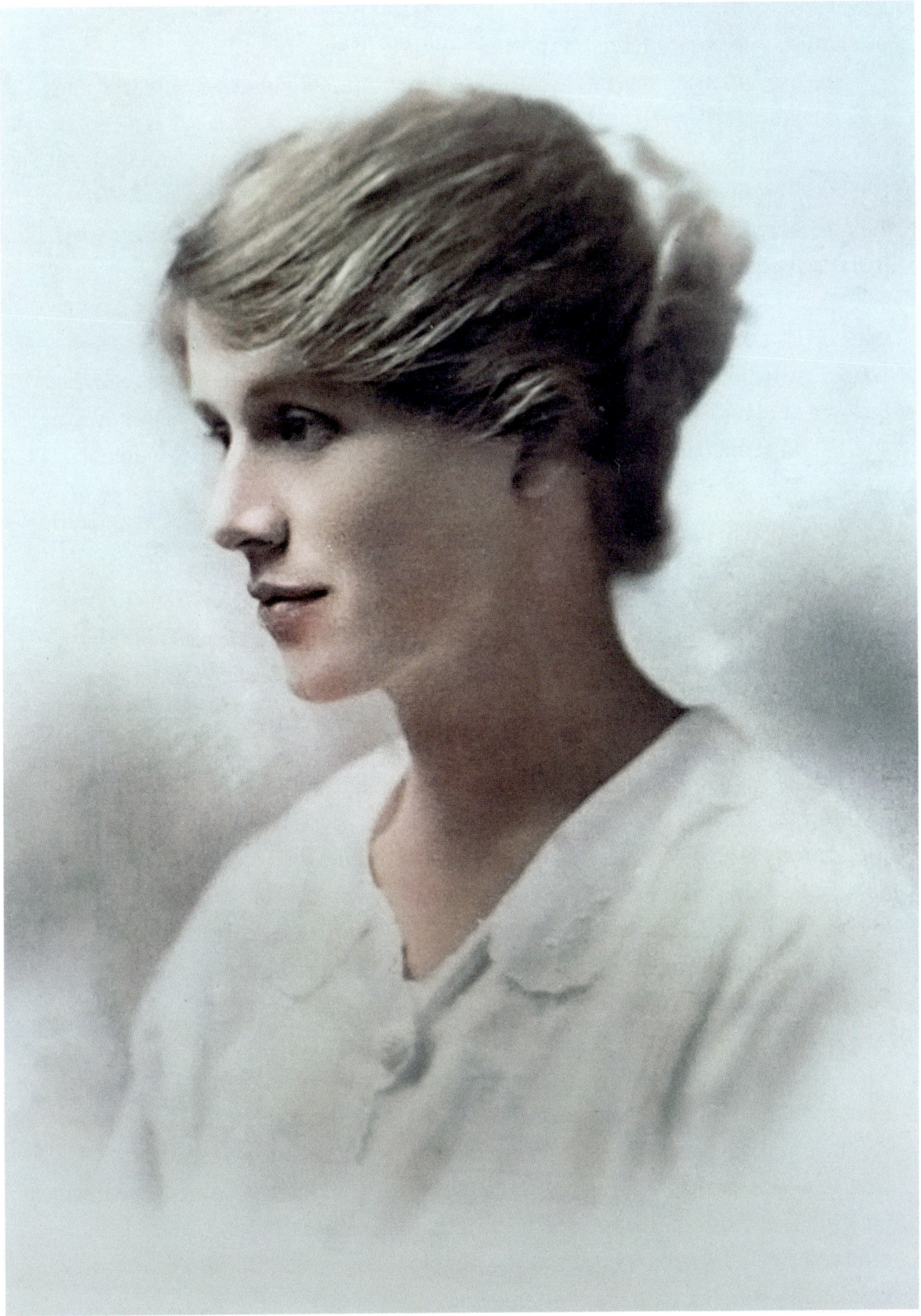

Emma Gertrude Atmore (née Applegate), c.1918. *Courtesy Tony and Chris Bush*

perhaps why she was offered this position so early in her career.[78]

In April 1922 she married Charles Frederick Atmore, an Ōtaki barrister and solicitor who also served as the town's mayor for nearly two decades.[79] Atmore set up and ran a busy medical practice from their home in Domain Road, Ōtaki, where she lived for the rest of her life. She was involved in the development of the Otaki Health Camp for children and worked there as medical officer on a volunteer basis in its early years.

She was also closely associated with the care of the large Māori population in Ōtaki. She focused on obstetrics in her practice, and during the Depression she helped birth more than 100 children — and was reputedly paid for only one of the births.[80] She would travel with her bicycle by train to Te Horo, 5 kilometres to the south, and Manakau, 5 kilometres to the north. After attending to her patients in these rural areas, she would cycle back to Ōtaki.

Life was busy: in addition to her duties as a GP, Atmore had responsibilities as a wife and a mother to her two children — Colin (born in 1925) and Lois (1929). She also supported her husband during his tenure as the mayor (from 1929 to 1933 and then again from 1938 to 1953), and took on the office of mayoress for 20 years, including during the Depression and the start of the Second World War. Her medical knowledge and wide acquaintance with the people of the borough made her ideally suited to discharge the social welfare duties of this public office.[81]

As mayoress, she was responsible for entertaining military personnel from the US Army camps (Camp McKay and Camp Russell) at what is now Queen Elizabeth Park. During the war she was chair of the Otaki Women's Emergency Committee, helping in its wartime activities, including organising parcels to be sent to troops overseas. In 1930 Atmore worked with Doris Gordon to establish the chair of obstetrics at Otago Medical School, and initiated an appeal for funds.

+++

Atmore's son-in-law, Richard Bush, a paediatrician who practised at Hutt and Wellington hospitals during the 1960s and 1970s, described her as 'a tall, statuesque woman with a quick intelligent mind and wide interests. She was an astute medical practitioner, with a large practice of devoted patients, as I found when I did a 9-month locum for her in 1955 when she went to Europe and Britain for an overseas holiday. She was a most memorable and lovely lady.'[82]

Atmore was diagnosed with breast cancer and decided to retire in December 1957 at the age of 64. She died at home on 24 February 1959. As a sign of the esteem in which the Ōtaki Māori community held her, she was given a tangi at Raukawa Marae before her church funeral. The tangi was one of the largest ever held at the marae, with Māori, Pākehā and Chinese mourners all paying their respects. After a short ceremony at the marae, her casket was draped in a korowai — an honour reserved for rangatira — before being taken to Rangiātea Church, which the iwi had offered as a fitting place to farewell her.

Atmore was greatly loved and esteemed by the Ōtaki community. In 1964, a clock tower was dedicated in her honour.[83] The entrance to the library has an inscription on a large stone that reads: 'Beloved physician for 37 years and Mayoress of Otaki for 19 years.' And the 'supper room' at the Memorial Hall in Ōtaki is named the Gertrude Atmore Lounge.

When Otaki College opened in 1960, the Atmore family made an endowment to create the Dr Gertrude Atmore Memorial to fund three annual prizes: for dux; for a junior student showing promise in science subjects; and for the Māori student showing the most promise during the year. Atmore's memory lives on in the community through these annual prizes.

The Otago Medical School third-year class of 1922. Second row, from left: Margaret Lemon (née Grater; 1926), Uriti Strack-Torrie (née Strack; 1925), Mary Russell (1927), Effie Morgan (1925), Muriel Bell (1922; by this point a lecturer), Felicia Walmsley (1926), Helen Deem (née Easterfield; 1924), M. M. Auburn (did not graduate), Catherine Anderson (1925), Alexandra Mathieson (1927). *Otago Medical School Archives*

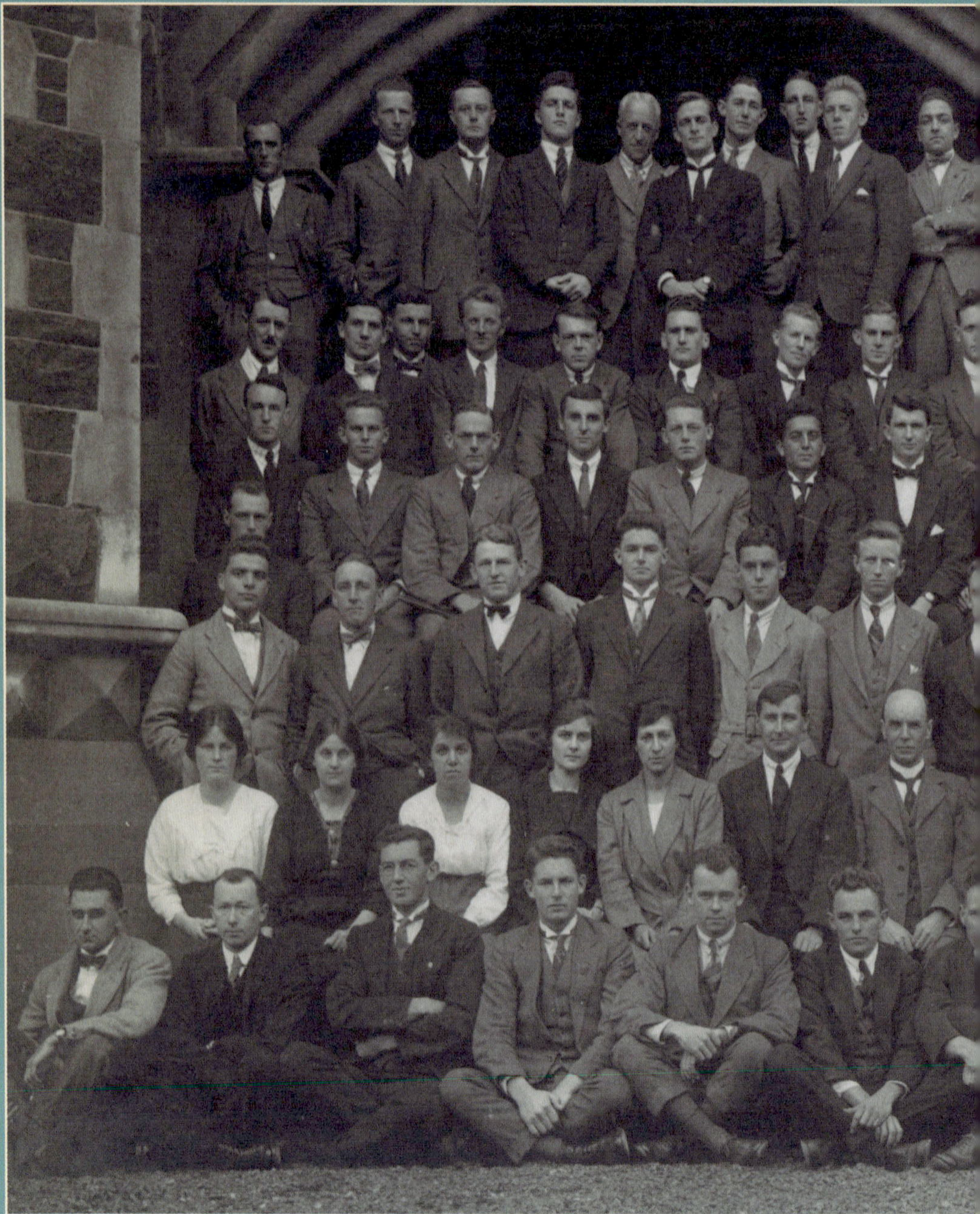

3. The interwar years 1920–1938

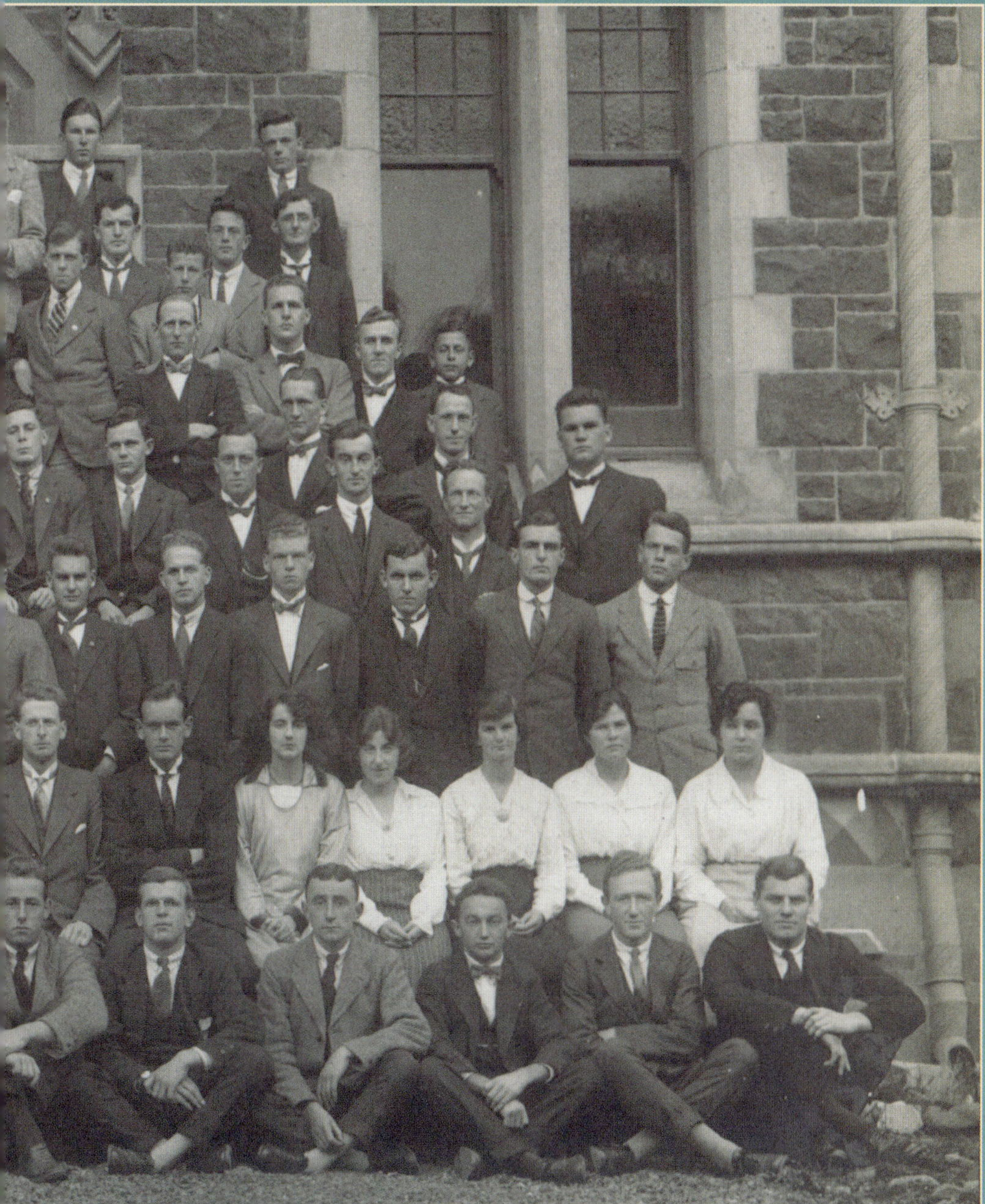

The period between the end of the First World War and the declaration of the Second World War was a time of great change in New Zealand. Cars and other motor vehicles arrived in droves; ships and shipping routes expanded, bringing more resources and people to the country; the dairy industry grew as farms mechanised; and cinemas sprouted in towns and cities, provoking fears of an 'American invasion' as Hollywood dominated the talkies.[1] Society's strict social mores relaxed: by the end of the First World War, young women were no longer expected to be chaperoned and unmarried women had unparalleled access to paid employment.[2]

But for all the seeming modernity, New Zealand's image of itself — and the image it depicted to the rest of the world — was still as a 'better Britain'. The sense of empire may have been tested by the experiences of the First World War, but it was enduring, and the country was continually neglectful of Māori and intolerant of non-white immigrants. In 1920, New Zealand denied people of Chinese birth or descent the right of permanent residence while allowing it for those of British or Irish birth. Intimate relationships and intermarriage between Pākehā and Māori became socially more acceptable but were still taboo between Māori and Chinese people.

A strong eugenics movement was popular among the social elite. Eugenics was initially perceived as a progressive social movement. With roots in social Darwinism, it was designed to control populations and selectively 'breed out' traits, diseases and disabilities deemed undesirable. Throughout the 1910s and 1920s, it was a frequent intellectual and political point of contention, with advocates for the movement on both sides of the political spectrum, including Emily Siedeberg and

Truby King, founder of the Plunket Society in 1907. When a short-lived eugenics board was established by the government in 1928, Ada Paterson was appointed to the board — a sign to women's organisations that women's voices were being heard on the issue.[3]

The number of women entering domestic service continued to decline as better wages and conditions became available in offices, stores and factories; and the number of jobs increased for women as teachers, nurses, social workers and — for a limited few — doctors.[4] Historian Barbara Brookes argues that in this period 'the focus on motherhood as the purpose of female existence was increasingly being contested by a new generation of women who experienced independent working lives in the growing towns. As one said, "All a flapper wanted to do was to have a jolly gay time."'[5] Brookes estimates that by 1921, 'over 50 per cent of young women between the ages of 15 and 24 were in paid employment, compared to about 39 per cent in 1891'.[6] Women's wages, however, remained lower than men in equivalent roles. Women working in the public service were frequently denied promotion, as male officials deemed them 'not fully suitable for higher positions'.[7]

The same was true for women doctors. By 1936, 110 women had completed the MB ChB at Otago Medical School, but as Michael Belgrave has noted, 'it was one thing to emerge with a medical degree and quite another to earn a living'.[8]

Although opportunities for women in medicine had improved during the war years, the difficulties of achieving hospital or practice placements returned in the 1920s as preference was given to male doctors returning from the war. Male doctors were often reluctant to share private practice patients with their female colleagues, and many patients were still suspicious of women doctors. Women often worked as locums throughout their early careers; others joined difficult-to-access rural practices. Because of the difficulties of purchasing or trading private practices, some women doctors felt their only choice was to join the School Medical Service (SMS), which was staffed predominantly by women and was largely seen as suitable for a 'lady doctor'.[9]

The SMS was established in 1912 in an effort to improve public health: doctors working for the service examined children three times throughout their school years. Many of the women who took positions at the SMS found that the job constrained their ability to move into other specialties later in their career.

Despite these obstacles, women graduates were able to make the most of the newly reopened world. Postgraduate qualifications were not yet available in New Zealand, but specialisation was becoming more prevalent in Western medical practice, and opportunities were opening up for postgraduate study in Europe and the United States.[10] Augusta Klippel, Kathleen Todd, Kathleen Pih-Chang (1929), Margaret Smith (née Riddell; 1936) and Alice Bush (née Stanton; 1937) all did further training in Britain, Austria or the United States. Some of them reunited while they were overseas. Vienna was a centre for postgraduate medical studies in 1925, and doctors travelled there from all over the world to enrol. The American Medical Association of Vienna was established to assist English-speaking doctors, and became a hub for expats. Kathleen Todd caught up with Augusta Klippel while they were both in Vienna for postgraduate studies, and Todd boarded with two other women doctors in Bloomsbury, London, while she was gaining surgical experience.

While opportunities were increasingly opening up overseas, in New Zealand the conditions of marginalised groups deteriorated during the Depression as wages dropped, unemployment rose and the country sank into an economic slump. Doctors such as Moana Gow (1921) often did not charge for consultations, or they allowed patients to pay in kind: according to her daughter and granddaughter, she could be paid in 'a leg of lamb from the farmers'.[11] Molly Smith (née Wagstaff; 1938) noted the effects of the Depression in her student years: in the boarding house where she lived, the landlord attempted to save money by airing his tenants' sheets on the line rather than washing them; he would then distribute the sheets at random back to the students. Smith decided she would rather sleep on her own unwashed sheets than someone else's.

A wave of women joined the workforce between 1930 and 1935, and there was a 30 per cent drop in the number of women enrolled in the medical school. As historian Dorothy Page noted, though class sizes grew during the 1930s, the proportion of women in those classes shrank.[12] The Depression may explain the decrease: reduced incomes left many unable to afford the fees. At the 1935 general election, Labour had promised that it would lift incomes to a level sufficient to provide a man and his family with enough to make a 'home'. Barbara Brookes notes that women and children were 'classed together as dependants, to be provided for

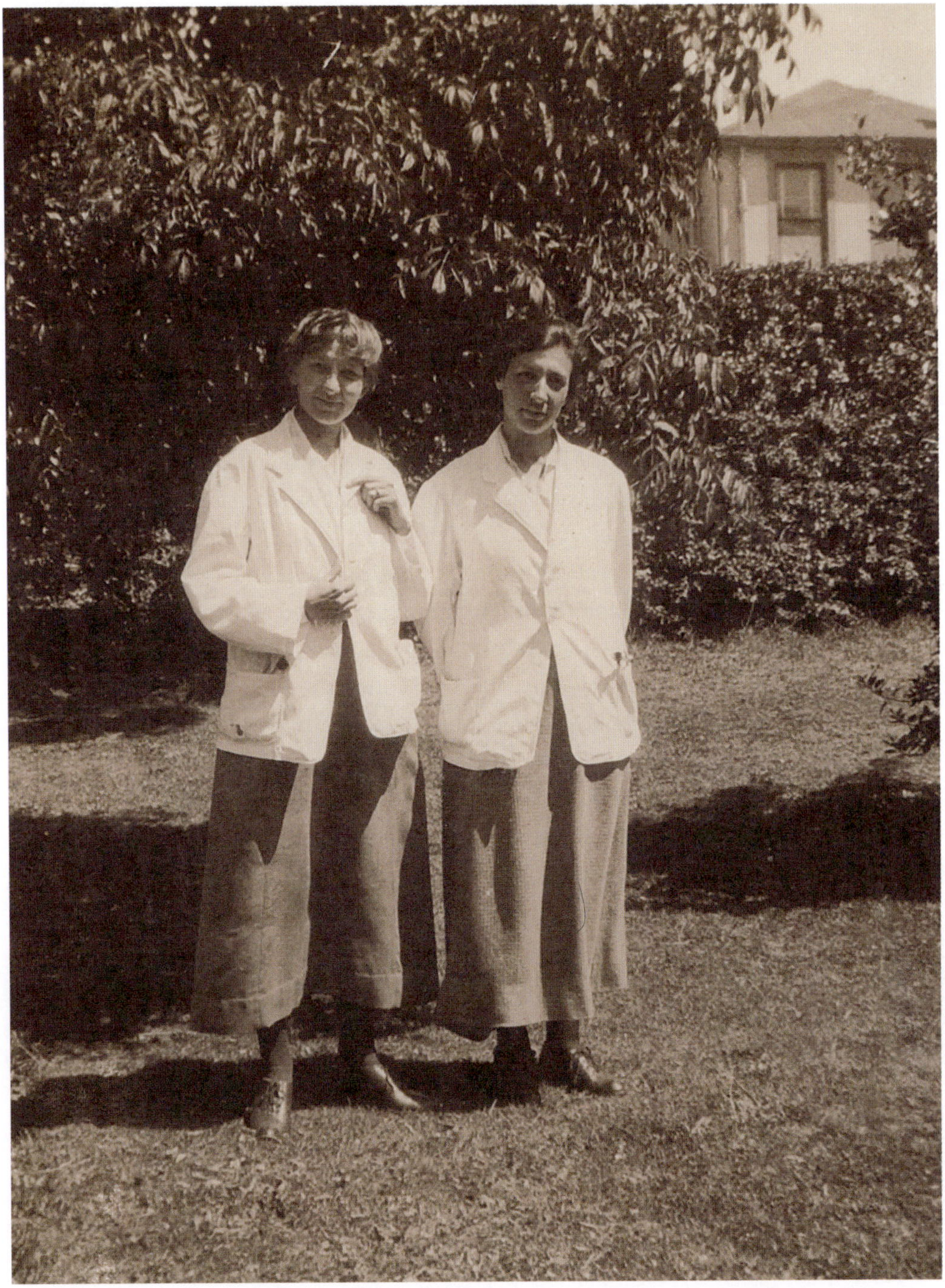

Students Elaine Gurr (left) and Muriel Bell, both 1922 graduates, working as hospital bursars in 1921. Bursars had to attend lectures and complete their practical work in addition to their hospital duties. *Houghton family collection*

by the male wage earner'.[13] This was reflected in the gender wage gap: men were still paid higher wages than women.

The Labour government introduced a minimum wage, the family benefit was increased, and the Social Security Act of 1938 made superannuation universal and hospital care free. Before these reforms, medical care had been provided on a 'user-pays' basis, with the cost mitigated by several charities. Alice Bush, like a number of other doctors, was reluctant to embrace the healthcare reforms as she felt they would turn doctors into salaried civil servants and would interfere with freedom of choice for both doctor and patient.[14]

Single women in the workforce may have been somewhat more socially acceptable by the late 1930s, but once a woman was married, she was generally still expected to devote herself to the home.[15] Women doctors would have felt the same pressure to conform with this push to support the household headed by the male. But many of those who stepped away from active practice after marriage remained involved in their local medical communities and often resumed practice once their children came of age. Molly Smith, for example, trained as an anaesthetist at Dargaville Hospital in the 1960s as her husband's health declined.[16]

Not all women doctors left medical work after they married. Alice Bush managed work and motherhood throughout the 1940s with the aid of nannies and her family while her husband, Faulkner, was serving in the Middle East. She was able to establish a private paediatric practice in the 1950s, and in 1955 she became the first New Zealand woman to be elected a Fellow of the Australian College of Physicians.[17] Likewise, with the help of their parents, Margaret Smith and her husband divided domestic duties so she could continue her medical career. She took pride in being a pioneer 'working mum', and her son remembers her as 'a great mum to the three of us who would often talk about interesting cases she had seen'.[18]

Despite the more flexible attitudes to women working during this period, women doctors had to navigate a heavily patriarchal society, and to fight for opportunities for having both a family and a career in the face of seemingly unending opposition.

AUGUSTA KLIPPEL (NÉE MANOY)

1922 graduate — first Jewish woman graduate[19]

Augusta Klippel was born in 1898 in Tukums, a small town not far from Riga, the capital of Latvia, at a time when Latvia was under Russian Tsarist rule.[20] The period of social and political unrest leading up to the October Revolution of 1905 was difficult for her family. Her father, Aaron Manoy, was forced to flee Tukums because a cousin was implicated in the riots that preceded the 1905 Bloody Sunday massacre in Russia. He went first to England, where some relatives had settled after previous pogroms, before moving to New Zealand, where an uncle had immigrated earlier. He decided to settle in Stratford, where he established a drapery shop.

In 1910, he finally had enough money to send for his family in Latvia. His wife, Yetta, and their three daughters escaped without passports or documentation and found their way to London, where they took a passage to New Zealand to start their new life in Stratford.[21] After a long and difficult journey Klippel, who was 12, found Taranaki a disappointment: 'It was like landing in a desert . . . the only beauty you could see in Stratford was Mount Egmont [Taranaki] but they had started to burn out the land and all you could see was burned out trees . . . and it was very depressing.'[22]

The early days in Stratford were humble beginnings for the Manoy family. Initially, their small house on Juliet Street lacked heating and had little furniture. There were only three other Jewish families in the whole of Taranaki, and they were very remote from the congregations; the nearest rabbi and synagogue were in Wellington.[23]

Klippel's family was horrified when she told them that she wanted to become a doctor — traditionally, the youngest daughter in a Jewish family would stay home to look after her ageing parents. Nevertheless, her family financed her to attend medical school. She entered straight after finishing high school in 1916 and only came home to visit her family in the summer holidays. She boarded at St Margaret's College where, as the first Jewish resident, along with two Catholic students she had to get permission from the matron to attend prayers and readings from the Old Testament only, despite constant threats by the college that they would dismiss her if she did not attend New Testament meetings as well.

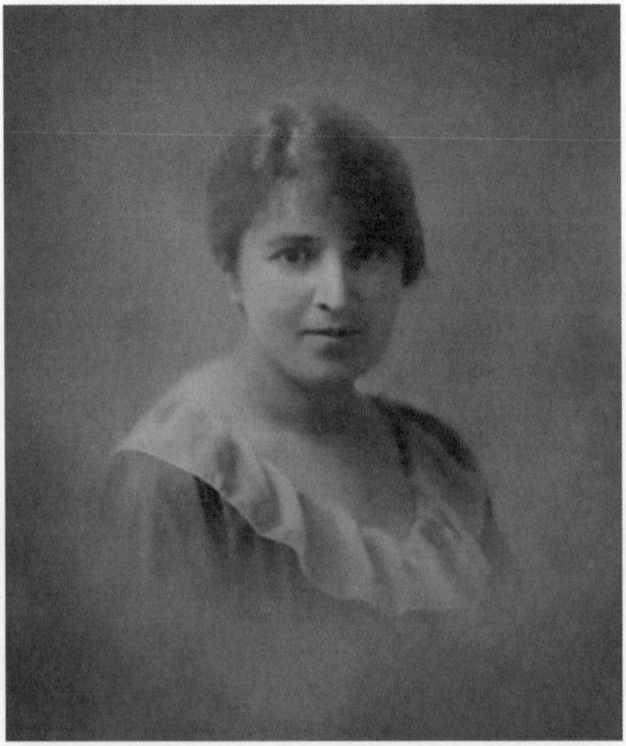

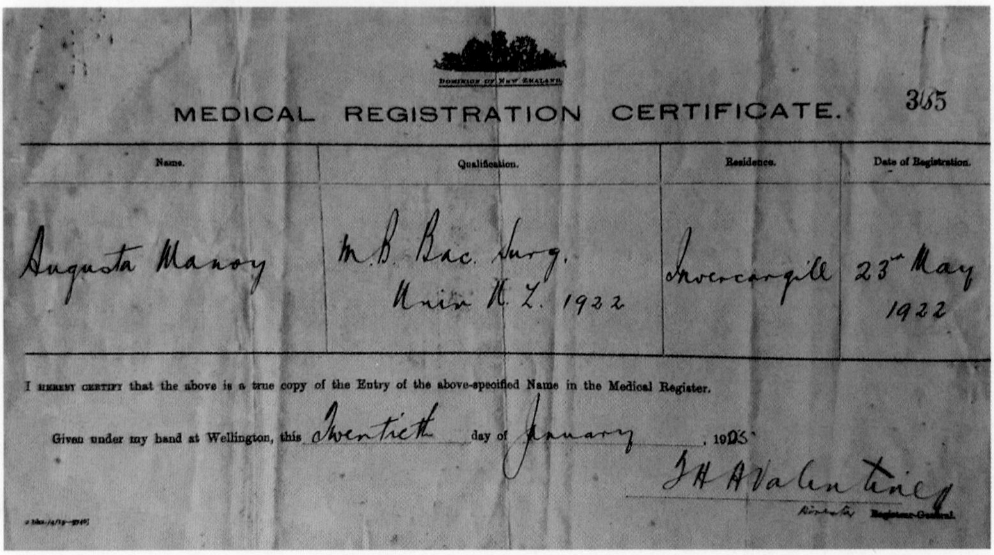

DOMINION OF NEW ZEALAND

MEDICAL REGISTRATION CERTIFICATE. 365

Name.	Qualification.	Residence.	Date of Registration.
Augusta Manoy	M.B. Bac. Surg. Univ N.Z. 1922	Invercargill	23rd May 1922

I HEREBY CERTIFY that the above is a true copy of the Entry of the above-specified Name in the Medical Register.

Given under my hand at Wellington, this Twentieth day of January, 1923.

T H A Valentine
Director Registrar-General.

ABOVE: Augusta Klippel's graduation photo, taken in Stratford, 1922.
She did not attend her capping ceremony or the ball in Dunedin. *Courtesy Ann Gluckman*

BELOW: Augusta Klippel's medical registration from May 1922. *Courtesy Ann Gluckman*

The first year of medical school was difficult: Klippel had not learned any science at high school, and she spent the first year catching up on other subjects she had not previously studied. Even so, she quickly became known for her diligence and intelligence: in 1919 she was awarded 'Keenest Lady Student' in Louis Edward Barnett's surgical class. She also had a very active social life.

In November 1918, at the end of her second year, the influenza epidemic reached Dunedin, and the second-year medical students were asked to work in the hospital. Klippel requested to be rostered on to the all-male Plunket ward. 'It was the most tragic six weeks . . . Night after night, I can't tell you what it was like, it was like a plague. The horror of it. Well we just stuck it out.' At the end of the year she came down with the flu, and went home to recuperate with her family in Stratford. When she returned to Dunedin, she was granted access to the viceregal compartment of the train, in the governor-general's coach, as a special reward for her work on the Plunket ward.

+++

In 1922, Augusta Klippel became the first Jewish woman doctor to graduate from Otago Medical School. Finding work was difficult, however: she claimed that Truby King wrote to all women who applied for a job at the Karitane Hospital until his retirement in 1927: 'I do not approve of women medicos . . . It's your job to get married and produce bonny babies.'[24]

Eventually she secured an assistantship in Tākaka for eight months under a Dr Woodward. Life as a rural medical practitioner was difficult and lonely. Woodward was the only doctor in the area, and he was always on call. When Klippel joined the practice, he hoped to 'make some scheme to work upon as regards being on duty so that each may be certain of having a "Spell" off duty . . . It is not the actual amount of work that kills. It is the horrible sensation throughout the whole 24 hours that one is likely to be called upon at any minute.' Despite describing her eight months in Tākaka as 'hard work' and a 'rough practice', she claimed that she 'learned a tremendous lot'.[25]

After two years as a house surgeon in Invercargill, Klippel moved to London for postgraduate studies in paediatrics, a field that had fascinated her while she was studying. During the stopover in Sydney, she stayed with the Kahn family, who were friends from Tukums, and met a young business associate of the Kahns,

Samuel Klippel. They spent 10 hours together before she boarded the ship and set off. When the boat docked again in Melbourne, there was a radio message from him: 'Will meet you in Adelaide, I'm coming by train.'[26]

He proposed to her in Adelaide and asked her not to go further, to which she replied, 'Not on your life. I worked eight years at medicine and I'm not going to abandon it now.' And so she carried on. During her time in England, Samuel Klippel bombarded her with messages asking her to come back. She finally agreed after fruitless attempts to find a job in London, but she attached conditions. First, she wanted to go to Vienna to complete her postgraduate studies. Second, he had to go to Stratford to formally ask for her hand in marriage and receive her family's approval.

At the end of 1925, after completing the certificate in paediatrics in Vienna, Klippel sailed from London to Adelaide. On 11 February 1926, the couple was married in the garden of the Manoy family home in Stratford before moving to Sydney, where Augusta worked in several hospitals. In 1927 they moved for a year to London, where Samuel bought textiles for his tie-manufacturing firm. Their daughter Ann was born in December that year. The family moved back to Sydney in 1928, and in 1930 their son Geoffrey was born. Klippel became ill during this time, and she never resumed medical practice. In 1934 the family returned to Auckland, where the children were largely looked after by a nanny.[27]

Although she was not actively practising, Klippel stayed heavily involved in medicine throughout her life. She served three terms as president of the Auckland branch of the Women's Medical Association, was a respected member of the Union of Jewish Women, a foundation member of the Friends of the Deaf, and raised funds for the much-anticipated National Women's Hospital on the slopes of Maungakiekie. Klippel died of kidney failure in October 1989 at the age of 91.

KATHLEEN MARY GERTRUDE TODD

1923 graduate — first woman child psychologist in New Zealand

Kathleen Mary Gertrude Todd was born on 19 November 1898 in Heriot, West Otago, the third of the seven children of Mary Hegarty and Charles Todd. She was a high achiever from the beginning: she was dux of St Dominic's Convent School for

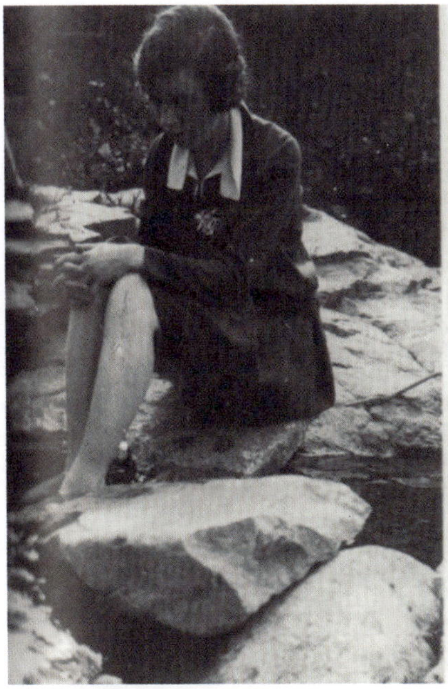

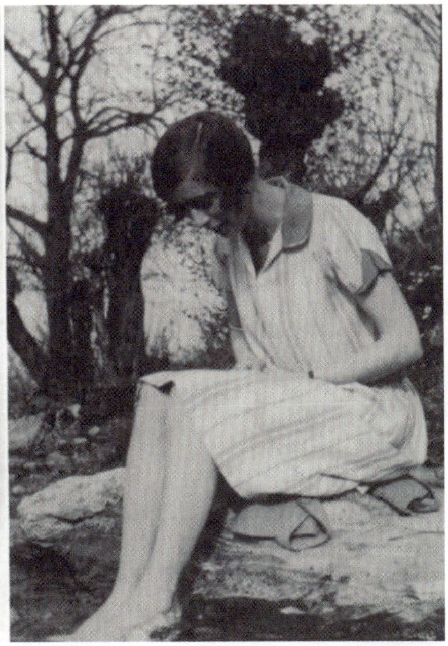

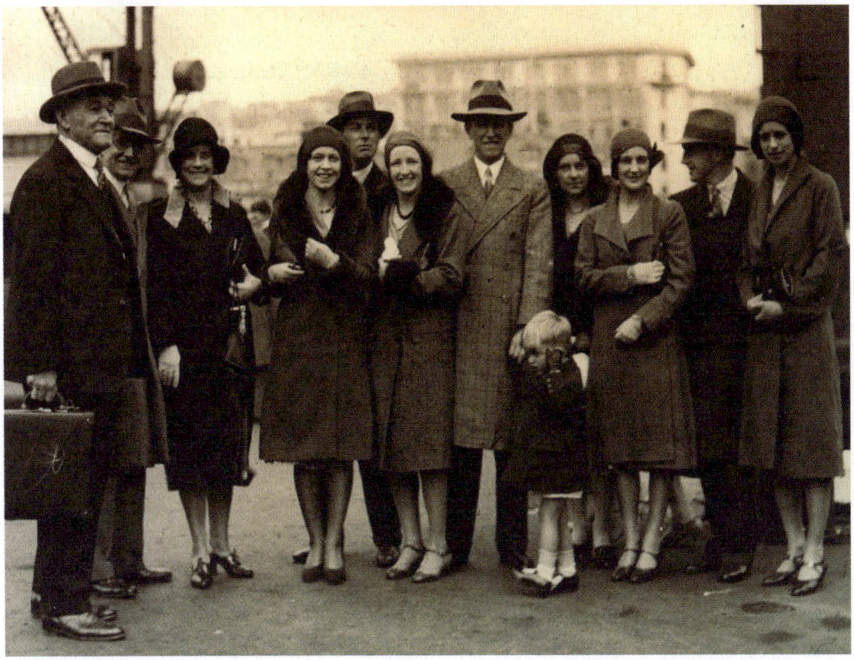

ABOVE: Kathleen and Moyra Todd in Italy in 1926. *Family collection*

BELOW: Kathleen Todd and her family reunited on Queens Wharf, Wellington, in 1930. From left: Charles, Bryan, Mary, Kathleen, Charles P., Bryan's wife Helen, Desmond with his son John and wife Rita, Sheila, Andrew and Moyra. *Ross Galbreath and Todd Corporation, Enterprise and Energy (2010)*

Girls in Dunedin, and passed the matriculation exam and the public service exam, which gave successful candidates an opportunity to be appointed to a position in the public service.[28]

But when Todd announced that she had decided to become a doctor her father, an auctioneer and founder of the Todd Motor Company, was astonished — he had been expecting that she would come and work with him in his office. Her mother, who came from an Irish family of doctors, including women doctors, was very supportive. Kathleen's sister Sheila remembered that their mother 'prayed all night for Dad to let her go to university rather than going into the office. Father gave in; Kathleen could go to university.'[29]

Todd entered her first year of medical school in the 1917 intake, which included an unusually large proportion of women. Although her achievements at school were many, she did not immediately succeed academically, a not uncommon situation for the many early women medical students who had not been taught physics and chemistry at their high schools.

Despite the rough start, Todd graduated in 1923 along with 11 other women doctors, the highest number yet at Otago. However, their medical degrees did not guarantee them a job. The few house surgeon positions Todd applied for all went to men, but fortunately she was offered a locum by George McCall Smith of Rāwene, Northland, and went to work in his general practice there in 1925.[30]

Later that year, Charles Todd offered to take the family on a world trip. Kathleen accompanied them until they reached Vienna, where she decided to stay while the rest of the family continued its travels. In Vienna, Todd reunited with her friends from medical school, Augusta Klippel and Sylvia Gytha de Lancey Chapman (1921), who were undertaking postgraduate studies in Vienna. She attended lectures and demonstrations in both the hospitals and at the university and joined the American Medical Association of Vienna, which assisted English-speaking doctors.[31]

In 1926, Todd and her younger sister, Moyra, left for London, where they stayed in a boarding house in Bloomsbury. She gained experience in surgical work and received clinical instruction as a house surgeon in London. At the same time, she was becoming increasingly interested in psychological medicine, and in 1928 she moved to the United States for further experience.

Todd first landed a position as a house surgeon at the Baby Hospital (now the Children's Hospital) in Oakland, California, which focused on maternal and child health. She then moved to Boston to work for the privately funded Judge Baker

Foundation, which focused on research and treatment of 'delinquency' in children. This research prompted her to return to London in 1929 to complete a Diploma in Psychological Medicine.[32] This involved several practicums at psychiatric institutions, including Maudsley Hospital, in Camberwell, and Tavistock Clinic, a voluntary psychotherapy establishment in Tavistock Square in Bloomsbury.

+ + +

In 1929 she returned to New Zealand and was offered a position that appeared perfect for her qualifications and interests. As part of the government's efforts to increase the health of the population, a Mental Defectives Amendment Act had been passed in 1928. Aligned with the eugenics movement, the intent of the Act was to improve the health of the population, but the legislation was abhorrent: it established a programme by which children could be classified as 'defective' and not fit for social life or procreation. The aim was to institutionalise them to prevent them from committing crimes. Psychological clinics, such as the one that hired Todd, were established around the country to conduct these assessments.

Todd's salary of £590 a year made her one of the highest-paid women in the public sector. Although high for a public servant, the salary was one of the lowest in the medical community. By 1935, frustrated at being passed over for promotion by men, she and Moyra returned to London, where they established a permanent home in Hampstead. Their home became a meeting place for New Zealand doctors travelling through London.

In London Todd soon returned to her 'beloved Tavi', the Tavistock Clinic. She also secured a position in the psychiatric clinic of Hill End Hospital for Mental and Nervous Diseases, and she opened her own private practice in Wimpole Street. She received great recognition for her work in London. In 1938 she became a member of the British Psychological Society, and she was appointed as a fellow in 1942. She became a Fellow of the Royal Society of Medicine in 1941, and was the first New Zealander to be admitted as a member of the Royal Medico-Psychological Association in 1943.[33]

At the end of the war, men were returning to their positions and there was a period of readjustment. Todd had health issues and so in 1946 she and Moyra decided to return to New Zealand so she could recuperate. However, her health deteriorated and she was diagnosed with cerebral arteriosclerosis. In 1949 she and Moyra moved to Wellington and bought a house in Melling, Lower Hutt. At first, they had plans to establish this as a children's home or psychiatric hospital but instead Todd renewed her New Zealand medical registration and opened up a private practice there. In 1962, Kathleen established the Todd Charitable Trust — a fellowship for young psychiatrists to pursue postgraduate studies in Europe. She died at home on 21 March 1968.

KATHLEEN (KAY) ANUEI PIH-CHANG (BI ZHEN-WAH) (NÉE PIH)

1929 graduate — first Chinese and first non-European woman medical graduate

Bi Zhen-Wah,[34] later known as Kathleen (Kay) Pih, was born on 10 June 1903 in Antung (now Linshui) in Jiangsu Province, northwest of Shanghai.[35] Her father was a scholar who worked primarily teaching Chinese to missionaries. One day he told Margaret Reid, a New Zealander who taught at the mission station, that his daughter was dying, and Reid offered to look after her despite having no medical training herself. The girl was unconscious and had a weak pulse, and Reid asked her father to sign a document saying that he would not blame her if his daughter died. She proceeded to revive her, feeding her milk from donkeys, water buffalo and goats, and glucose water. It took a whole year for her to recover.[36]

In 1907 Reid received a letter from her own father asking her to return to New Zealand: his health was declining. She did not want to leave Pih-Chang until she was stable, so her brother John suggested that she bring the girl to New Zealand with her. His personal request to the governor-general, Lord Plunket, helped speed up the application, which was usually a protracted and complex process given that people from China were considered 'restricted entry aliens' in New Zealand.[37]

The boat left from Shanghai, and Pih-Chang's father travelled with them from Antung to see her off. This was the last time she saw her father. Reid and the young Pih-Chang arrived in Wellington in February 1908. They settled at first in Dunedin and then moved to Waimate in South Canterbury after Reid married Charles Russell, a farmer. Russell had two daughters with whom Pih-Chang got on well, but life was difficult for her.

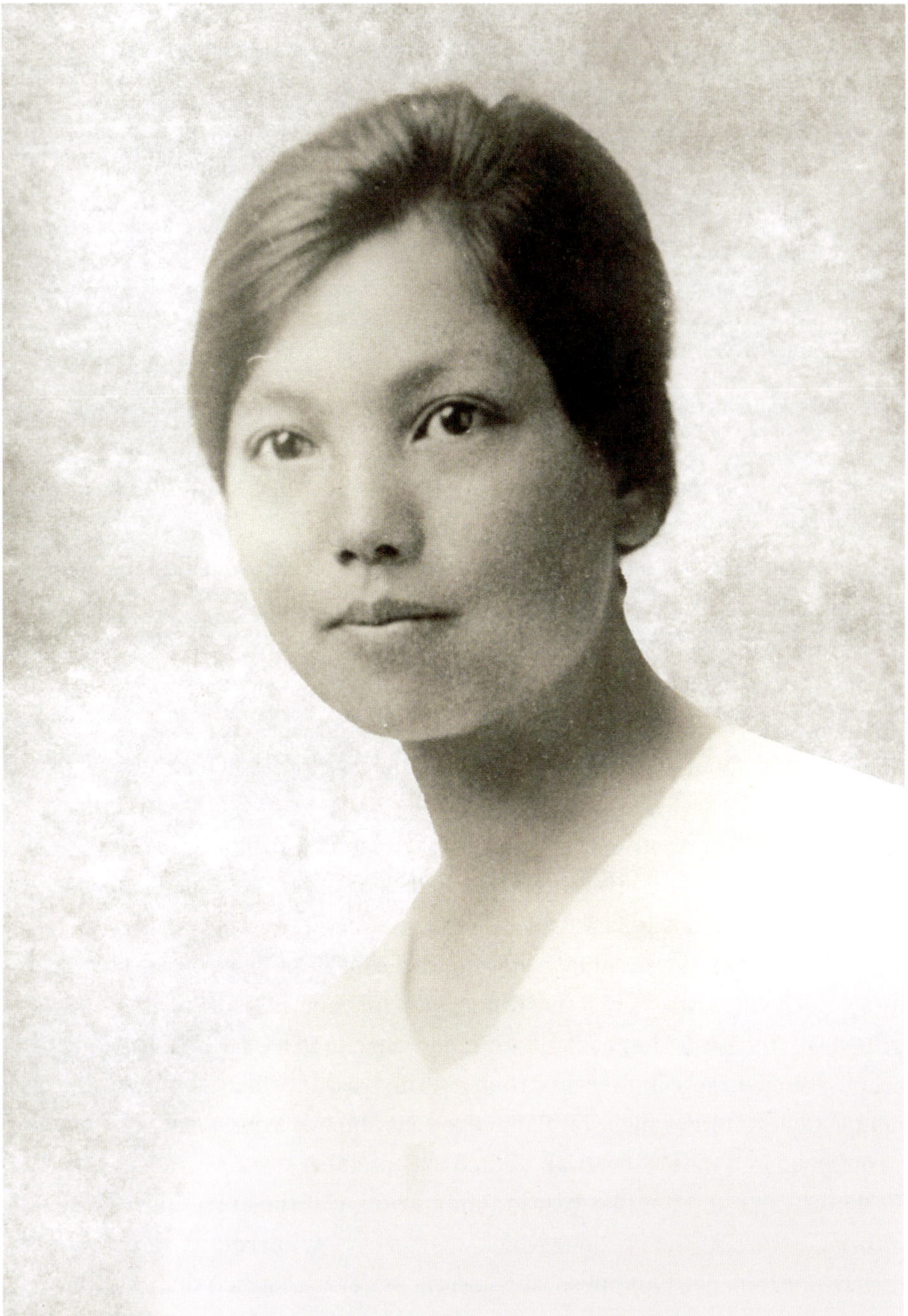

Kathleen Pih-Chang, 1929. *Hocken Collections Uare Taoka o Hākena, University of Otago Medical School, Alumnus Association Inc. records, MS-1537/690*

> In those days it was really hard to be a Chinese person in Otago. It was quite demeaning . . . Of course I knew I was Chinese. I wished I wasn't. It was all right when I was on the farm. But then in 1915 my aunt wanted to send me to the best girls' high school in Otago. I was the only Chinese. They looked down on me, but in those days I would say that 99.99 per cent of people in Dunedin looked down upon the Chinese anyway . . . In those days in Dunedin there were a lot of Scots. Very few of them, I think, would feel that the Chinese were their equals . . . In the girls' school, the girls were just not too friendly. In the university too, the medical girls were really arrogant. There were so few girls, and they came from good families, from the moneyed class, and they really looked down on the Chinese. They were not nice to me at all.[38]

Her father wrote to her throughout her childhood, and her decision to become a doctor was highly influenced by Reid's aid work in China.

+++

Little is known about Pih-Chang's medical school years, but we do know that she graduated early in 1929, and in June that year the Waitaki Hospital Board confirmed her appointment as a house surgeon at Ōamaru Public Hospital. Here, she found the same racism she had encountered at medical school. The male doctors were unfriendly, so she mostly kept to herself. Some of the patients were no better: 'When I started as a house surgeon at Oamaru Hospital, some of the patients said, "We are not going to stay here if that Chinese doctor comes." At the beginning I was terrified, just terrified. They got to like me later on.'[39] In 1930, Pih-Chang completed her house surgeon appointment and then returned to Dunedin to attend Missionary Training College, after which she planned to visit China as a missionary doctor. She was ordained into the Presbyterian Church in September 1930.

Pih-Chang spent her first year in China working at the Kong Chuen hospital north of Canton city (Guangzhou), which was run by New Zealand's Canton Villages Mission. She took five Cantonese language classes every day in order to learn it as quickly as possible. Her medical work was quite taxing, and she was always aware of the gulf between her comfortable life and the struggles of those she was caring for. Her wages were paid by the Presbyterian Church, while many of her patients made their living growing rice, peanuts and yams, or farming fish.[40]

The district covered by the hospital included around 100,000 people, and Pih-Chang was the only fully qualified medical practitioner. Because she was a woman, Chinese regulations meant she was not allowed to head the hospital itself. Nevertheless, because she was the most qualified, she found herself doing procedures that were unfamiliar to her: she pulled teeth without anaesthetics, she amputated limbs after untreated sarcomas had made their way to the bone, and she delivered countless babies. Most of the time, local mothers gave birth at home with the help of a midwife, but when there was a problem, the mother and baby were sent to the hospital. Many babies died of tetanus if the midwives had used a dirty piece of tile or glass to cut the umbilical cord — but they had to use what was there. She recalled later:

> I am really glad that I went back to China. As a girl, I did not like being Chinese at all. The people that I admired were the Scots. I accept that I am Chinese now, but I was very sensitive about it when I was young. Going back to work in China in the 1930s was really good for me, otherwise I would always have felt so sorry for myself for being born Chinese. Only after working in China did I find my Chinese identity.[41]

In 1936 Pih-Chang left Kong Chuen for London for postgraduate study. In July she passed the preliminary examination for postgraduate studies in ophthalmic surgery at Royal London Ophthalmic Hospital.[42] She was awarded a Diploma of Ophthalmic Medicine and Surgery (DOMS) in 1937, and she then returned to China. She continued her missionary work in Guangzhou and remained there until she married fellow doctor K. S. Francis Chang in August 1938. She then moved to Shanghai to join him as a staff member at St John's University.

The couple remained in Shanghai throughout the Second World War, the Chinese Civil War and the subsequent Communist takeover — though they did spend 1946 in New Zealand to have a break from the tense conditions. They fled to Singapore a month before the Chinese border closed in 1948, leaving all their belongings behind. Their escape was fraught: 'Back in Shanghai, no one had realised that we had escaped . . . From [Singapore] we sent a telegram and all hell broke loose. They went into our apartment and took all our things, searching for incriminating evidence. We lost most of our possessions.'[43]

They spent five years in Singapore, during which time her husband was invited to return to Hong Kong to take up a position as professor of anatomy at Hong Kong University. The couple spent 14 years in Hong Kong, where Pih-Chang taught at the university, ran her own clinic and worked as a missionary doctor for two clinics run by the Brethren Church. Most of her work was with refugees from Canton.

In 1969, when Francis Chang turned 60, the couple retired and moved back to New Zealand. They settled in Tauranga, and he spent a lot of time developing their garden. When he died in 1978, she attributed his early death to his bad habits: 'He used to smoke over a hundred cigarettes a day and drank coffee from six till after midnight.'[44] Pih-Chang continued living in their home until her death on 22 February 1991, aged 87.

FLORENCE AILEEN CRAIG AND TERESA IMELDA THOMPSON (NÉE CRAIG)

1932 graduates

Florence Craig and her twin Agnes were born in Wellington in 1905, and their younger sister Teresa Craig (later Thompson) was born in 1908.[45] Florence and Teresa attended Wellington Girls' College, and both received university national scholarships at the end of 1922. In 1923, Florence passed the medical intermediate examinations in biology, organic and inorganic chemistry and physics at Victoria University in Wellington. Some time in the late 1920s, she and Teresa were accepted into Otago Medical School. At the end of 1928, Florence passed her first professional examination, and Teresa passed physiology. In June 1932, they both graduated with MB ChB.

Florence spent at least some of her house surgeon training at Christchurch Hospital, and Teresa was based at Palmerston North Hospital. Both sisters then spent some time in 1934 at Greymouth Hospital before going to Britain, where Florence obtained a Diploma in Public Health and Tropical Medicine, and Teresa a Diploma in Public Health.

By 1940, Teresa was registered in the *New Zealand Gazette* as living at North Hummock Estate, Klang Selangor, Malaya (now Malaysia). The following year, she

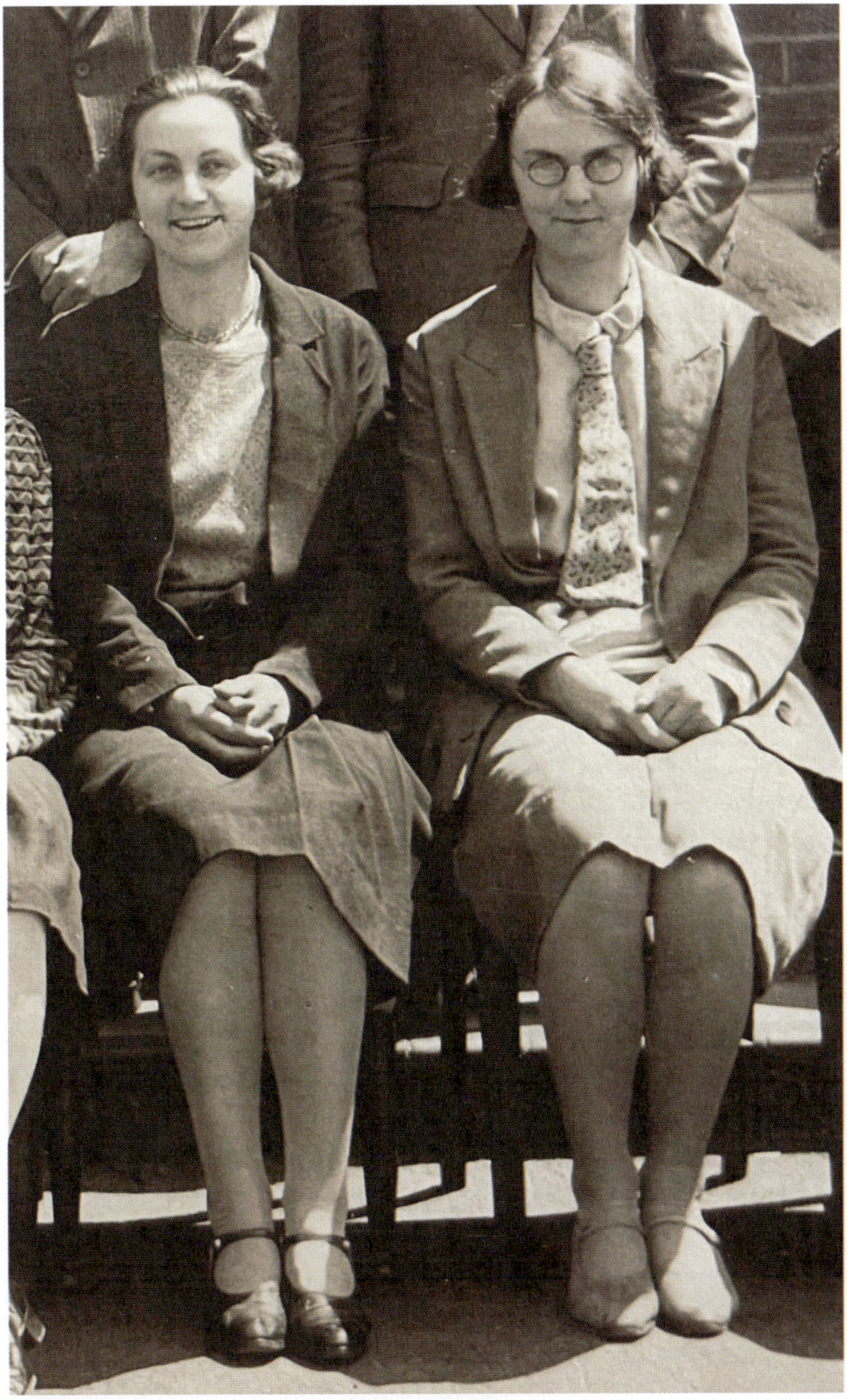

Florence Aileen Craig (left) and Teresa Imelda Thompson (née Craig), 1931.
Otago Medical School Archives

married Francis Scott Thompson, a barrister who worked for the North Hummock Rubber Company in Klang. Florence, meanwhile, was a medical officer with the Malayan Medical Service in Ipoh.

In the late nineteenth to mid-twentieth century, the Malay Peninsula was a British colony and, by the turn of the century, was a source of cheap raw materials, particularly rubber and tin. Western medicine and health practices were established to service the needs of the growing population, and great effort was put into eradicating infectious diseases, especially malaria.[46] From the start of the twentieth century, but particularly in the 1920s and 1930s, New Zealanders were a key part of the expatriate community in the Malayan Peninsula, referred to as the Federated Malay States (now Malaysia and Singapore).

+++

When the Japanese invaded Northern Malaya on 8 December 1941, their advance down the peninsula was swift. Thousands of civilians crowded south to Singapore, but by the second week of February, the Japanese were advancing across Singapore Island. Government propaganda had assured residents that 'Fortress Singapore' would never fall. When the delayed evacuation was eventually ordered in February, a flotilla of vessels set out for Sumatra in what is now Indonesia.

Florence and Teresa were evacuated to Singapore from their locations further north and were put in charge of first-aid hospitals, working day and night under constant bombing, while their sister Agnes worked as a nurse in the soldiers' hospital.[47] All three sisters were on the SS *Kuala*, which was bombed on 14 February 1942. Survivors had to swim to nearby islands. Florence sustained injuries that left her paralysed, bleeding and with her internal organs smashed. She was evacuated by launch to the Indonesian island of Sangeang, where she died on 17 February 1942.

Teresa and Agnes survived the bombing of the *Kuala*. They made it to Pompong Island, then boarded the rescue vessel SS *Tanjong Pinang* with several hundred other women and children. When the ship was shelled and sank on 17 February 1942, both of the sisters died.

Florence is buried in the Kranji War Cemetery in Singapore. There are no recorded graves for her sisters Teresa and Agnes.

MARGARET STUART SMITH (NÉE RIDDELL)

1936 graduate

Margaret Stuart Smith was born in 1912 in Wellington to Edith May Yarr and John Riddell.[48] She attended Chilton House School in Wellington, a private boarding and day school established in 1897. Like most girls' schools of the time, Chilton House did not teach science, which was required for medical school, so she persuaded her father to employ a private tutor to teach her chemistry and physics. When the exam marks were posted, she had come second in all of New Zealand for chemistry.

Smith enrolled at Victoria University for the medical intermediate year and transferred to Otago in 1931. Her son Rodney remembers her telling him why she went into medicine. When she was about eight years old, her friend had become very sick with diphtheria. The doctor was called but took a long time to arrive, and her friend died of an obstructed airway. From that time, she decided to become a doctor: she wanted to make a difference.[49]

During her third year, her father, who was in his fifties, died while on holiday with the family. His will set aside money for Smith and her brother Claude to complete their medical degrees and travel to England for postgraduate studies. She graduated from Otago Medical School in 1936.

Smith spent 1937 and 1938 working as a house surgeon at Wellington Hospital before postgraduate study in London. In Wellington she worked with Eric Anson, New Zealand's first specialist anaesthetist, and decided to pursue anaesthesiology as her postgraduate specialisation.[50] To qualify for the new Diploma in Anaesthetics at Guy's Hospital in London, she was required to perform 1000 anaesthetic procedures, including 500 for major operations, each of which had to be certified by a supervisor at Wellington Hospital.

She achieved this milestone early in 1939 and set off for London with her mother and Evelyn Stonewigg, matron of Wellington Hospital, with whom she had developed a friendship while working on her ward. She gained her Diploma in Anaesthetics from the Royal College of Surgeons and Physicians in London in 1939.

+ + +

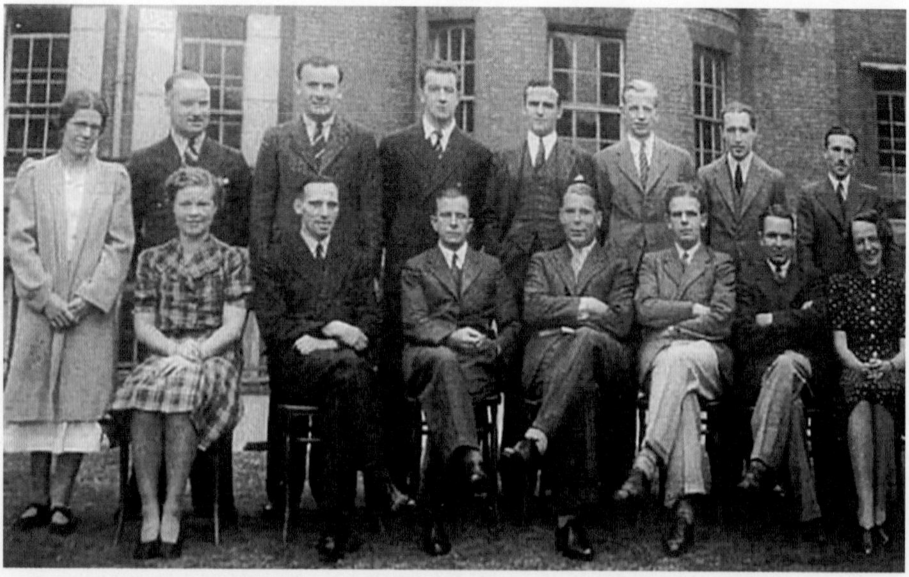

The graduating class for the Diploma of Anaesthetics, 1939. Margaret Smith is seated on the left in the front row. *Courtesy Anthony Smith*

By the time Smith completed her diploma, the Second World War had begun. She was summoned to New Zealand House by the high commissioner, who suggested that it was safer to remain in England than to try to return home as merchant ships were being attacked in the English Channel by German U-boats. He also told her that the war was expected to be resolved within six weeks. She took his advice and stayed.

Smith was appointed as senior resident in anaesthesia and surgery at the Leicester Royal Infirmary for one year, and then in 1940 went to Edinburgh Royal Infirmary, where she met fellow New Zealander Harold Gillies, a plastic surgeon and consultant to the Ministry of Health. Gillies asked her to set up an anaesthetic department for the New Zealand plastic surgeon Archibald McIndoe, who worked for the Royal Air Force at the Bangour Village Hospital, midway between Glasgow and Edinburgh. Smith worked with Gillies and McIndoe as a specialist anaesthetist in emergency medical service. She said of her experience:

> Bangour Hospital was a large psychiatric hospital which was being turned into a surgical hospital for the three forces — so for three months

> I bought equipment from Gillies and Boyles, machines, to spinal needles and planned the anaesthetic department and theatres. Here I worked with Sir Harold Gillies, AB Wallace, Henry Wade, Tommy Millar, and Noel Gray. They operated on airmen with severe burns, army and naval personnel for routine and emergency procedures as well as German prisoners. These men could speak no English and thought I was going to kill them.[51]

Smith remained at Bangour Hospital until 1945 and assisted plastic surgeons there, working on facial reconstruction in soldiers with battle wounds, including many pilots who had suffered horrific burns. Her next appointment, in 1946, was as a senior resident anaesthetist at the Great Ormond Street Hospital for Sick Children (now the Great Ormond Street Hospital) in London. This appointment confirmed her intense interest in paediatric anaesthesia.[52]

Smith returned to Christchurch in late November 1946 to become a visiting consultant specialist in anaesthesia to the North Canterbury Hospital Board, a position she held for the next 30 years. She was initially turned down for this position on the grounds that she was 'Wellington trained and a woman', but her future husband, Carl Smith, whom she married in 1948 and who owned a menswear shop, met the medical superintendent, Hugh Acland, and persuaded him to appoint her. At the time, anaesthetists were largely self-trained and used a limited range of techniques and drugs. However, during Smith's first 10 years in Christchurch there were many developments in the field of anaesthesia, and she led their implementation on the local scene.[53]

In 1952, Margaret Smith was awarded the Foundation Fellow of the Faculty of Anaesthetists, Royal Australasian College of Surgeons, for services to anaesthetics, particularly for children. She was the last remaining foundation fellow at the time of her death in 2007. In 1977 she was awarded the Queen's Silver Jubilee Medal for services to the community, and in 1990 she was awarded an OBE for her services to medicine, especially to anaesthesia and the community, and for her work in England during the Second World War. In 2002, at the age of 90, she was awarded the Australian and New Zealand College of Anaesthetists Medal: only one is awarded each year.

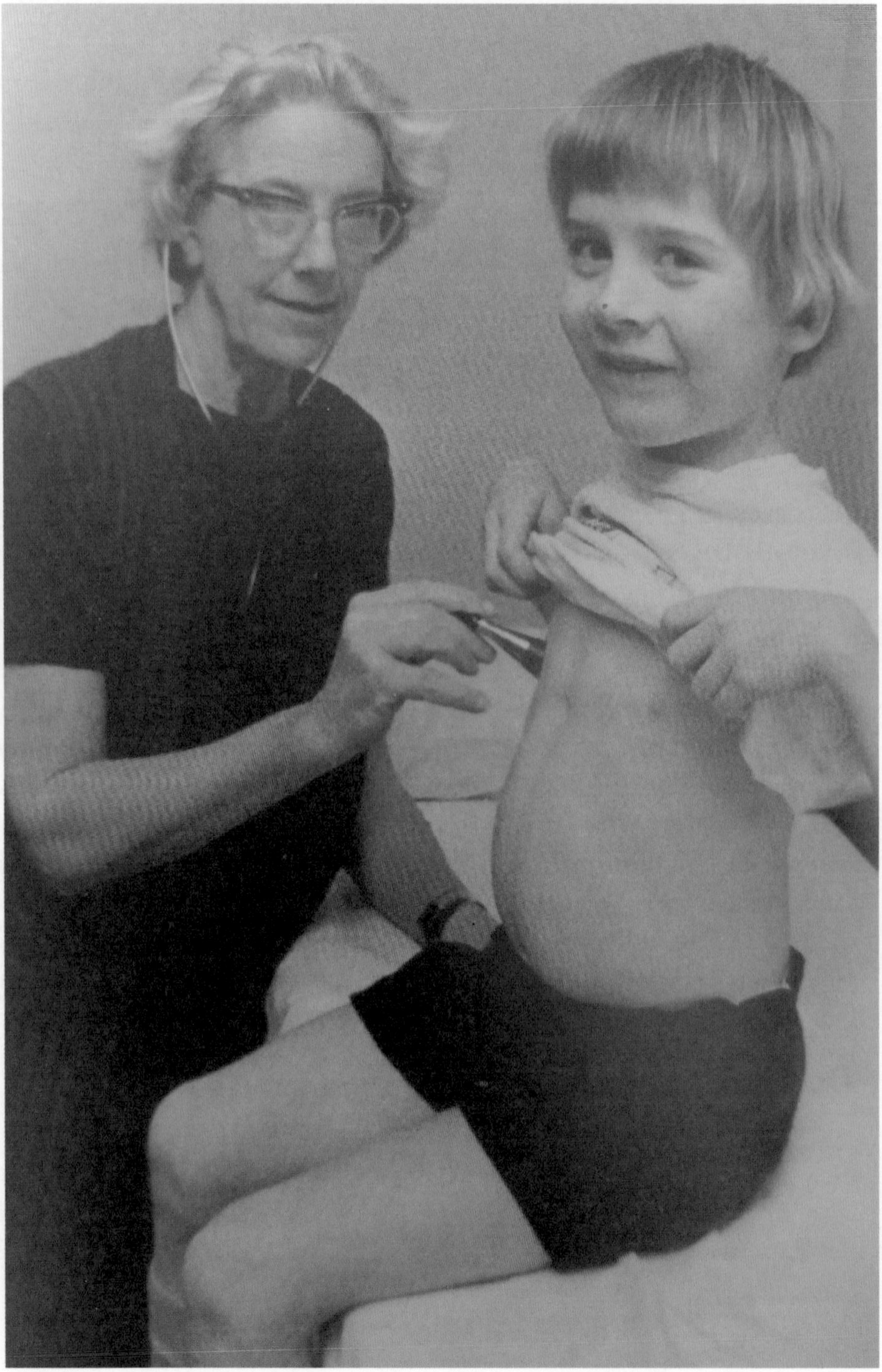

Alice Bush and a young patient in the early 1970s. *New Zealand Herald, courtesy Fay Hercock*

ALICE MARY BUSH (NÉE STANTON)

1937 graduate — first New Zealand-trained woman to gain membership of the Australasian College of Physicians and first New Zealand-trained woman to be elected a Fellow of the Royal College of Physicians in London

Alice Mary Bush was born in Herne Bay, Auckland, in 1914. Her father, Joseph Stanton, was a prominent lawyer, and her mother, Marjorie McMaster, was from an affluent family. In 1921 the family moved to Mountain Road in Epsom, and Bush attended the private girls' schools Hill Top and Diocesan High School. She completed her medical intermediate year at Auckland University College in 1932 and began her studies at Otago Medical School in 1933. She said that it had been her goal to pursue medicine since she was a girl. It helped that she came from a family who were able to support her financially over the six years of study.

Bush was an active participant in university life at Otago, and eventually became vice-president of the Students' Association and chair of the Women Students' Club. In 1934 she received the Scott Medal, awarded to the student with the best knowledge of human anatomy — she had passed with 85 per cent. Traditionally, the medal recipient was offered an appointment as a graduate demonstrator in anatomy on completion of their degree. However, Percy Gowland, head of the anatomy department, took Bush aside and told her that although the staff had great respect for her, the appointment would go to a man.[54] In 1937, her sixth year as a medical student, she was appointed to Auckland Hospital, where the medical superintendent, J. W. Craven, noted that she was probably the most brilliant student the hospital had that year.

As with so many other women medical school graduates of this period, the Second World War reduced the prejudice they would otherwise have faced in the workforce. Bush found herself in an opportune position. Late in 1939, she contracted with Edward Sayers (a visiting physician at Auckland and Karitane hospitals, later dean of Otago Medical School) to be his locum for the duration of the war. She was bound to work in his practice in Epsom, Auckland, for the rest of the war, or until Sayers returned. If he did not return, she would have the option of buying his equipment and carrying on under the same arrangement for two years, after which time the practice would become hers entirely.[55]

Bush took on the responsibilities of Sayers' practice with diligence. Her work there developed what was to become a lifetime interest in the diagnosis and treatment of asthma and allergies — one of Sayers' interests. The war years also steered her into the field of sex education, because of an increase in sexually transmitted diseases and pregnancies outside of marriage; she gave lectures at the Auckland YWCA on 'Men and Women's Relationships in Wartime'.

Sayers returned from his war responsibilities towards the end of 1944, and they negotiated a second three-year partnership. Bush, by now married to Faulkner Bush, a teacher at a country school north of Taihape, continued in full-time medical practice and planned to specialise in paediatrics. She then started making plans to travel to London as a candidate for Membership of the Royal College of Physicians (MRCP).

The Bushes' son Peter was born in September 1947, and the family sailed for London in late 1947, accompanied by a Karitane nurse. Bush failed her first MRCP exams in early 1948 but was successful on her third attempt in January 1949. She also studied and sat for a Diploma in Child Health, at that time the only formal qualification in paediatrics, at Great Ormond Street Hospital in London.

+++

In 1949 the couple returned to New Zealand, where Alice Bush resumed private practice in Auckland, and Faulkner went back to teaching. In April 1952 she became physician-in-charge at an allergy clinic at Auckland Public Hospital. She also contributed to teaching sixth-year medical students on behalf of the branch faculty of Otago Medical School at Auckland Hospital.[56] Her reputation as an allergist helped attract patients to her private practice, located in a residential block in Whitaker Place, off Symonds Street. Her patients were mostly children, but some adults also presented with allergy and asthma problems, as well as for counselling and contraceptive advice.

Alice Bush believed that the impacts of a child's early environment, both physical and emotional, are far-reaching, and only when those were understood would it be possible to improve life in the community.[57] She had strong ideas on raising children and believed the worst thing a doctor could do to a mother was to make her afraid of looking after her baby; the mother, she believed, was the one who would know her own baby best. In the 1950s, firm control of children was considered a virtue, corporal punishment was legal, and early toilet training was the hallmark of maternal success. Bush challenged these concepts. She believed, for instance, that a good father spent time with his children and shared equal responsibility for parenting.

From the 1940s, Bush became more involved in the Family Planning Association (FPA). Conditions during the war years had made generalisations around contraception difficult. In a 1944 national executive meeting, she raised the question of what attitude to adopt when young people who were about to marry sought contraception advice: the association decided that the medical advisor should use their own judgement.[58] Bush was increasingly concerned that the wider medical profession had chosen to ignore women's quest for information on contraception based on scientific knowledge.

By 1960 she was an active member of the Auckland division of the Medical Association and the Auckland branch of the Medical Women's Association. In 1970 she was elected a Fellow of the Royal College of Physicians in London, the first New Zealand-trained woman elected to this position.[59]

Bush continued to work at Auckland Hospital, Karitane Hospital and in private practice until her early death in February 1974, aged 59. Had she lived longer, she would no doubt have received an honour that recognised her important contribution as a physician, paediatrician and activist for family planning services and abortion access. The Alice Bush Memorial Prize was established by the NZMWA in 1976 and is given to the best performance in undergraduate paediatrics during their MB ChB Part V year at the Auckland School of Medicine.

After Bush's death, it was suggested that a new national children's hospital, for which she had campaigned, should bear her name, but this was rejected by the hospital board. The long-awaited hospital, known as Starship Children's Hospital, was not established in Auckland until 1991. In 1980 Faulkner Bush wrote of his wife: 'She was tremendously determined . . . In real terms, any "sacrifice" I made was minimal, and immeasurably recompensed by the life I was able to lead with this supreme woman.'[60]

MOLLY SMITH (NÉE WAGSTAFF)

1938 graduate

Molly Smith was born in 1916 in Wellington and moved with her family when she was young to North Otago, where her father, John, worked as a farm inspector.[61] She travelled each day by train to Waitaki Girls' High School in Ōamaru, and as a result missed the first and last lessons of the day, which were often focused on domestic chores such as sewing and cooking. As an adult, she joked that this explained why she was such a poor homemaker.

She was close to her father and despite the academic ability she showed at high school, her dream was to follow in his footsteps and work in farming. Her mother, Edith, a schoolteacher, realised her daughter's potential to succeed academically in a male-dominated society. Under their parents' direction, both Smith and her older brother Ron entered medical school, although neither was particularly passionate about the career choice.

Smith was accepted into Otago Medical School at the age of 16, although her mother insisted that she first repeat the sixth form so that she was old enough to attend university. She was one of only three women to begin their studies in 1932. She felt uncomfortable entering university at such a young age and felt intimidated by some of the other students, many of whom came from upper-class families. She felt the differences in social class were emphasised by her clothes, which were often handmade by her mother. She was particularly embarrassed by her underpants, which her mother made — as many did during the Depression — from old flour bags; although she had bleached them, the 'FLOUR' stamp was still visible when they were drying on the clothesline.

After graduating in 1938, Smith completed her house surgeon training in Wellington and then worked as a junior doctor in New Plymouth, where her family was living and where her fellow graduates Jean Sandel (1939) and Dorothy Spence-Sales (1938) were working.

+++

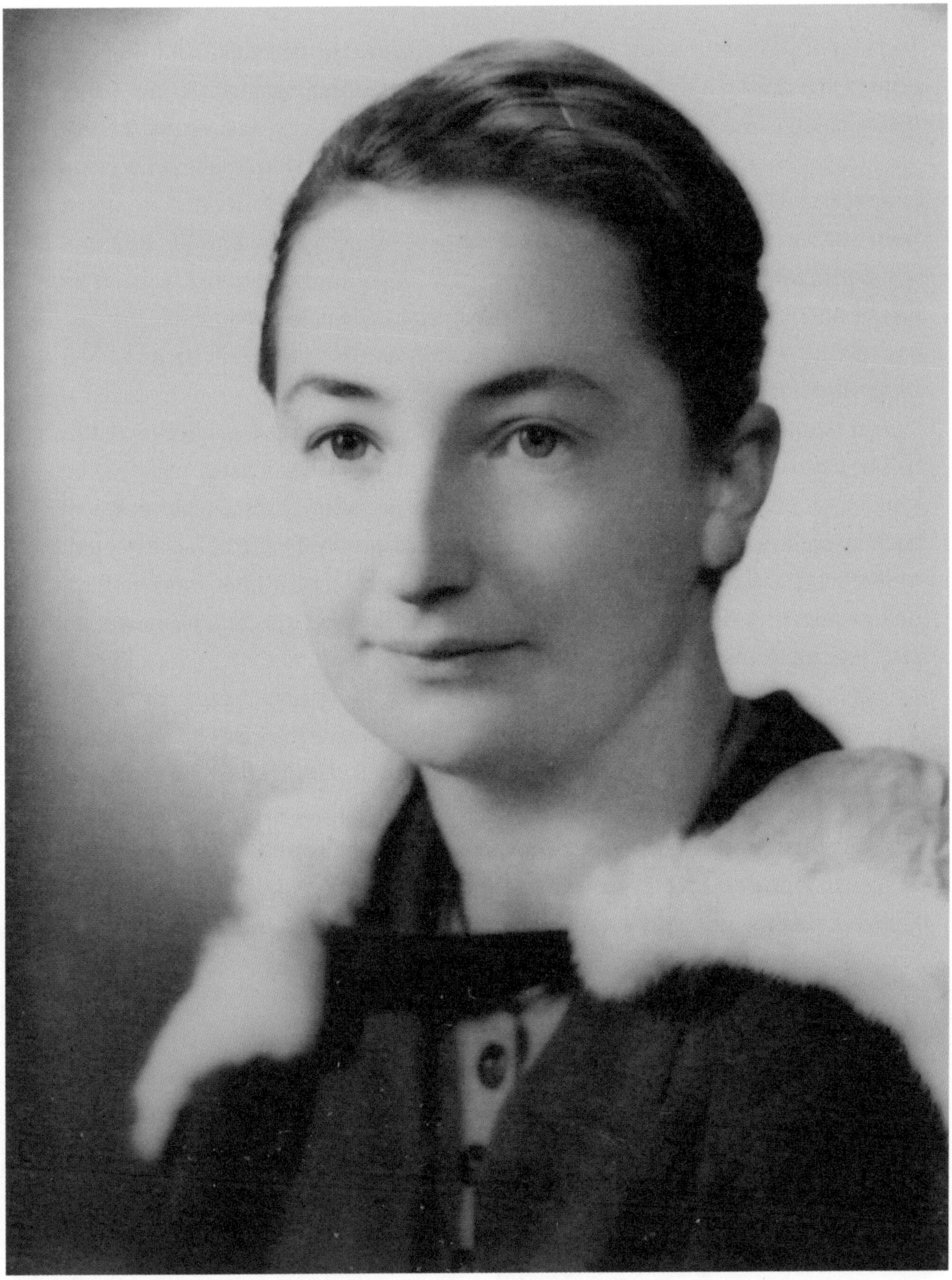

Molly Smith (née Wagstaff) on her graduation day in 1938. *Courtesy Ruth Newton*

The loss of so many doctors to the armed services in the Second World War had opened the door for women to fill their place and Smith became a locum GP in Waihi, taking over a practice from Frederick Barrowclough and working there until the end of the war. After the war ended, Barrowclough returned from serving overseas, and Smith secured another position through her brother Ron, who had been working at a GP practice in Dargaville.

Smith settled in to Dargaville, where she worked for the next five years as one of only two GPs in the area. She soon became a much-loved member of the community, where she was known universally as 'Dr Molly'. A display in the Dargaville Museum pays tribute to her work delivering babies.

In 1950, travel to the maternity annexe in Te Kōpuru was a challenge: Smith had to navigate seven miles down the river on rough roads, often at night, while avoiding wandering cattle. Without any modern specialist training in obstetrics or back-up facilities, Smith and the other GPs would simply do the best they could. In one instance, she was able to recognise Rhesus disease (which was relatively unknown at the time) in a newborn baby, and she sent the infant straight to Auckland Hospital for a blood transfusion, saving its life.

In 1950 she married Bertram Gisborne ('B. G.') Smith, a much older man, who was a builder and joiner. The mores of the time dictated that married women should be homemakers, and as she always did the 'right and proper thing', she sold her practice immediately to Maurice Matich. Their two children were born in 1951 and 1953. Tragedy struck when their four-year-old son was diagnosed with leukaemia; he died in 1957. Eventually, not wanting to leave their remaining daughter, Ruth, as an only child, the Smiths privately adopted a second daughter, Colleen.

+++

By the 1960s, Bertram Smith was winding down his business, and Molly started working part-time, this time as an anaesthetist. At first, she trained 'on the job' at Dargaville Hospital, although she soon received formal training from Preston Calvert at Whangārei Hospital. Her approach had some quirks: even after newer anaesthetics came into common usage, she preferred using ether, arguing that it was safer, even though the patients suffered from nausea in recovery.

Later in life, when her husband's health began to fail, Smith retired and looked after him until he died in 1982. She continued to work for the community. She was the medical officer for St John for 40 years. In her retirement years, she volunteered for Save the Children, delivered Meals on Wheels and helped at the Dargaville Museum. Near the end of her life, her daughter Ruth tried to convince her to record her life story, but she refused, believing that no one would be interested. She was not the sort of person to focus on her own achievements — but she would be proud to learn that her granddaughter was inspired by her grandmother to become a nurse. Molly Smith died in 2013, aged 97.

The Otago Medical School third-year class in 1944. Third row, from left: Diana Montgomery (1948), Miss James, Helen Florence Wood (née Salkeld; 1950), Miss Mawson, Judy Ann David Wilson (née Collins; 1947), Maire Jean Smith (née Tait; 1947), Dorothy Field Potter (née Usher; 1948), Miss Farris, Diana Marcia Smith (née Morton; 1947), Jean Boyd (née MacDonald; 1947), Mary Alice Theodore Tolley (1947), Winifred Mary Staple (née Croke; 1947), Mary Hanafin (1948). Second row, from left: Marianne Fillenz (1948), Nancy Margaret Saunders (née Salmond; 1947), Barbara McLeod Allen (née Graham, 1947), Mrs Alan, Helen Rarity McCreanor (née Young; 1947), Rina Winifred Moore (née Rōpiha; 1948). Those for whom no date is recorded either did not graduate or were members of staff. *Otago Medical School Archives*

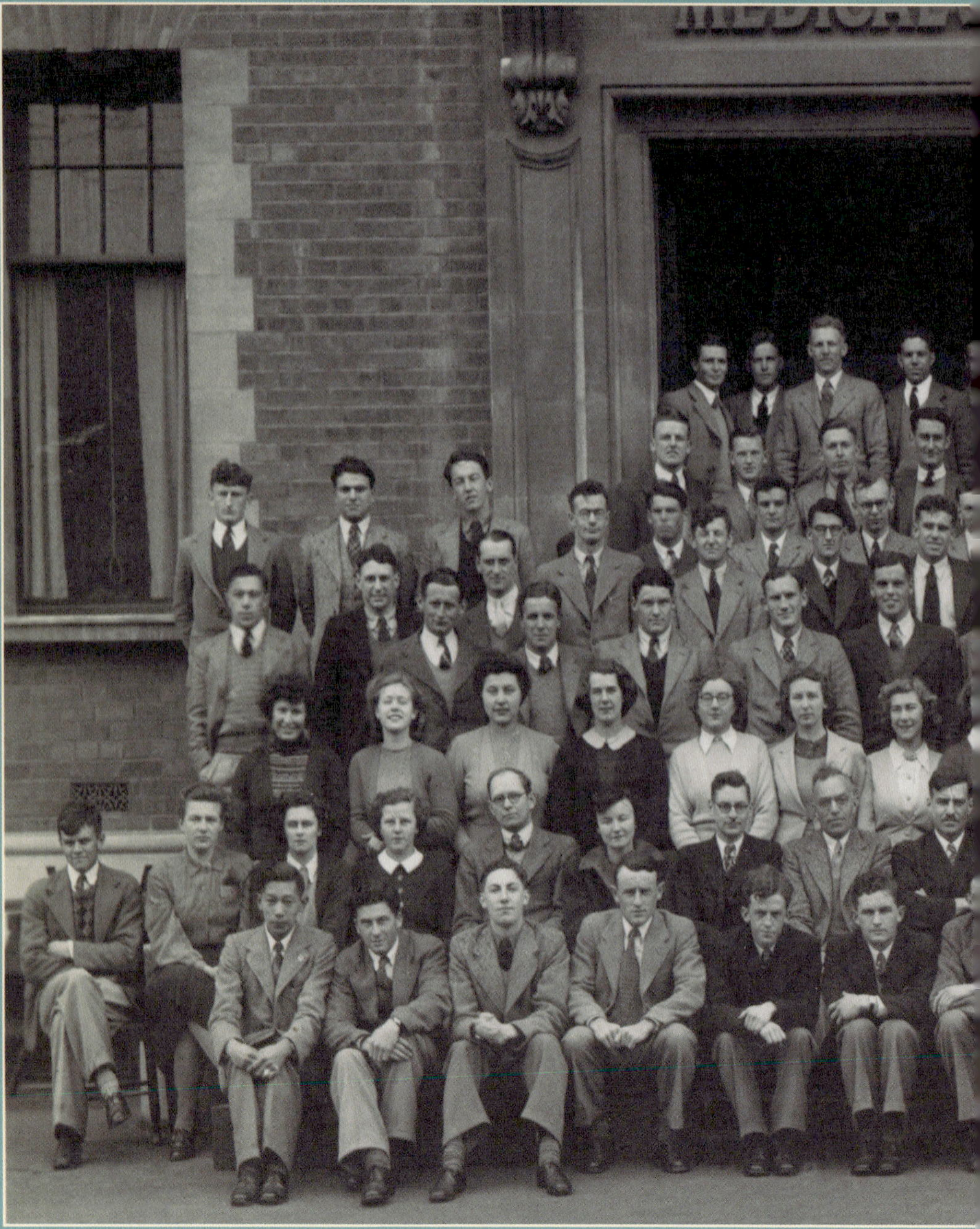

4. The ‘privilege of being students’ 1939–1948

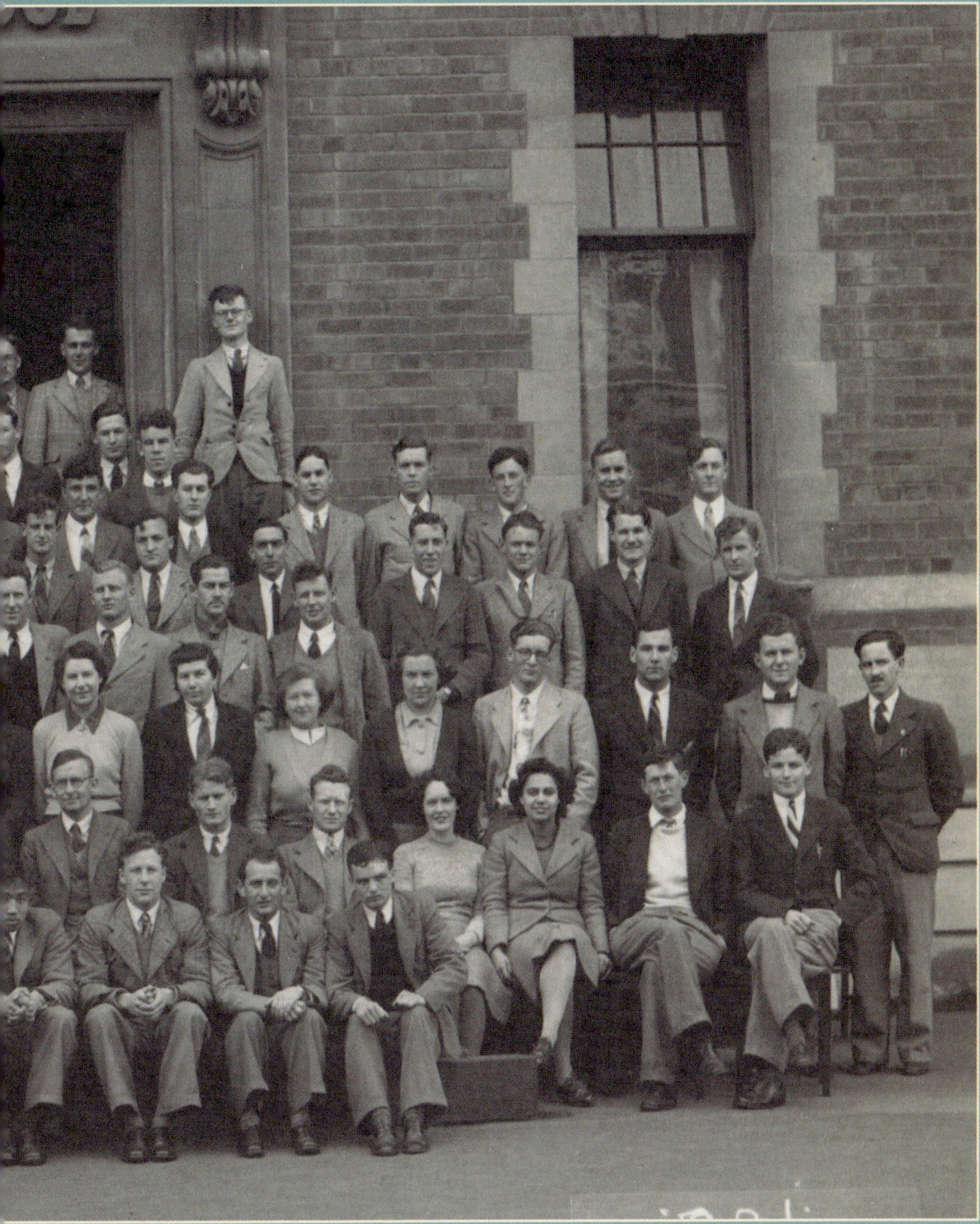

More women than ever trained to become doctors during and after the Second World War. By 1949, over 200 women had graduated with a degree from Otago Medical School, 94 of them between 1939 and 1950.[1] The war changed the fabric of university life, and women doctors training or starting work had to confront the questions the war raised about femininity and gender roles.

The academic pressures on women medical students continued, but a nationwide shortage of doctors meant that men and women medical students encountered further pressure in the final years of their degrees and the early years of practising. Medical students were being put into clinical practice earlier than ever, and new graduates found themselves with greater responsibilities in the absence of mentors.

Barbara Heslop (née Cupit; 1948) recalled that on her first day of medical school in 1943, her professor reminded the class that 'we were all exempt from military service and that we were never to forget that New Zealanders were dying overseas while we enjoyed the privilege of being students'.[2] This privilege occupied the thoughts of many medical students throughout the Second World War. Student life was relatively stable, but the impact of the war was felt everywhere. As Heslop said, 'in the circumstances, it would have been almost subversive for any of us to have complained of our lot'.[3]

Judy Wilson (née Collins; 1947) agreed, recalling that 'you weren't allowed to be seen to be having too much fun'.[4] She remembered the 'food rationing, night blackouts, restricted travel, restricted campus activities, [and] army training camps' that pervaded her time in Dunedin.[5] In the wider Dunedin community, there was a

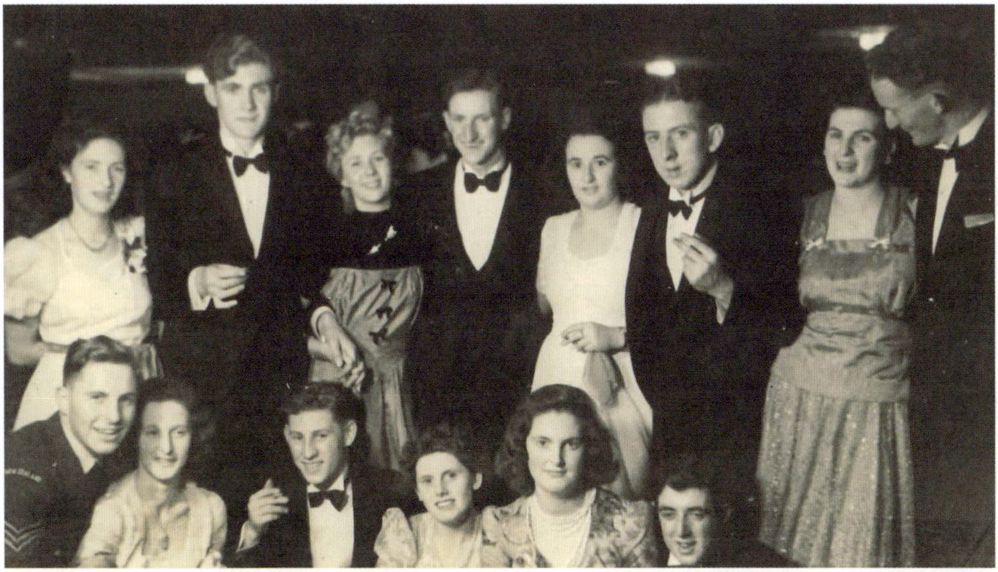

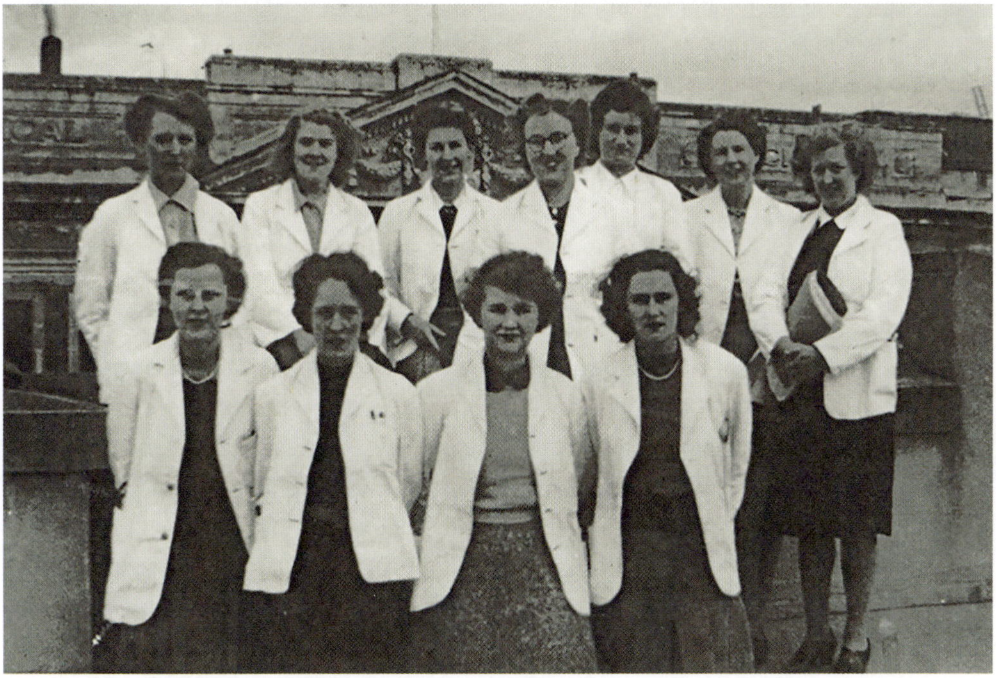

ABOVE: University of Otago Capping Ball, 8 May 1945. Medical students Meredyth Gunn (left) and Beryl Howie (third from left) are in the back row. *Family collection*

BELOW: Fifth-year Otago Medical School students, 1946. Back row, from left: Maire Tait, Judy Faris, Diana Montgomery, Judy Collins, Diana Morton, Jean Macdonald, Winifred Croke. Front row: Barbara McLeod Allen (née Graham), Helen Young, Sally Fitzgerald, Margaret Salmond. *Courtesy Chrissie Kershaw*

perception that male medical students should have enlisted, and attitudes towards the students could be hostile.[6]

By April 1940, nearly 35,000 New Zealand men had volunteered for military service, and by July of the same year volunteer corps of women were training throughout the country. By two years later, about 43 per cent of the country's paid workforce had been mobilised into the war effort,[7] and by 1946, a total of 650 nurses had served outside of New Zealand and 682 Otago Medical School graduates had participated in the war.

The Second World War had a lasting impact on gender relations in New Zealand.[8] Eligible women aged under 40, including medical students between semesters, were 'manpowered' into what the government deemed to be essential work in industries, such as clothing and shoe factories and in hospitals, as part of conscription regulations from 1942. Deborah Montgomerie has argued that 'rather than overturning accepted ideas about women's place and women's work, government mobilisation tended to conform to convention'.[9]

Her research demonstrates how, despite the prevalence of women entering essential services from 1942 and single women being taken seriously as participants in the workforce by the end of the Depression, married women were still expected to perform unpaid labour in the home (as would continue to be the expectation for decades after).[10] During the 1940s, activists began campaigning for equal pay for men and women, a campaign that gained traction in the 1950s.

In 1944, secondary education was made free and compulsory up to age 15. This had a definitive impact on opportunities for girls, as parents could 'no longer argue that secondary education for their daughters was a waste of time'. Student numbers in girls' secondary schools exploded in the ensuing decade, and as the baby boom started more schools were required. The number of women employed in professional occupations such as lawyers, dentists, librarians and, of course, doctors rose noticeably as a consequence.[11]

Alongside the greater proportion of women working in medicine during the war, there was increasing acceptance of women at the medical school. Few women graduates during the war years described instances of discrimination while they were students. Women were no longer reporting that they had to sit at the front in lecture theatres, or that they were separated from the men in laboratory sessions.

Rather than all the women students in an anatomy class having to work on one body during dissections, they intermingled and worked alongside the male students. At hostels such as St Margaret's they became involved in sporting and social activities, as there was less pressure on them to focus solely on their studies in order to prove their right to a position in medical school.

Even so, some social events — in particular, the fifth-year class dinner hosted by the professors — still excluded women.[12] This restriction continued through to the early 1960s, when Carol Shand (1962) famously organised a protest, only to discover that 'the reason they couldn't have the women come was because the lecturers liked to tell dirty jokes and they couldn't tell them in front of the women. That was the last year that women were excluded, we made so much fuss.'[13]

Joan Walton (née Robertson; 1945) claimed that the 11 women students in her year did not ever talk to the male students, as 'that was considered fast behaviour'.[14] Walton used to bring her knitting along to lectures until some of the male students decided to wind her wool throughout the lecture theatre in what they thought was a hilarious prank.

Diana Mason (née Shaw; 1945) reported that even if there was less personal gender discrimination, there was constant pressure to outperform her male classmates in order to justify her right to be there. Despite the increasing number of women in the programme, there seemed to be no chance of getting a common room bigger than a cupboard. But the real trouble, according to Heslop, began once they started work.

Typically, the final year of their medical studies required students to work as trainees in hospitals. This changed during the war years, when women medical students could be manpowered in the summer months to work on farms, make rural deliveries or serve as orderlies or nurses in hospitals. As soon as the final academic year began in March many were placed in general practice clinics around the country to relieve the shortage of GPs, many of whom were in service overseas.

The clinics were often in rural areas, and only male doctors were given cars; the women had to find whatever transport they could. Diana Mason found herself utterly overwhelmed in her final year in 1944. She developed a system whereby she would 'take a [patient's] history, say, "Excuse me, I hear the phone", and dash into the consulting room next door to look up the appropriate book of medicine, surgery, or gynaecology'.[15]

Even with the war on, placements during their final year and house surgeon positions after graduation meant dealing with varying degrees of animosity from locals towards newly trained female doctors, particularly if those doctors were married and had children. Few husbands were accepting of the idea of a working wife and mother. The children of Maire Smith (née Tait; 1947) recalled that their mother 'found life pretty hard as a suburban housewife . . . she was always quite interested in science and the latest this and that and the other thing'.[16] Judy Wilson had planned to go overseas for postgraduate study after her house surgeon years but, according to her son Nigel, this all changed once she met and married her husband, John, who did not believe that she should work while raising their children, and 'so she stopped work'.[17]

There were many other women doctors, though, who felt a moral obligation to put their training into practice. Judith McCann (née Faris; 1947) put it simply: 'because I've done medicine and it's a privilege . . . I need to work'.[18] Those who chose to work throughout were on the receiving end of a degree of animosity. Caroline Stenhouse (1923) was an ophthalmic consultant to the New Zealand Army during the war and a founding member of the Ophthalmological Society of New Zealand (OSNZ). On one occasion, when the annual society dinner was held at the gentlemen-only Christchurch Club, Stenhouse was obliged to attend at a different venue with the wives.[19]

Women who were mothers and who chose to continue working were still expected to perform the many duties of the housewife. In 1943, representatives of women's organisations met with government ministers to demand more domestic help, as 'the emancipation of women . . . has been rather unevenly distributed. The one to receive the least benefit has been the seven-day-week worker — the mother.'[20] Those who could employed a housekeeper or, if it was available, sought family support to assist with childcare.

Rina Moore (née Rōpiha; 1948), the first Māori woman graduate of Otago Medical School, spent her clinical sixth year at Wellington Hospital while living in Nelson: she commuted from Nelson during the week while her husband and two-year-old daughter stayed with his mother. Yet while some husbands continued to put pressure on their wives not to work outside the home — a pressure that increased in the 1950s, during the baby boom — the mindset was slowly shifting.[21] Diana Mason's husband, Bruce, often looked after their children while she was working full-time; the children got a lot of 'flack' from their peers for coming from such an unusual household.[22] Other women found ways to keep a foot in the door, or returned to work once their children were older. Judy Wilson joined the Department of Health in Upper Hutt in 1965 and volunteered for the Red Cross, and Margaret Wishart (née Moore; 1942), who had six children and had recently been widowed, took up pathology in 1961.[23]

When the war was over, finding a job became harder for women medical graduates. As had been the case after the First World War, hospitals gave preference to returned servicemen. Working as locums in schools or setting up their own practices and having local support networks were some of the ways women doctors could work long-term after graduating.[24] Norma Benson (1940) eventually set up a practice in the Auckland suburb of Mount Roskill with Nira Dorset as practice nurse. General practices were still often family affairs: Dorset's brother Norman made some of the furniture for the practice.[25] Mavis MacDougall (née McClymont; 1941) set up her own practice on Sandringham Road, Auckland, in October 1944 when she was just 28; and Judith McCann and her husband became the sole GPs in the rural town of Bulls in the Rangitīkei in 1948, when their baby was just three weeks old.[26]

Dorothy Potter (née Usher; 1948), later the first woman president of the OSNZ, agreed to marry her husband and move to Masterton on the condition that she would not be expected to do the housework and could keep her maiden name. According to Bruce Hadden, who wrote the first comprehensive history of ophthalmology in New Zealand, 'the people of Masterton could not handle the latter so in 1965 she took her married name'.[27] It would be a long time before such a notion became anywhere near normal.

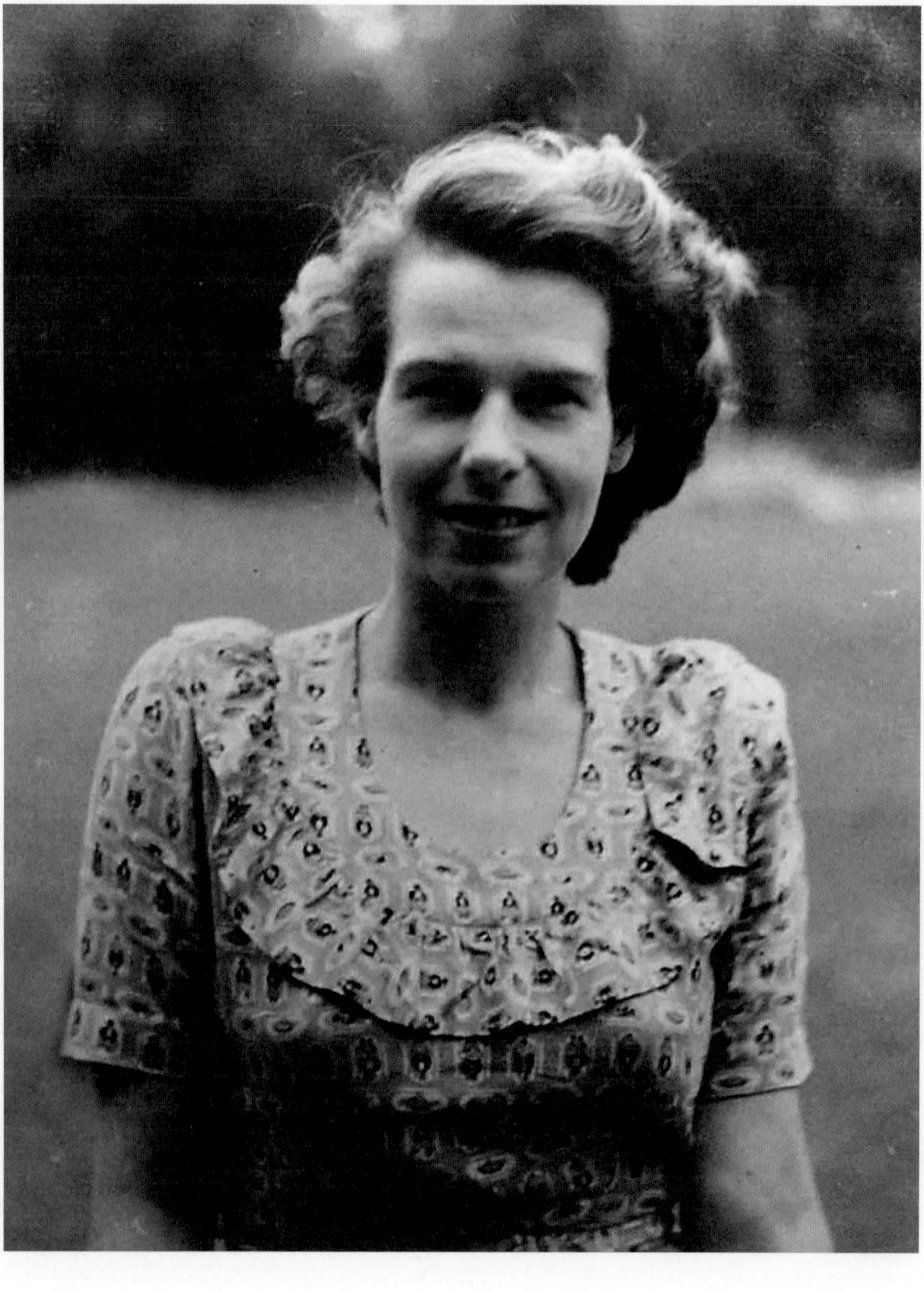

Isabel Wishart (née Moore), c.1940. *Family collection*

MARGARET ISABEL WISHART (NÉE MOORE)

1942 graduate

Margaret Isabel Wishart was born in 1918 at the home of her grandmother in Mount Eden, Auckland. Her parents were both teachers and had married in 1917. Her father Rupert died in the First World War in 1918, so he never met his daughter Isabel (as she was known).[28]

Wishart enrolled for her medical intermediate year at the University of Otago in 1936 and lived at St Margaret's College during her five years at medical school. As was often the case with women students, her schooling at Epsom Girls' Grammar School had not given her a good grounding in chemistry and physics, so she found that first year hard work. Her children remember her commenting occasionally that a couple of the lecturers were particularly tough on the women medical students.

She was involved with the women's tramping club and enjoyed going to university balls with her friends. Two of her close friends were Elizabeth (Betty) Macready (née Cuttle; 1942) and Roma Roberts (née Chatfield; 1942); they maintained a close 'telephone' friendship into their late eighties.

In 1941 Isabel married Paul Wishart, who was in the medical school class of 1940; he was 31 and she was 22. Their three daughters, Anne, Catherine (Kitty) and Judith, were born between 1942 and 1945. During that time, Wishart completed her sixth year and spent her two years of registration at Auckland Hospital. Her graduation certificate indicates that she finished her examinations in 1942, but the certificate was not signed until July 1944. Meanwhile, Paul Wishart was posted to the 2nd New Zealand Expeditionary Force in January 1942 and was appointed regimental medical officer to the 37th Battalion in February 1942.[29]

These would have been extremely challenging years, dealing with her husband being almost immediately posted overseas for war duty, completing her studies and her sixth-year hospital work, as well as three pregnancies in quick succession. She moved back into the family home in Mount Eden with her mother Roberta, who gave her the same support she herself had once received from her own mother, Isabella. In around 1944–45, Roberta bought a house on a large section with an orchard on Cockle Bay Road in Howick, and she, Isabel and the children moved out there.

After Paul Wishart was discharged from the army in 1945, the family moved to

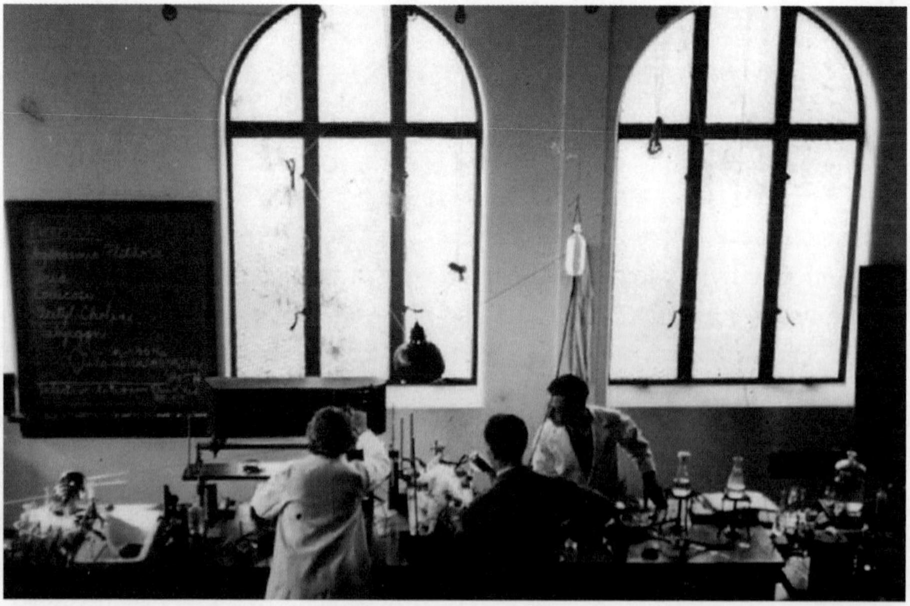

Isabel Wishart working in the chemistry laboratory at Otago Medical School, c.1938. *Family collection*

Tauranga, where he worked for two years at Tauranga Hospital and then went into private practice. His consultation rooms were in the family home. It was hard work with long hours and a lot of travel into the surrounding countryside for deliveries and to attend accidents.

Their fourth child, John, was born in 1948. In 1949, the three girls stayed in Howick with their grandmother while Isabel and Paul and baby John went to Britain for 18 months, where Paul pursued his postgraduate studies. They lived in war-torn Croydon, in what Wishart later described as a 'tip of a place': they were subject to food rations, and she remembers using a 'lot of lard'. Paul was in London much of the time studying, and she spent long lonely days and nights, missing her girls and her mother back in New Zealand.

+++

They returned from England in 1950, and Paul became physician and radiologist at Tauranga Public Hospital. When their youngest child was five, Isabel Wishart started working part-time at a private laboratory run by her old classmate Graham

(Slim) Somerville, doing allergy testing at first and later more varied work. She unexpectedly became pregnant again in 1958, at the age of 41. Her older children described their younger brother, Guy, as her 'sunshine child'.[30]

Paul Wishart died of a heart attack in October 1959, just before his fiftieth birthday, leaving Isabel with six children ranging in age from one to 17. The oldest, Anne, soon left home for teacher training in Auckland, and Kitty went to university the following year. One-year-old Guy joined the next-door neighbours' one-year-old while Wishart worked, and Kitty looked after him during the university holidays. The family tradition of one generation supporting the next came into play again when her mother moved from Howick to Tauranga to live with the family and help with childcare and cooking until her death in 1976, aged 91.

Science teachers were always in short supply, so Wishart taught for a year at Tauranga Girls College in 1960 — her first year as a widow — but she decided teaching was not her forte. The following year, Somerville again offered her a job at his laboratory and provided on-the-job training to become a pathologist. The children remember her diligently studying at home in the evenings. She was on the Medical Register in 1961, but the only evidence of a formal qualification is a certificate from 1974 for membership in the International Academy of Cytology. She eventually handled a wide range of work: in a regional town in that era, all pathologists were generalists. She did postmortems and gave evidence in court cases: she was proud of this work, as it was harder than working behind a microscope.

Isabel Wishart faced many challenges throughout her life, but she met them with stoicism and good humour. She forged a pathway that incorporated the medical skills from her earlier training. She had interesting interactions with the medical profession over the years: she once argued with an emergency doctor when he was not convinced by her diagnosis of a ruptured appendix (she was right).

When she was 91 and had developed breast cancer, the surgeon was reluctant to do a mastectomy under general anaesthetic because of her age and general health; instead she insisted on having it done under local anaesthetic, as 'she did not want to die of brain metastases'.[31] Her children said this toughness was characteristic of her. She was a favourite patient for case studies when she was in hospital — the combination of having had rheumatic fever as a child, chronic obstructive pulmonary disease and living into her nineties was unusual. She died in 2013 at the age of 94.

DAPHNE PHYLLIS ADAMS (NÉE MORRISON)

1944 graduate

Daphne Adams was born in 1921 in Tapanui, a small town in West Otago, and spent her early years on her parents' dairy farm in a Presbyterian environment of service to family and society and education for all. The family moved to Dunedin in 1927, when she was six.[32]

Adams attended Otago Girls' High School, where she was head girl and dux in her final year. She continued to excel in ballet and, at one stage, contemplated following her contemporary, Rowena Jackson, to a career in ballet. However, her parents recognised that she had an intellect that should not be wasted and asked their dour Scottish lawyer for advice. Should she pursue a career in law or medicine? 'Oh no,' he replied, 'there is no place for women in the law.'

With the decision made, Adams entered Otago Medical School in 1939, just as the Second World War was beginning. She was the first in her family to go to university, and she lived at home in Dunedin while she studied. There were few women in her medical school class, but they stuck together, even though they were not all in the same year level — they would retreat to the separate women's common room where they could socialise. Four women students who became lifelong friends were Shirley Juliette Dowding (née Appleton; 1945), Molly Joan Woodroffe (née Boyes; 1943), Mavis MacDougall and Shirley Tonkin.

After graduating in 1944, Adams applied for a house surgeon position at Waikato Hospital, one of the few hospitals that would take female graduates and also one of the few that would take medical officers returning from the war. Here she met one such young medical officer, Butt (Albert) Adams, who looked after her when she was hospitalised with scarlet fever. They were married in Dunedin in March 1946 and soon after travelled to Auckland, where her husband had been invited to join his colleague and friend Vic McGeorge in general practice in Mount Eden.

Although Adams had entertained ideas of a career in anaesthetics, having worked in this field at Waikato Hospital, the birth of her first daughter, Jenny, in 1947 meant this was put on hold. When Jenny was just a baby, Butt left for paediatric specialist training and exams in Edinburgh, while Adams returned to work as a pathology registrar. She presented a paper at the Auckland branch of the NZMWA

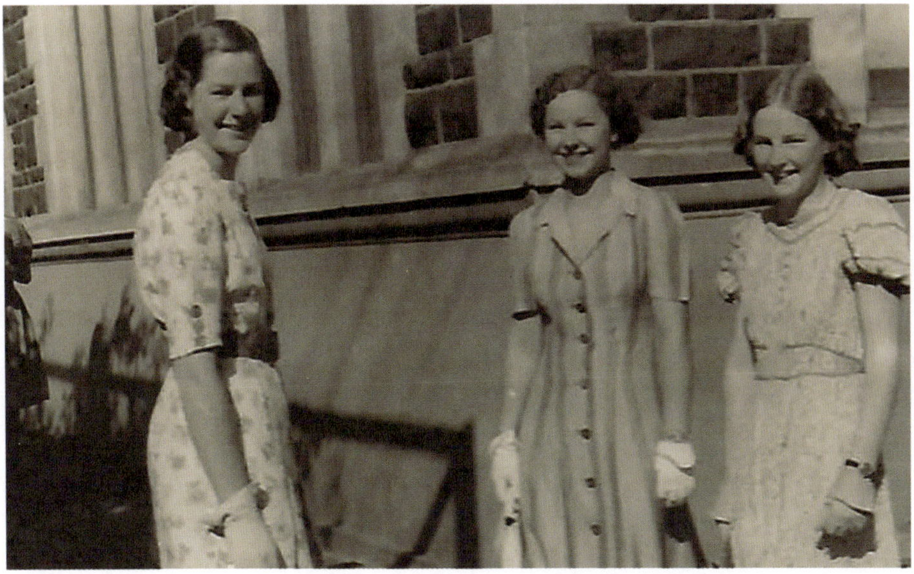

The first day of university, 1939. From left: Margaret Cameron, Daphne Adams (née Morrison), Gwen Buchan. *Adams family collection*

in 1948 titled 'Pathology and Hygiene of Housework'. Her work was again put on hold when she and Jenny travelled to Britain to join Butt. They holidayed in Europe for some months, then returned to New Zealand, where he rejoined the practice in Mount Eden.

+++

Adams then joined the Ministry of Health as a school doctor. Her second child, John, was born in 1953, and Margaret in 1958. She continued to work as a school doctor based at the ministry's Mount Roskill office, with trips to the main department at the Marinoto Clinic in town, which provided mental health assessment and therapy for people under the age of 20. Such roles were important in the 1950s and 1960s, a time when many women medical practitioners gave immunisations and cared for the health of children referred by their schools. She also worked at the government-run health camps.

The NZMWA was a strong organisation, and Adams and her colleagues were committed members from 1948 onwards. In 1971, as Auckland branch president, she planted a tree in the Auckland Domain on behalf of the NZMWA to mark Auckland's centennial year. She spent many hours preparing submissions on health policies, such as the Abortion Law Reform Bill and submissions to the Royal Commission of Inquiry into Contraception, Sterilisation and Abortion (1975–77), and the government's white paper on health (1975).

After leaving the school doctor service, Adams joined the Family Planning Association and became a long-serving doctor at its Newmarket branch. She also joined her husband for a short time in his practice until they both retired in the mid-1980s. Daphne Adams died in 2010, aged 89.

DIANA MANBY MASON (NÉE SHAW)

1945 graduate

Diana Shaw was born in Wellington in 1922.[33] When she first told her parents that she wanted to be a doctor, her father thought she was being silly and that she must have meant nursing. 'In leapt my mother, ambition rampant — "Nonsense, Charles, the child must do what she wants, no matter what the odds",' she said in an interview in 1998.

Mason was just 16 when she began the medical intermediate at Victoria University College in Wellington in 1939.[34] She entered the course thinking the academic work would be no trouble to her since she had graduated as dux of Samuel Marsden Collegiate School. But this proved not to be the case: 'Physics was Chinese to me, both chemistries not much better. At the first term exams a result of 19 per cent in physics was such a shock that I dragooned a childhood friend who was repeating medical intermediate to give up his first term holiday to coach me in the basics of physics. Nothing in my life was to be such hard work as those next two terms.'[35]

She would wake up at 4 am to study, often continuing to work late into the night after her classes in order to keep up. Despite starting with little experience in the sciences, she was rewarded with an offer to study at Otago Medical School the following year and, after taking a year off in Australia with her mother, moved to Dunedin at the beginning of 1941.

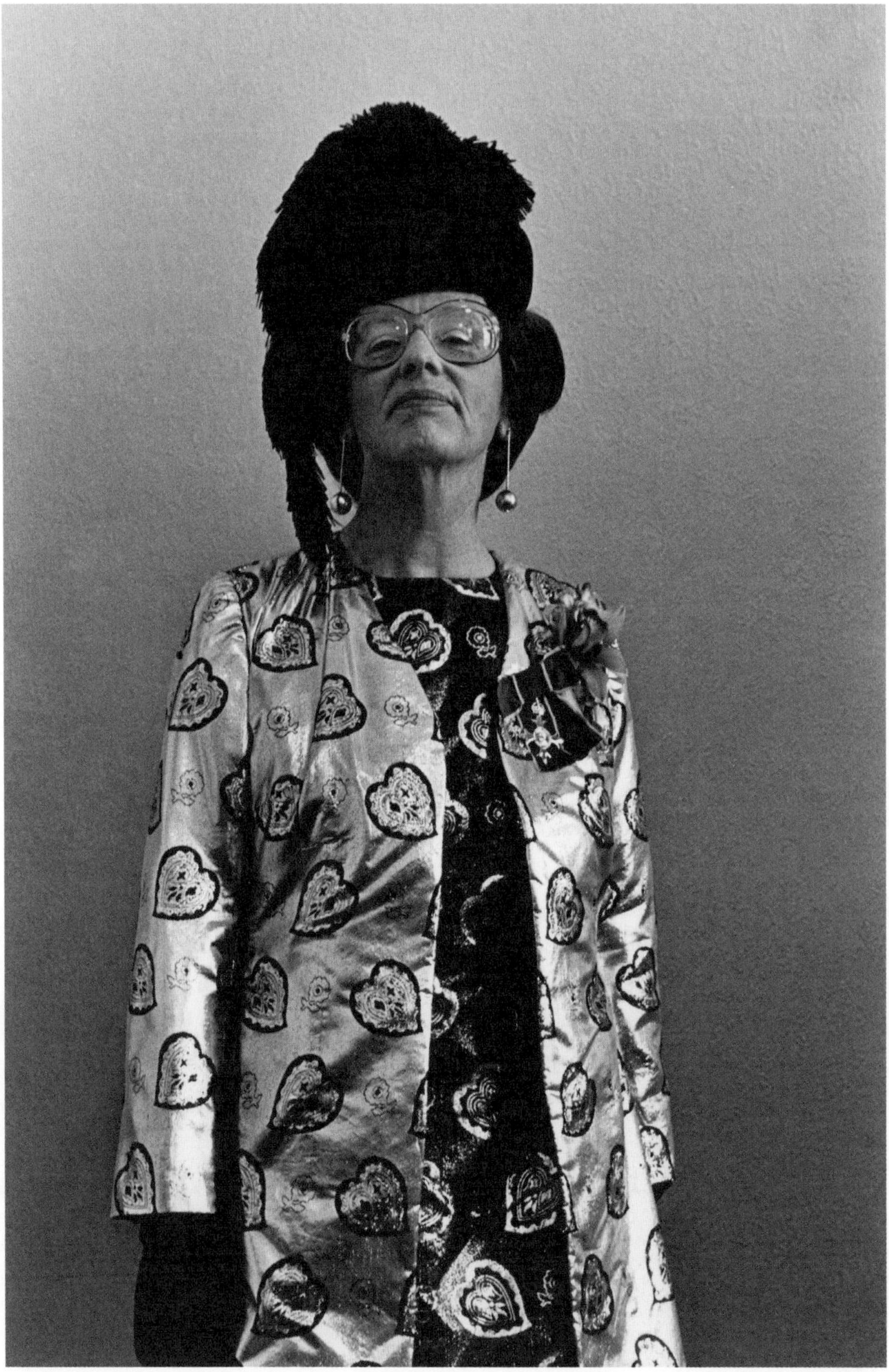

Dr Diana Mason photographed by Peter Black in Wellington in 1978. This was her favourite photo. *Museum of New Zealand Te Papa Tongarewa, O.003073*

When Mason began her medical degree she was one of nine women in a class of 100 — there was a smaller intake of students that year because of the war. She never felt discriminated against for being female but she did feel a constant pressure to outperform her male classmates. Towards the end of her career she acknowledged that 'after a lifetime in medicine I realise that you "make it" in the eyes of your colleagues, regardless of sex or colour, only if you show you can do it. If not, discrimination is certainly the name of the game.'[36]

Mason claimed that she and her fellow students were not taught about contraception, sexuality or sexual health. Their few lectures on obstetrics were read from a textbook, and she did not remember learning about gynaecology. They were also not taught how to relate to patients; and even their psychiatry training was rudimentary — it involved only a visit to Seacliff psychiatric hospital.

In her fifth year, Mason was given temporary registration and sent to Te Puke as part of the wartime placements to relieve GPs who had not had a break during the entire war. She was put in charge of a clinic that covered the whole area between Tauranga and Rotorua. 'I didn't know the first thing about anything, absolutely nothing except bookwork. I certainly had no idea of how to handle patients and I didn't know how to recognise clinical conditions.'[37] She came face to face with this lack of hands-on experience when a woman who worked on a dairy farm came in with a foul-smelling bandage on her lower leg: the wound was crawling with maggots. 'I rushed into the lavatory, where I vomited violently, all the while asking myself whether I was not entirely deluded in my belief that medicine was what I wanted to do.'

She did not experience any explicit discrimination for being a woman doctor while she was at the clinic, but she did find the practice nurse and the midwives at Tauranga Hospital quite antagonistic. At the end of the year she was thankful to return to Dunedin, where all of the fifth-years compared notes and shared how out of their depth they had felt.

Diana Mason graduated in December 1943. Three days later, she married playwright Bruce Mason, with whom she had been in a relationship since 1940. The couple spent their first two years of marriage in an old flat in Thorndon while she was completing her junior and senior house surgeon years at Wellington Hospital. Bruce obtained a position at the Alexander Turnbull Library and the War History Branch of Internal Affairs. She described these years as being full of hard work, poverty and joy.

+ + +

After two years as a house surgeon, Mason decided that she wanted to pursue paediatrics, for which she would need to complete postgraduate training in England. Bruce Mason was also interested in moving to London and trying to break into the West End. They did not have enough money to fund the trip, and so in 1948 Mason went to work for a practice in Newtown, a low-income, multicultural inner-city Wellington suburb, that was looking for a young woman graduate. The practice was run by an older GP, William (Bill) Shirer, who believed that 'one never turned anyone away and never refused a call twenty-four hours a day seven days a week'.[38] The position was well paid and, unusually, included a car. Along with her regular hours, she worked every other night and every other weekend, something that was very common for family doctors at the time.

The area was quite rough, and in later years Mason marvelled at how she would walk into houses at 1 or 2 am without a backward glance: 'I felt somehow protected by my invisible professional cloak.' She found that it was often the poorest who were the most grateful; they would pay in prized food like a chocolate bar or a can of sweetened condensed milk.

After a year at the Newtown clinic, Mason became pregnant, and the couple decided to move to England once she had given birth to their daughter Belinda.[39] She had delivered so many babies at the clinic that she believed she would have no trouble with the birth, but she ended up having a painful 30-hour labour that resulted in an emergency caesarean section. This 'produced feelings of guilt and failure, feelings that I have since seen reproduced countless times in my patients,' she said in 1998. '"Having a baby is natural," we all say, and we resent nature letting us down. We question ourselves as to how and where we went wrong.'[40] It was experiences like this that led to her being widely loved as a GP obstetrician later in life.

The Mason family arrived in London at the height of the summer of 1949. They reconnected with Richard and Edith Campion, friends from their theatre days in Wellington, and flatted with them in a house in Chelsea for two and a half years.

Diana Mason enrolled in the six-month postgraduate paediatrics course at Great Ormond Street Hospital. Three other Otago women graduates were in her class: Juliet Carleton Harrison (née Williams; 1945), Shirley Lyford Tonkin (née Curtis; 1945) and Patricia Hunter Cook (née Will; 1945). The Masons hired a nanny for Belinda so that Mason could study. On the course, she felt discriminated against for being a woman in medicine for the first and only time in her career: the male students were referred to by the title of Doctor, but the women students were called Miss or Mrs. 'I seethed but ascribed it to the conservatism of the Brits versus the liberalism of the Kiwis.'[41]

In 1952, back in New Zealand, Mason returned to work for Bill Shirer, and the family moved into the flat above the surgery on Riddiford Street. Bruce Mason, who later described himself as New Zealand's first house husband, started working from home so he could help look after their now three children. Mason became very busy very quickly. She started in paediatrics but soon realised that she preferred obstetrics. Shirer gave her all his maternity patients, and she worked closely with other GP obstetricians in the area, such as Ken Pacey, T. F. Corkill and Gordon Findlay. She worked days and alternate nights whenever she was required for a delivery. Over the rest of her career, she delivered on average 300 babies a year.[42]

+ + +

In 1958, Mason was offered the position of superintendent at Alexandra Hospital and the Alexandra Home for Unmarried Mothers. The private hospital in Wellington had been opened by the Wellington Ladies Christian Association and was later taken over by the Women's Temperance Movement to look after girls around New Zealand who had become pregnant outside of marriage, impoverished women and women prisoners. Her responsibilities were delivering babies, holding a clinic every week and teaching midwifery to the nursing staff.

Looking back on it later, she thought that the adoption process was extremely traumatic for the girls. The babies were removed from the mothers quite soon, usually after 10 days, which was just enough time to see if the baby had any congenital disorders. Even then, for those 10 days the babies were handled primarily by the nursing staff and the mothers had very little contact with them. Only a small minority kept their babies. Most of the adoptions were organised privately, and the rest went through the welfare department.[43]

At the same time as she was working at the Alexandra Hospital, Mason established a student medical service at Victoria University, where she worked as an obstetrics and family planning advisor. She was a strong proponent of family planning and was renowned for providing unmarried women with contraception.

At Alexandra Hospital, she was approached by the members of what would later become known as the Society for the Protection of the Unborn Child (SPUC) — now known as Voice For Life. Through her work as a GP obstetrician, she developed an 'abhorrence' for abortion.[44] She received a lot of criticism from colleagues and friends, who felt this contradicted her otherwise liberal opinions.

Mason officially retired from obstetrics work in 1988 after more than 30 years, but she remained involved in the medical community. In 1973, she was elected the second woman president of the Wellington division of the New Zealand Medical Association (NZMA), of which she had been a member since its inception, and she was also a founding member of the College of GPs. She died on 5 June 2007, aged 84.

JUDY ANN DAVID WILSON (NÉE COLLINS)

1947 graduate

Judy Ann David Wilson was born in 1923 to David and Sybil Collins in Wairarapa, where they had a sheep farm.[45] She attended the local school, riding her Shetland pony bareback, then transferred to St Matthew's School in Masterton. She attended secondary school as a boarder at Woodford House in Havelock North, which she remembered as particularly cloistered. She decided to study medicine in her final years at school. When the headmistress asked her if she would be continuing with her music studies when she left school she was surprised. She had been playing piano for five years, but for the last two years she had been preparing to follow in the footsteps of her father and grandfather and enter medical intermediate. 'No, Miss Holland', she replied. 'I am going to be a doctor!'[46]

Once she had announced her decision to pursue a medical career, the school excused her from dressmaking classes and instead arranged for her to be tutored in Latin and mathematics, subjects that were required for medical school entry. She picked them up relatively easily.[47]

During her medical intermediate year at Victoria University College in 1941, she boarded in Seatoun with the wife of a vicar who was serving overseas.[48] She did well and was accepted into the medical school intake for 1942. She made several lifelong friends in her five years in Dunedin — they bonded through their shared

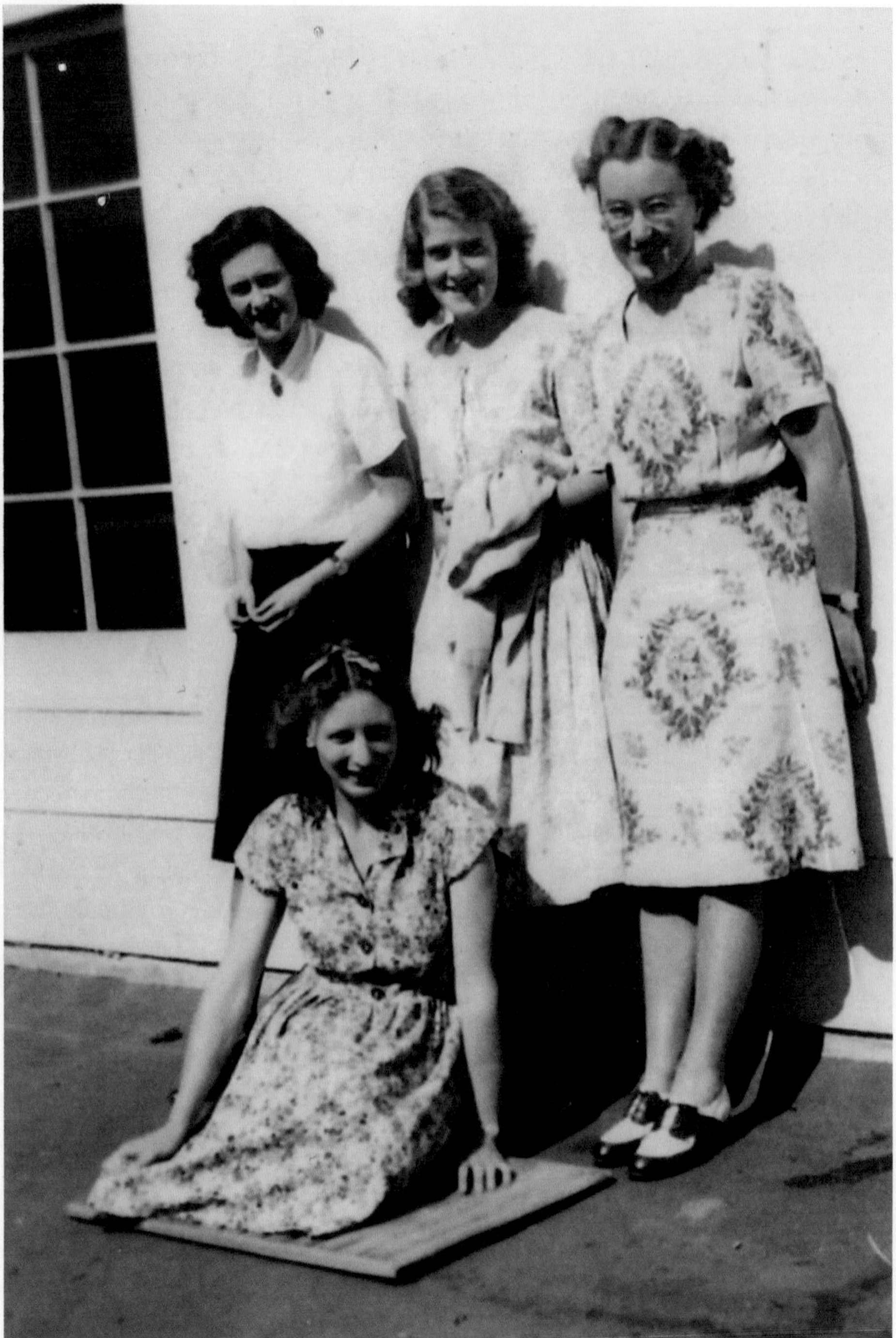

Fourth-year medical students in Dunedin, 1945. Standing, from left: Margaret Saunders, Judy Faris and Judy Wilson (née Collins). Seated: Maire Smith (née Tait). *Courtesy Michael Kelly*

learning, sports, and the food rationing, blackouts and restrictions on travel and campus activities imposed on them by the war.

For her final year, Wilson returned to Wellington, where she had been offered live-in accommodation at Wellington Hospital — an offer open only to the highest achieving students. After she graduated, she took up a house surgeon position at the hospital, first in the eye, ear, nose and throat department, and then in casualty. She completed her house surgeon years at Silverstream Hospital in Upper Hutt, which had been built by US marines during the war to treat their casualty patients from the war in the Pacific.

+++

Wilson's plans to apply for postgraduate training in England changed when she met John Wilson at a ball in Wellington around 1947. John had trained as a lawyer before spending three and a half years as a prisoner of war under the Japanese. After a two-year relationship, they married in Upper Hutt in 1949.

John Wilson was conservative — in his opinion, his wife should not work while she was raising children — so when their first child was born in 1951, Judy stopped work. By 1955, the couple had three sons, and as they grew up, she did not even tell her children that she was a doctor; her son Nigel remembers being surprised when he went to the letterbox one day when he was around 10 or 11 to find a letter addressed to Dr Judy Wilson. But although the children did not know, the local Silverstream neighbourhood certainly did. 'People would arrive and ask, "What do you think about this, Judy?"' Nigel recalls.

During her pregnancies, Wilson took in unmarried pregnant women — a common practice for women doctors at the time. She offered them care and support, and, in return, they helped her with the children and the housework. One of the four women they fostered, Jean, became a close friend of the family and they remained in contact for the rest of their lives.[49]

In 1965, with all her boys now in boarding school, Wilson decided to return to part-time work with the Department of Health in Upper Hutt. She started in the Plunket clinics but soon expanded out to working with public health nurses in schools, the Society for Intellectually Handicapped Children (IHC), and various kindergartens. She came across many child health issues that the Plunket nurses had to be convinced to address. She argued that most infant cot deaths (now termed sudden unexplained death in infancy syndrome [SUDI]) 'were a result of tiredness, travel, and respiratory infections resulting in suffocation when babies were put down to sleep on their tummies'.[50] She based this on four specific sudden cot deaths that she had investigated. When she presented on this topic to the local hospital, the paediatrician present, Rodney Ford, was disparaging of her observations. Interestingly, some years later Ford was co-author of a landmark New Zealand study led by Edwin Mitchell that found sleeping on their tummies was indeed a risk factor for cot death in babies.[51]

In her role, Wilson was asked to conduct a survey on obesity in children: the survey found that 'the children who went to school with no breakfast were often the obese ones'.[52] She also worked with plastic surgeon Cecily Pickerill (née Clarkson; 1925), arranging referrals for patients with cleft lips or palates.

Alongside her work, Wilson volunteered for the Red Cross: twice she was president of the Upper Hutt branch, she was a patron from 2008 to 2011, and was later made a life member. She offered free preschool babysitting to tired, stressed mothers to give them a break, and in 1976 she assisted the relief team after massive flooding in the Hutt Valley, arranging a welfare caravan and the distribution of food and relief funds.

In 2011, Wilson broke her hip. Her health gradually deteriorated, but her sons and health carers helped her to stay in the family home in Silverstream. She died in January 2016.

RINA WINIFRED MOORE (NÉE RŌPIHA)

1948 graduate — first Māori woman graduate

In 1948 Bishop Frederick Bennett, the first Māori bishop of Aotearoa New Zealand, commented on Rina Moore's graduation from the University of Otago:

> New Zealand's first Maori woman doctor will take her degree next month . . . an illustration of the ability of members of the Maori race to succeed in any pursuit. Bishop Bennett said Mrs Moore studied hard to within a few days of having a child and went back to her studies as soon

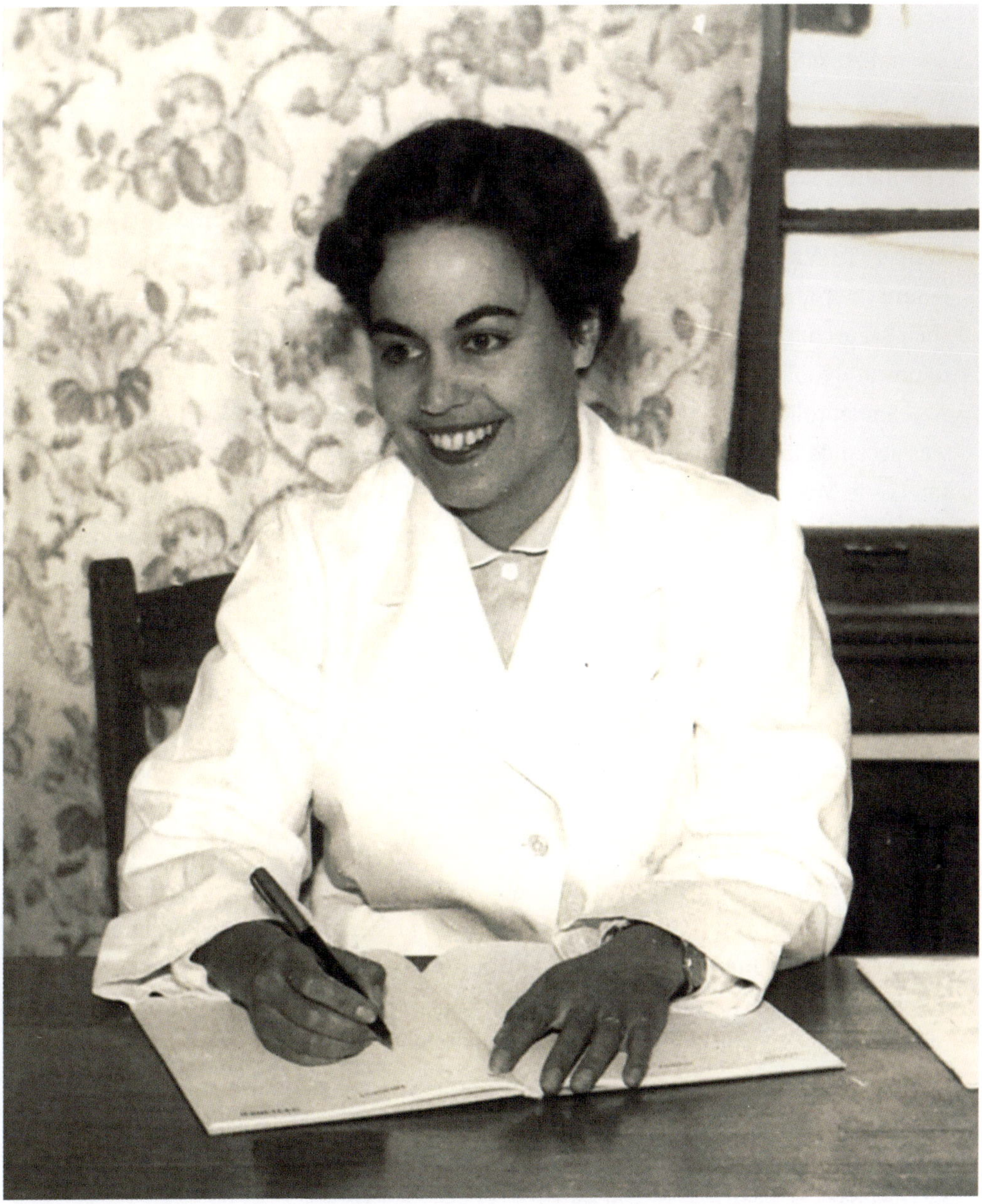

Rina Moore (née Rōpiha), c.1950s. *Archives New Zealand*

as possible afterwards, leaving her husband to look after the baby on the Plunket system.[53]

Rina Moore (Ngāti Kahungunu, Te Whānau-ā-Apanui) was born in 1923. Her father, Tipi Tainui Rōpiha (Ngāti Kahungunu, Rangitāne), was the first Māori secretary of the Department of Maori Affairs, and her mother, Rhoda Winifred Te Tūruki Walker (Te Whānau-ā-Apanui), had worked as a nurse among Māori in rural areas before their marriage. Rina and her brother Peter were brought up detached from their Māori heritage. They lived in Remuera, Auckland, where Rina had an English nanny and took lessons in elocution, ballet, ballroom dancing and piano.[54]

She enrolled at Otago in 1941, passed her medical intermediate subjects and was accepted into medicine in 1943.[55] At the start of her second year, she married Ian Leslie Moore, a law student from Nelson; his family was an old Nelson family who established the law firm Pitt & Moore. The couple's first child, Karin, was born in August 1945. Finances were stretched, but both families provided support and practical assistance. Rhoda Walker stayed in Dunedin for six months to help while her daughter continued her studies. Afterwards, Moore's husband and two-year-old daughter stayed with her mother-in-law, Ruby, in Nelson. She and Ian had three more children: Christopher, Nicholas and John. In 1949, Moore began working as an assistant medical officer at Ngawhatu Psychiatric Hospital in Nelson, primarily with female patients.

Moore was intelligent, bold and articulate — qualities that meant she was sought after as a public speaker. In the late 1950s she was invited to participate in a series of hui with young Māori leaders discussing issues such as urban migration, high crime rates, mental health and education. Like many Māori migrants to the cities, she realised that she had missed out on much of her Māori heritage. Despite many attempts, she never mastered te reo Māori. In 1960 she was one of five speakers to the first South Island Conference of Young Maori Leaders in Christchurch, where she spoke on the topic 'Health Trends in Modern Maori Society'. Later that year, she was made an inaugural member of the Maori Health Committee formed by the Board of Health — one of only two Māori doctors.[56]

Moore was outspoken on the controversial issue of family planning. She advocated strongly for education about sex and relationships in schools, and she was one of the first doctors in New Zealand to prescribe the contraceptive pill in the early 1960s.[57] In 1961 she prepared a paper on family planning to present to the influential Māori Women's Welfare League (MWWL). They did not endorse the paper; instead, they told the Maori Health Committee that although the MWWL was concerned about the high infant mortality rate, this was more a matter of health education.[58] Moore was also actively involved in promoting higher standards of education for young Māori. In 1962, as the Māori representative on the Nelson district committee, she helped organise a national campaign to raise funds for the Maori Education Foundation.

In 1963, after 15 years at Ngawhatu, Moore resigned. During these years, men had been promoted over her, her health was poor and her career prospects were restricted by the lack of a postgraduate degree, which would have required training overseas — impractical when her husband was tied to his Nelson legal practice and she had four children. Instead, she set up a private psychiatric and counselling clinic in the family home. Her children would come home from school to find their playroom (now the waiting room) full of patients and Moore in consultation in the living room.

In 1966, Moore was diagnosed with cancer of the breast and lymph nodes. She decided not to have a mastectomy, which was the norm at that time, but she did have the tumour removed, followed by radiotherapy treatment. From that time onwards, she was fearful of dying in pain and suffered periods of depression. In 1975 she had a mild stroke, and shortly after it became apparent that her cancer had returned, this time in her brain. She died in November 1975 at the age of 52.

The third-year Otago Medical School class of 1958. The women pictured (front row, from left) are: Janis Oliver (née Sutherland; 1961), Phyllis Charlton (née Taylor; 1961), Margaret Sparrow (née Muir; 1963), Pauline Blue (née Ellis; 1961), Lucy Chung (née Chan; 1964), Lorraine Smith (1962) and Mirdza Palmer (née Robins; 1961). *Otago Medical School Archives*

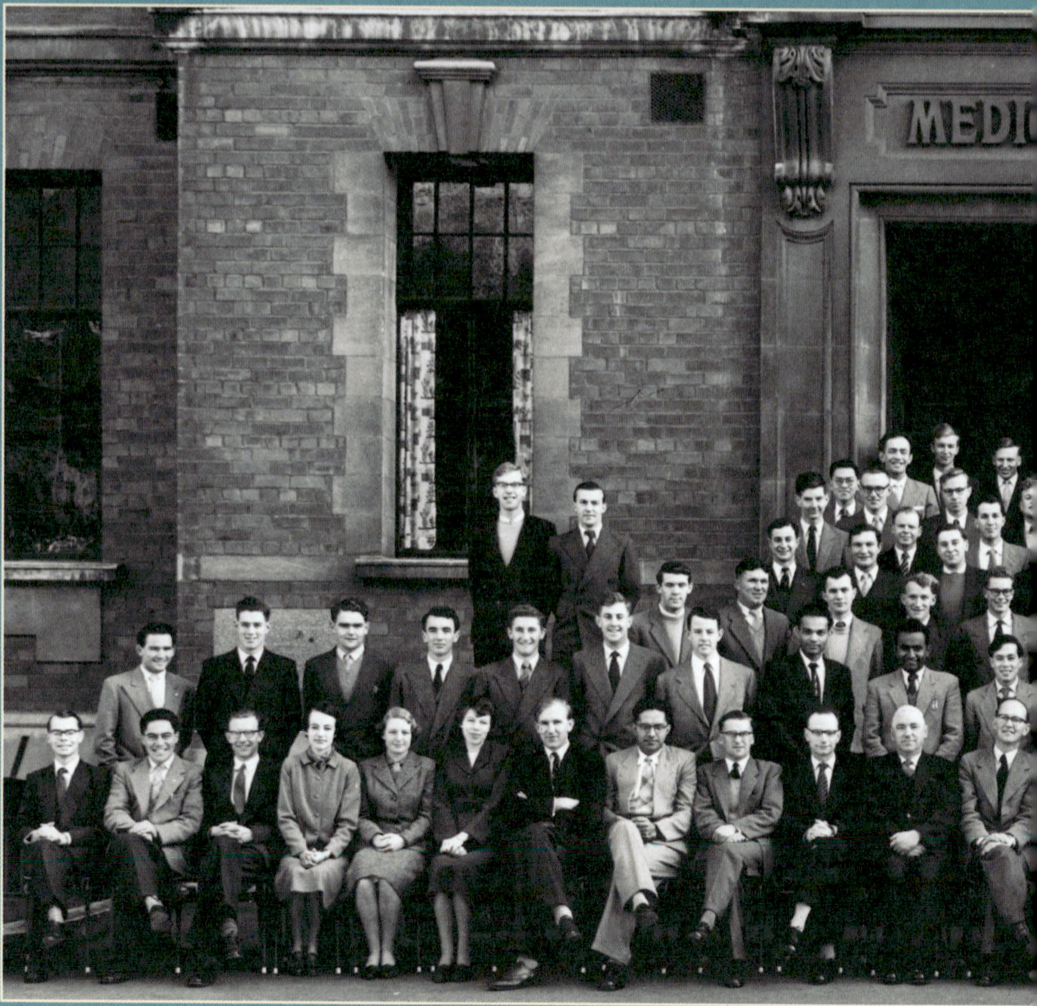

5. Refugees of war 1941–1967

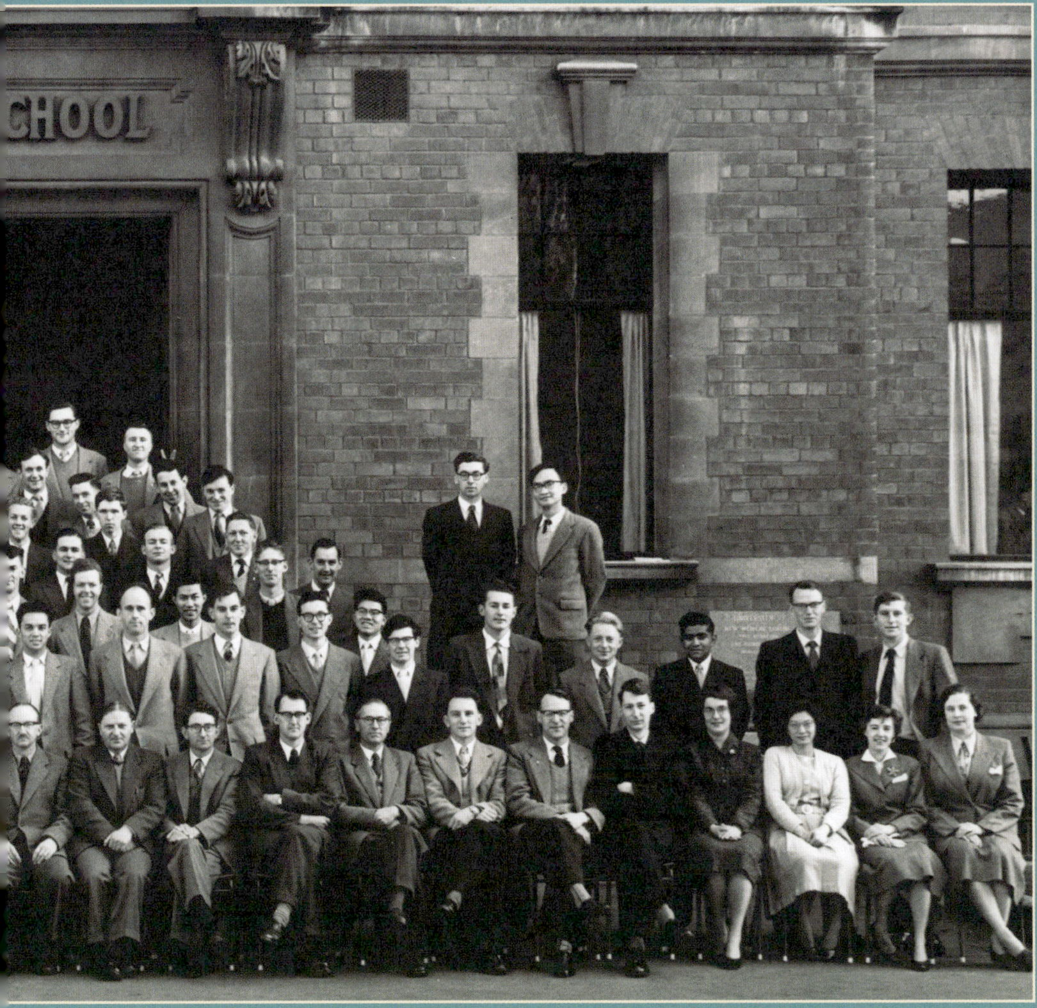

Adolf Hitler began his campaign against the Jews in 1933 in Germany. Violence against Jewish people started almost immediately, with attacks on banks, family stores and places of trade. Yet it was not until 1936, when the Nazi party legalised its acts of 'Aryanisation' (the transfer of Jewish-owned property to non-Jews) and began the coordinated violence that sparked popular anger against Jews that many feared for their future in Europe.[1] A wave of emigration followed as not only Jews but also other displaced peoples sought to get as far away as possible from the danger.

The international community needed to accept these refugees, but many countries expressed concern that those who arrived would end up being a drain on their economies.[2] Yet, with so many men away at the front lines, countries such as New Zealand were short of labour. Refugees were willing to fill these positions, but mistrust, anti-Semitism and racism kept many out of the country, as well as out of the workforce and the war effort.[3]

New Zealand took a strict approach, stipulating that applications for entry would be decided on a case-by-case basis. Those of British birth or descent were allowed to enter on a free permit, but all others had to obtain a visa — an approach some historians have argued was in keeping with New Zealand's early twentieth-century aims of restricting the entry of certain races.[4] In the end, only 1100 refugees were accepted to New Zealand during the war years; by comparison, Australia accepted 170,000 displaced persons over five years.[5]

Medical practitioners were among the educated professional refugees preferred by the New Zealand government, but they were still subject to distrust, limitations on travel and a lack of opportunity after they arrived in New Zealand.

Five women doctors who were Jewish refugees — Olga Wilhelmine Lina Semon (1941), Katharina Newman (née Weisz; 1941), Hilda Fleischl (née Barber; 1942), Rachel Munk (née Beneraf; 1948) and Zelma Ronigar-Hahn (née Ronigar; 1953) — were admitted to New Zealand and given the opportunity to retrain within the British system in a 'special' three-year training course at the Otago Medical School.

In addition to these five, nine Jewish women graduates had been displaced by the war, and arrived in New Zealand either as children or as young adults — Marianne Fillenz (1948), Edith Ruth Black (née Blumenthal; 1952), Eva Ruth Seelye (née Hersch; 1953), Irene Therese Valentine (née Abrahamsohn; 1954), Susanna Williams (née Lemchen; 1957), Miriam Frank (1960), Dorothy Jean Kral (1962) and Marion Joan Boock (née Kral; 1964).[6] They all completed the six-year course. Marianne Fillenz's sister Liselotte was also enrolled at the Otago Medical School but died in an accident only months before sitting her final examinations.[7]

These women had arrived while young, but even so these nine felt that their experience in New Zealand was shaped by their status as refugees. On arrival in New Zealand, Munk, Ronigar-Hahn and Newman anglicised their names, and all records relating to them thereafter refer to them as Rachel Monk, Selma Ronigar-Hahn and Catherine Newman.

Hendrika Waal-Manning (née Waal; 1957), Viola Palmer (née Heine; 1959) and Mirdza Palmer (née Robins; 1961) were all displaced by the Second World War but were not of Jewish descent. Since Waal-Manning and Viola Palmer (not a relative of Mirdza Palmer) arrived as children, they entered the New Zealand schooling system.

These 16 graduates had very different experiences at Otago Medical School and in their subsequent careers than their New Zealand counterparts. The way the medical school and, later, their colleagues treated them reflected the evolving attitudes towards refugees, particularly women refugees, and much of it was patronising, fearful and unkind. Some of the women felt so indebted to their adoptive country that they decided to dedicate the rest of their careers and lives to giving back. Others did not ever manage to get past the cultural dislocation and returned to Europe not long after completing their studies.

Although medical refugees were more welcome than those of other backgrounds, obtaining a visa to New Zealand was still extremely difficult. Refugees had to pay their way into New Zealand, but they were not allowed to arrive with any goods or equity. Instead, they had to provide proof of a sponsor or guarantor should they require financial help.[8] The Lemchen and Hersch families were among these early refugee families who found a sponsor. Others came across sponsors purely by luck.[9] Hilda Fleischl, along with her son and soon-to-be husband, had escaped to Switzerland in 1938.[10] While in Lausanne, her son Peter made friends with an English boy. One day, when they were swimming in Lac Léman, the boy almost drowned, but Peter, who was a strong swimmer, saved him and brought him back to shore. Out of gratitude, the boy's mother offered to help the family obtain documentation to emigrate to New Zealand.

After the first wave of refugees arrived in New Zealand, the wider public and government officials became anxious that refugee numbers could escalate. The medical community shared the view that New Zealand would be 'overrun', and the New Zealand branch of the British Medical Association (BMA) put pressure on Otago Medical School to close places to refugees.[11] A perception developed that refugee doctors were taking the places of New Zealand's own.[12] In 1939, when it was announced that 13 'foreign medical practitioners' had been admitted to the medical school,[13] the BMA lodged a protest with the Customs Department, which had been informing refugees with medical qualifications that if they were accepted to New Zealand they would be given the opportunity to retrain.[14]

The chancellor of the university stated that since the medical school was staffed for only around 100 students and the numbers were 'swelling' with refugees, the intake would be capped from 1941: only 100 places would be available, and only three refugee doctors would be admitted each year. In the heightened environment of the war years, this was a further blow to refugees.

Those refugees who managed to arrive after the Second World War did so under very specific conditions. As the newly established International Refugee Organization (IRO), a specialised agency within the United Nations, placed pressure on all countries in the Commonwealth to increase their refugee intake, New Zealand created a racial hierarchy based on the Immigration Restriction Amendment Act of 1920 to determine who New Zealand would accept.[15] As always, at the top of the list were those of British birth or descent.[16]

Beyond that, the racial hierarchies that had developed over the war years and that were already present in New Zealand's immigration processes persisted. Refugees from Estonia, Lithuania, Latvia and Western Europeans who were not of Jewish descent were preferred because it was believed they would assimilate more easily. At the bottom of the list were Jews, particularly those displaced by Hitler, and people from Asia.[17]

Selma Ronigar-Hahn was born in Gablenz, Czechoslovakia, in 1901 and was a concentration camp survivor. She received her degree from the University of Prague in 1935 and then worked for three years in medical and surgical hospitals. Her medical licence was revoked before the war as she was Jewish. During the war years, Ronigar-Hahn 'doctored, if it can be called that, in concentration camps'.[18] We are not sure which camp she was in but we know that her parents and husband died at Auschwitz. After the war, Ronigar-Hahn offered her services to the British Army in the British occupation zone of Germany, and this eventually led her to New Zealand late in 1949.[19]

Hendrika Waal-Manning, who was of Dutch descent, was living in Bandung, Java (now known as Indonesia), when the Japanese invaded in 1942. In 1943 Waal-Manning, then aged 11, and her mother and her sister were taken to a prison where they remained until 1946, when the Allied forces freed Indonesia from Japanese control. During these years, her mother continued to educate the two girls using one piece of paper on which they would write their notes; at the end of each night, they would erase the notes so they could use the paper again the following day. At the end of the war the family was offered a place in New Zealand: they arrived in Wellington in late 1946.[20]

Mirdza Palmer and her mother were able to gain permits to New Zealand because, as Latvians, they were on the list of preferred refugees.[21] When the war ended, the family were all sent to a displaced persons camp, where Palmer and her sister finished their high school diplomas. Palmer's father died there in 1946. They then applied for refugee status. In July 1951 Palmer and her mother were approved for a visa, and they arrived in Wellington on 13 August.

Ruth Black left Czechoslovakia with her parents and grandparents as a young teenager and the family stayed in England for a short time before they emigrated to New Zealand.

There is very little information on Irene Valentine, who also arrived after the war. She and her mother and brother managed to escape capture, but her father, Albert Abrahamsohn, died in October 1943 in Berlin. The family is listed in

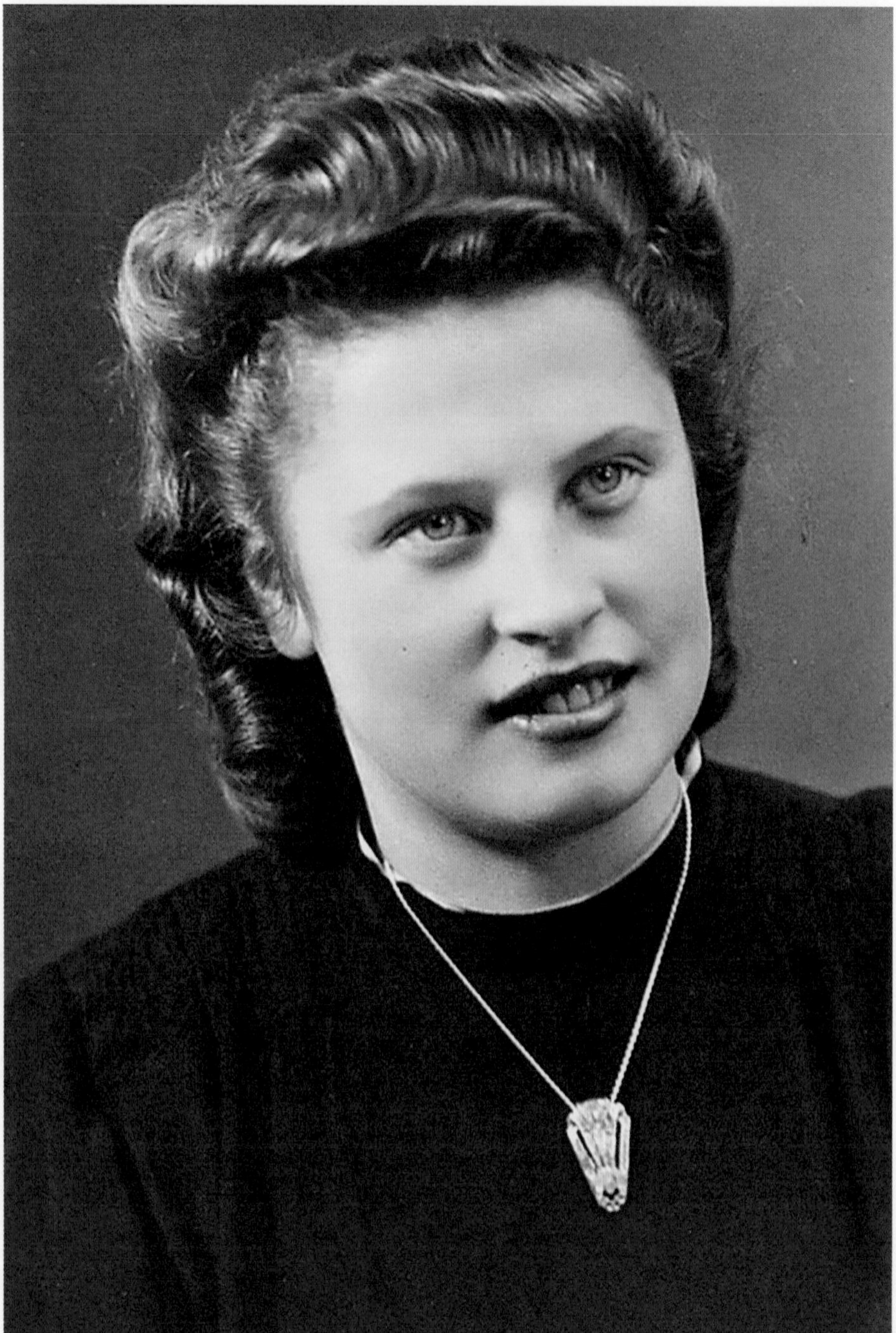

Mirdza Palmer as a teenager. *Summerset Scene Summer Edition, 2017*

shipping records as entering New Zealand in October 1948 on the SS *Derna*, which they boarded in Marseilles, France.[22]

Depending on the date of their arrival in New Zealand, the refugee families encountered different experiences in their new country. Some found relatively large refugee communities to attach themselves to, but others felt that their only option was to integrate into New Zealand culture as quickly as possible. For many, this meant changing their dress and mannerisms and attempting to lose their foreign accents. No matter how hard they tried, though, most refugees reported feeling some degree of cultural dislocation, isolation and racism. However, they would remind themselves that what they experienced in New Zealand was better than the alternative.

Susanna Williams and her family had arrived in New Zealand before the declaration of war, but as soon as the war started they were regarded with suspicion.[23] The family lived near the army base at Trentham, and Williams had to walk past the base on her way to school; often, the men would call out 'Dirty Huns' as she walked by.[24] Because of this hostility, the family created 'a little cocoon' for themselves.[25]

Heavy restrictions further isolated refugees. They were not allowed cameras or radios or to travel further than the town centre without first alerting the police.[26] Their status as enemy aliens denied medical refugees the ability to join the BMA, making it impossible for them to obtain malpractice insurance. This put many doctors out of work.

Many avoided socialising with other refugees in order to integrate into New Zealand society, but there were a few exceptions. Marion Boock recounted that even though her parents did not fully integrate into any specific refugee groups in Christchurch, where they settled, the Christchurch refugees would collect at announcement boards that reported who had survived the war and who had not.[27]

Even those who arrived well after the war had ended were viewed with suspicion, so most made a concerted effort to integrate into New Zealand society. When Miriam Frank arrived in New Zealand as a child in 1948, she lived with her aunt and cousins in Christchurch. As Jewish refugees seeking to escape the Nazi Wehrmacht, her family had moved between Spain, France and Mexico, constantly staying with different families who were willing to hide them.[28] In comparison to these places, Christchurch was an intense cultural shock. As with many refugees dealing with 'severe cultural dislocation', Frank's aunt, with whom they first lived, decided that the best way forward was to put the past completely behind them.[29] She insisted that the family adopt British mannerisms and clothing as quickly as possible, and that they speak only English at home.[30]

Sometimes, the switch was forced on refugees. When Hendrika Waal-Manning arrived in New Zealand at the age of 17, her family knew no English. She was sent to Wellington East Girls' College, where the headmistress believed that the best way for migrants to settle into life in New Zealand was to separate them all. Each migrant child was placed in a different classroom so that they were forced to meet New Zealanders and learn to speak English. Waal-Manning described her first three years in New Zealand as 'living in a mist . . . not really quite sure where I was or what I was doing'.[31] The 'mist' only started to clear in the fifth form, by which point she was able to sit and pass the school certificate examination.

Initially, those with medical qualifications from overseas needed to complete only a one-year training course to transfer their qualification.[32] But as the situation in Europe deteriorated, New Zealand turned into one of the most difficult places to retrain as a doctor. In 1938, an influx of medical refugees 'triggered a heated debate on a new three-year qualification'.[33] British historian Paul Weindling argued that the increase to a three-year course, two years more than any requirements in Britain, 'was effectively a bottleneck preventing professional activity in New Zealand for most or all of the war'.[34] The three-year course was approved, and started in 1939.

Hilda Fleischl, Rachel Monk, Catherine Newman and Olga Semon were in the first two intakes of the new course, and they faced varying degrees of racism and sexism along the way. The students entered into the fourth year of a standard medical programme and had to complete all four parts of the professional examinations. This could take a varying amount of time, depending largely on their knowledge of English.[35] Newman and Semon sat their final examinations in 1941, Fleischl in 1942 and Monk in 1943.

They could now practise, but their degrees were not conferred until 1947. This delay may have been on account of naturalisation, which had been halted for the duration of the war: Monk had become naturalised in May 1946, Newman in August

1946, and Fleischl and Semon in April 1947.[36] The only record of the women's experiences of this three-year course is from Hilda Fleischl, who was supported by her husband, Mario, while she studied: he worked 16 hours a day to keep the family running.[37]

Selma Ronigar-Hahn also retrained in New Zealand, though at a later date. She arrived in New Zealand late in 1949. Though this was after the war, presumably the 'special' course was still on offer for medical refugees, as she graduated in 1953. According to historian Ann Gluckman, Ronigar-Hahn had 'great difficulty in coping when she had to requalify in anaesthesia in Otago' because of the trauma of working as a doctor in the concentration camps.

> It was a struggle for survival. Any form of rejection or criticism, deliberate or implied, by staff or students revived memories of the fears, punishments and dangers associated with disapproval by the non-Jew in the camps. Her survival techniques made her unpopular with those students who lacked understanding. Once she was her own master, when she was no longer in what, to her, was still a hostile and threatening environment, she was much happier.[38]

The situation was slightly improved by the time the younger generation of refugees came to study at Otago. Hendrika Waal-Manning, Miriam Frank, Susanna Williams and Viola Palmer had attended school in New Zealand, and so were eligible for bursaries and scholarships that were not available to earlier refugees. Marion Boock did not receive a national scholarship from her school examinations, but she did receive one from the University of Otago directly after her first year of study. Marianne Fillenz attended Christchurch Girls' High School and achieved well in the national scholarship examinations, with a score of 1386; however, the newspaper reported that she was 'not eligible' — meaning she was disqualified. No reason was given for this.

Fillenz was not the only one to be disqualified. Marion Boock stated that she left school a year early because of the anti-Semitism she experienced there. She attended Rangi Ruru Girls' School in Christchurch, where she was told that even though she was top of her class she would not be made head prefect at the school because she was Jewish.[39]

Hendrika Waal-Manning entered the medical intermediate course at Victoria

University College, Wellington, in 1951. This year was intensive, but she decided to keep her head down and focus on her studies as much as possible.[40] She spent her six years at medical school with the same mindset. Despite many stressors, including the sudden death of her father, she graduated in 1957 aged 27.

Eighteen months after Mirdza Palmer moved to Wellington with her mother, she applied for the medical intermediate course at Victoria University College, where her international high school certificate was accepted. She gained entry on her second attempt and graduated in 1957.

Eva Seelye had a similar experience. When her family arrived in the late 1930s, she was enrolled in her local high school, even though she spoke no English: 'Her schooling was very much that of teach yourself, having been given a copy of Dickens and a German/English dictionary, and sat at the back of the class.' Eventually she completed her schooling through correspondence and matriculated at the age of 16. Seelye applied for and was accepted to study medicine at Otago Medical School, but her father, who had just completed the course, believed she was too young, so she first enrolled in a BA at Auckland University College, graduated from there in 1948, then went straight to Otago to do her medical studies, which she completed in 1953.[41]

It was relatively common for refugees to first complete an undergraduate degree before entering medical school. There were several reasons for this, including their age, as in the case of Eva Seelye. Ruth Black, in comparison, enrolled in medical intermediate but her marks were not high enough to win her a spot at medical school. She went on to do a BA at Auckland University College, then obtained a place in Dunedin in 1948. Black was in the same class as Liselotte Fillenz, who also took a bachelor's degree at Auckland University College before going to medical school in Dunedin. Black graduated MB ChB in 1952, but Fillenz only completed the first section of her third professional exam in 1953. Perhaps she had to repeat some years of her medical degree.[42]

While some struggled to acclimatise to studying in their new country, others thrived. Marianne Fillenz was a dedicated student who achieved many academic awards. She was top of her sixth form class at high school, and though she did not qualify for a university national scholarship, she was awarded a Mickle Scholarship directly by the University of Otago. She continued to do well and was selected to complete the one-year BMedSc. High-performing students were offered the opportunity to delay their medical studies by one year in order to focus on a

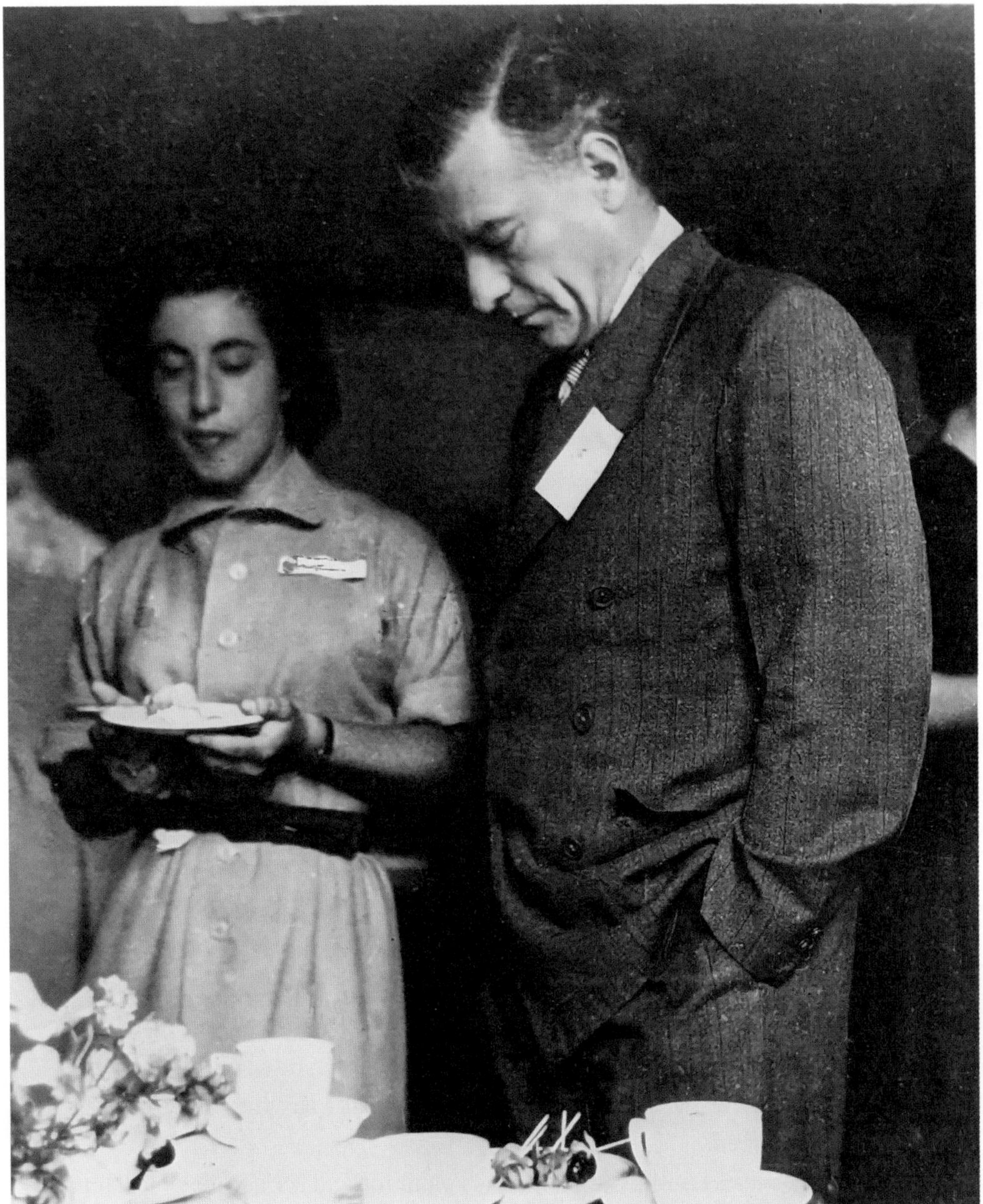

Miriam Frank with Bill Adams, professor of anatomy, at an event to welcome the women students in their first year at medical school, 1955. *Courtesy Miriam Frank*

research project, which was supervised by one of the professors at the medical school. She was encouraged to publish her research, and it was accepted by the *Journal of Neurophysiology*.[43]

Having completed their studies at Otago Medical School, the women medical graduates were faced with a decision: what to do next. The majority decided to stay in New Zealand and practise. Many felt, as Hendrika Waal-Manning did, that they had to: 'I had benefited from the education that New Zealand had given me, so it was up to me to repay to the best of my ability.'[44] She held fast to her father's request, barely speaking about her life before moving to New Zealand.

Mirdza Palmer also felt indebted to New Zealand. She told the EMWoNZ project in an interview, 'I'm so thankful to New Zealand and to the tertiary education sector for accepting me and for the education that I received. I do not feel that I would have achieved as much in any other country.' A part-time clinical assistant position in rheumatology was created for her at Otago Medical School while she raised her three sons.[45]

Viola Palmer married fellow student Phil Palmer after she completed her degree. The couple moved to England for postgraduate study, and Viola completed a Diploma in Anaesthetics at Kingston on Thames and the Royal Free Women's Hospital. When they settled in Tauranga she retrained as a GP.[46]

Eva Seelye returned to Auckland to take over her father Hans Hersch's practice after he died in 1954. This did not last long, however, as she did not enjoy the career path of general practice. Instead, she did postgraduate studies in anaesthetics, achieving three different fellowships with the Royal College of Anaesthetists in Britain, Australia and New Zealand between the years 1961 and 1992. She spent the rest of her career as a specialist anaesthetist at Greenlane Hospital in the surgical cardiology department.[47]

Ruth Black became an advocate for family planning and worked for almost four decades at the Family Planning Association (FPA) in Auckland. In 1995, she gave a presentation to the Auckland Medical Historical Society titled 'From Disreputable to Respectable — Family Planning'.

Hilda Fleischl worked as a GP in the Wellington region. Her patients were mainly women, and this naturally led her into family planning. She died suddenly at the age of 51 from a cerebral bleed. Her obituary read: 'New Zealand and its quiet democracy meant much to her, and she served her adopted country faithfully and well.'[48]

After her house surgeon years, Susanna Williams went to England for postgraduate study and found the environment much more welcoming for women. When she sat her Diploma in Child Health while six months pregnant, no one questioned her.[49] She later remarked, 'I don't think I would have dared to attempt an examination in New Zealand while pregnant.'[50] On her return to New Zealand, she stayed in the Wellington region: she ran a practice with her father in Upper Hutt for 15 years, then she obtained a position in gerontology at Silverstream Hospital, where she was later appointed superintendent.

Catherine Newman supported many young doctors and fellow refugees during her medical career. Shortly after she graduated, she went into practice with D. Cummack in Worcester Street, Christchurch; then in 1955 she joined the practice of another Otago graduate, Phyllis Brass (1953). She assisted younger doctors in setting up their practices, was on the committee of the NZMWA, and was a member of the FPA. She was a foundation member of the British Royal College of General Practitioners and of the Canterbury branch of the same college, which was formed in 1957. On 11 July 1960, Newman was murdered by a patient. Her obituary described her as 'a woman who stood high in wisdom and knowledge of her profession. The warmth of her nature and her joyous and unfailing generosity went out to one and all who came to her for advice and help.'[51]

Little is known about the career of Rachel Monk apart from the information her husband, Frank, submitted to the Holocaust Centre of New Zealand. After Rachel received her degree from Otago, the Monks moved to Pukemiro, a mining town northwest of Hamilton. She held clinics at Tūrangawaewae, where she met Princess Te Puea, who was struggling to get adequate medical care for her people. She and Te Puea established a close relationship that continued through to Monk's retirement. The regular clinics ended in 1946 when Monk moved to Auckland, but Māori patients from the Waikato continued to visit her there.[52]

Selma Ronigar-Hahn settled in Blockhouse Bay, Auckland, and opened a general practice there after completing her retraining course.

Not all of the medical graduates decided to remain in the country that had given them refuge. According to the Stolpersteine (Stumbling Stones) Project, which seeks to remember the victims of the Nazi regime through commemorative plaques and family histories, Olga Semon moved to Waitākere in West Auckland after she graduated and attempted to establish a practice there, but without much success.[53] In 1954, she moved back to Germany and opened a practice in Bremen, which also failed. In that same year, she was also listed in the New Zealand Medical Register as living in England. She opened another practice in Kent, which also failed because of her worsening mental health. She received treatment at the Eppendorf Psychiatric University Hospital in Germany, and later moved back to England.[54] She died at the age of 90 on 20 December 1993 in St Martin's Hospital, Canterbury.

After completing her two years of registration at Auckland Hospital, Miriam Frank left New Zealand for postgraduate study and did not return. In her 2010 autobiography she wrote: 'I was finally ready to leave New Zealand. I had been afforded refuge, given a nationality and trained in a profession in this country with its tradition of hospitality and a just social order. Yet I was riddled with uncertainties and incongruities. I needed to find out who I was.'[55] Apart from short trips back to New Zealand, such as for medical reunions, she has spent her life and career in England and Europe.[56]

After completing her registration, Marianne Fillenz enrolled in a DPhil in physiology at Somerville College at the University of Oxford.[57] She went on to have a highly successful career in research at the university and remained there until her death in 2012.

Neither of the Kral sisters remained in New Zealand, even though their father continued to practise in his adopted country. Marion Boock moved to Israel directly after she completed her house surgeon years. In her interview, she admitted: 'I'm very ashamed to say I went straight to Israel . . . New Zealand gave me a bursary that I studied on. I should have at least given that a year. But I felt that the only important thing was for the Jews to have a country. I was very zionistic. I therefore felt that I wanted to come here.' Boock completed a one-year internship in Israel and then decided to specialise in ophthalmology. She travelled to London and studied at the Moorfields and Royal Free hospitals, then returned to Israel. She maintained her New Zealand medical registration until the 1970s.[58] Dorothy Kral, on the other hand, moved to New South Wales, Australia, in 1964. She specialised in psychiatry, achieving membership to the Royal College in 1973. She eventually settled in Sydney. Unlike her sister, Boock maintained her New Zealand registration for her entire career.

Across the 1950s, New Zealand slowly liberalised its policy towards refugees. This resulted in a sizeable increase in refugees from Central and Eastern Europe, as well as, finally, Asia. Many of these refugees took medical studies at Otago Medical School. Rosalie Davida-Horvath (née Davida; 1959) arrived with her husband, Csaba Henry Horvath, and their two children, in the 1950s. The Horvaths were Hungarian doctors who had 'escaped through the "Iron Curtain" after the Hungarian revolt'.[59] They retrained together at Otago Medical School, graduating in 1959. Natalia Venetz (née Pachomov; 1954) and Tatyana Hillerby (née Godyaew; 1961) arrived with the 1950s wave of Russian immigrants to Australasia.

Despite the heavy restrictions on Chinese immigrants, more were granted access to New Zealand during the 1950s. Among them was Lucy Fong King Chung (née Chan; 1964), who arrived with her parents, Yip Chong Chung and Hop Yeen Chun, from Canton.

In spite of the strict and often contradictory nature of New Zealand's acceptance of refugees, these women and their families managed to find refuge in a country on the other side of the world and were given a chance to build new lives for themselves. Equally, the contributions made by these women have enriched their adopted countries, and their journeys provide valuable lessons in resilience, adaptation and the ongoing struggle for acceptance and integration.

HILDA BERDACH FLEISCHL (NÉE BARBER)

1942 graduate

Hilda Fleischl was born in Vienna, Austria, on 2 June 1910 to Rosalie Freund and Arnold Barber. She had one brother, Heinrich, born two years later. At the age of 15, Fleischl met a young man, Karl Berdach, at the Grinzinger Bad on the northeast coast of Italy. A teenage holiday romance resulted in an unplanned pregnancy. On the advice of the family paediatrician, they married and lived with Karl's parents. Their marriage did not survive, and they divorced in 1928.

Fleischl took her bachelor's degree in Vienna and entered straight into a medical degree. Her university years were overshadowed by the growing influence of Nazism and the increasing presence of anti-Semitism.[60] After the Nazi occupation of Austria on 13 March 1938, the local Sturmabteilung 'hoodlums' came to their home and confiscated valuables. Fleischl, who was three months away from graduating with her medical degree, was no longer able to pursue her studies because she was a Jew.

On 26 August 1938 she and her son, Peter, escaped by train to Italy, where they were soon joined by her long-term partner, Mario Fleischl. They left Italy after two weeks with a three-week visa to Switzerland. While there, Fleischl was accepted by the medical school in Lausanne and earned her MD in 1939.[61] After Peter's heroic lake rescue led to them obtaining a visa, the couple decided to marry to make entry into New Zealand easier.

They arrived in New Zealand in 1940, just as the rules for overseas doctors other than those from Britain changed. Hilda Fleischl was required to study for a further three years at Otago Medical School in order to transfer her registration. After she completed this course, the family moved to Wellington, where Fleischl worked at Wellington Hospital as a junior doctor. Peter Fleischl later recalled that from the time they settled in Wellington, his parents made a conscious decision to live as New Zealanders and stopped speaking German altogether.

Fleischl began working as a GP in 1943 at the age of 33. She and Mario became well known for their soirées, for which she would cook her famous goulash. They maintained a wide circle of friends among the European refugees. Her practice in downtown Wellington served mainly women, which may have led to her active participation in the FPA from 1950 to 1961. Mario set up practice as a psychoanalyst and later became a part-time lecturer in abnormal psychology at Victoria University.

Hilda Fleischl died suddenly from a cerebral bleed at her Karori home in 1961 at the age of 51. Her health had been a concern over the previous two years, but she was in active practice until the day before her death. She left a lasting legacy to her family, in particular her love of medicine and music. In 1949, the New Zealand composer and professor of music at Victoria University David Farquhar wrote 'Waltz for Hilda Fleischl'. One of her grandsons, Peter Jr, a retired doctor in Taupō,

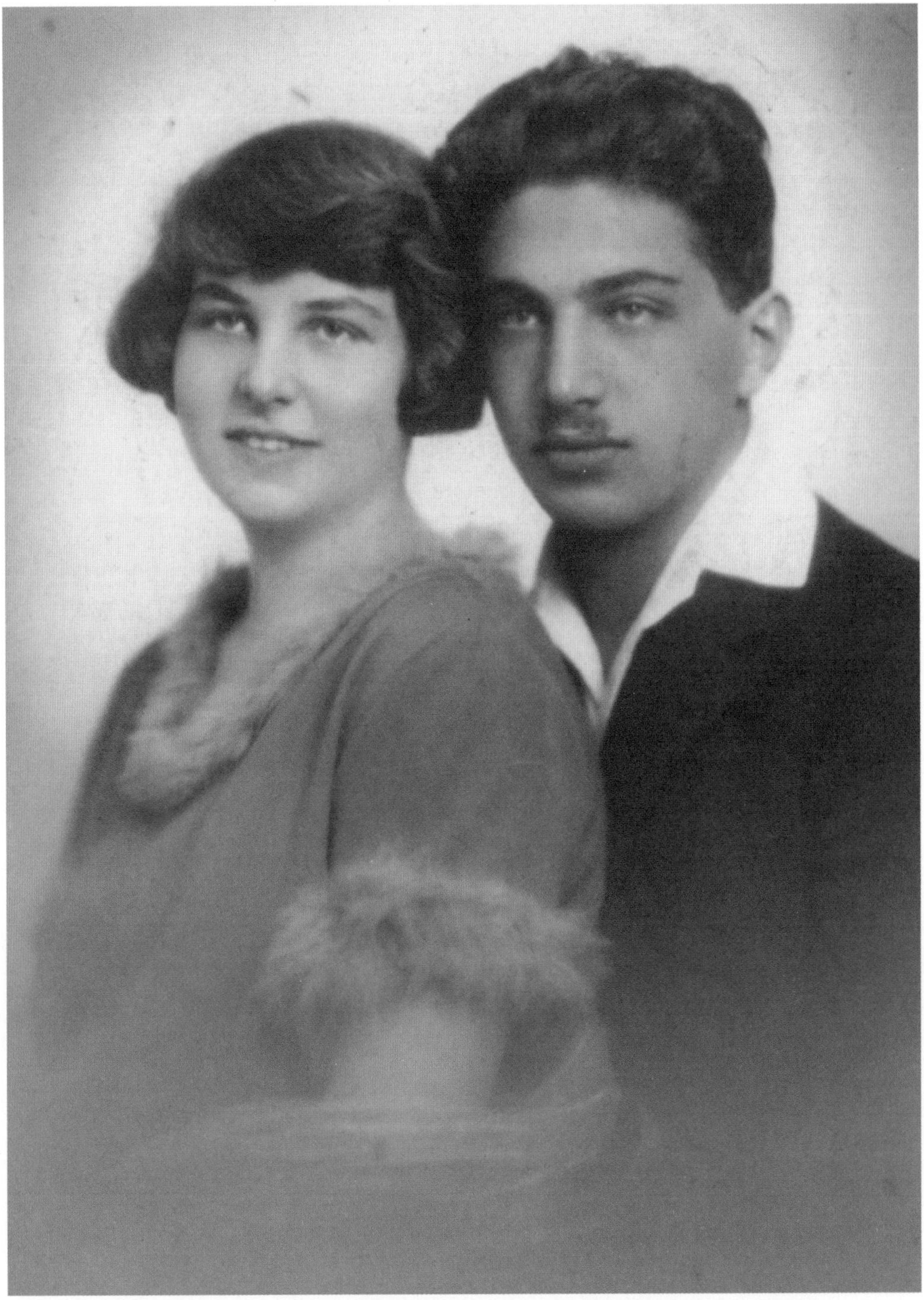

Hilda and Karl Berdach in 1926. *Courtesy the National Fund of the Republic of Austria for Victims of National Socialism, Fleischl family collection*

inherited his grandmother's musical ability and plays in different orchestras and chamber music groups around the country.

EDITH RUTH BLACK (NÉE BLUMENTHAL)

1952 graduate

Ruth Black left Czechoslovakia with her parents and grandparents as a young teenager and stayed in England for a short time before they emigrated to New Zealand. They settled in Auckland, and Black completed her secondary education at Epsom Girls' Grammar School. She became a naturalised New Zealand citizen in 1947. Black attended Auckland University College, from where she graduated with a BA in 1948 at the age of 23 (she had to resit the medical intermediate). After completing a BA she gained acceptance to Otago Medical School, and graduated in 1952.

Little is known about Ruth Black's time at Otago Medical School. However, she did recall the annual fifth-year lecture on contraception, where the medical students found it hard to find a seat because of 'interlopers from other faculties'. The lecture was 'hilarious, largely historical and mildly informative'.[62]

Black became one of New Zealand's pioneers in the FPA and worked in their clinic until the mid-1990s;[63] in her memoir she mentions that the FPA was 'helpful in that it provided part-time work for women doctors'. At that time there was opposition to the FPA from the New Zealand branch of the BMA. Black fostered the clinic's advisory role and promoted the contraceptive pill. She learned to be innovative, as family planning clinics had little funding. Together with Alice Bush, then president of the FPA, and a few others, she battled for funding. From 1963 to 1974, she was chair of the New Zealand FPA medical advisory committee.

She was a council member of the International Planned Parenthood Federation (IPPF) of South-East Asia and Oceania in 1964, and was the first New Zealand delegate at its regional council meeting. Black combined her FPA responsibilities with work at the University of Auckland student health service from 1959 to 1991, and at Carrington Hospital (a former psychiatric hospital) from 1976 to 1990.[64]

In 1973, Black was appointed to the board of the New Zealand Broadcasting

Corporation and later the board of TV2. During the first few fundraising 'telethons', the board and director-general asked her to suggest suitable recipients of the donations — these included St John Ambulance, NZ Child Health Research Foundation and the Mental Health Foundation. In 1986, Black was awarded the CBE for her public service, especially in the field of medicine.[65]

Black continued her early interest with Zionism. She was involved in the local Jewish community and one of her interests was Shalom Court, the rest home and hospital in St Johns, Auckland. She served on the Auckland committee of the United Israel Appeal for 10 years.

Jackie Edmond, chief executive of the FPA, wrote in Black's obituary: 'Ruth was a Family Planning doctor for many years and advocated for Family Planning doctors to be accepted by the New Zealand medical establishment in the 1960s. She helped make family planning available for hundreds (if not thousands) of New Zealand women.'

HENDRIKA JACOBA WAAL-MANNING (NÉE WAAL)

1957 graduate

Hendrika Waal-Manning was born in 1932 in Bandung, Java (now Indonesia).[66] The town was primarily filled with Dutch immigrants and Indonesians, who lived either in the village with the locals or in servants' quarters. She had an uncomplicated childhood until 1939, when the Japanese invaded Indonesia during the Second World War. During the war years, her family were made prisoners of war and lived in a prison cell for six years. This was when she decided she wanted to become a doctor. Every day they watched coffins being carried out of the hospital — a building adapted to house sick people from the camp — to be buried outside of the town. 'It was a very naive thinking . . . It was just a constant procession of coffins. And a naive thinking that, "Oh, doctors can do something about that."'

Her mother was a teacher and gave Waal-Manning and her sister daily lessons. They had limited supplies but they made it work: 'We rubbed out what we did during the day and then started again the next day . . . We had to rub out what we had done in order to maintain the supply.'

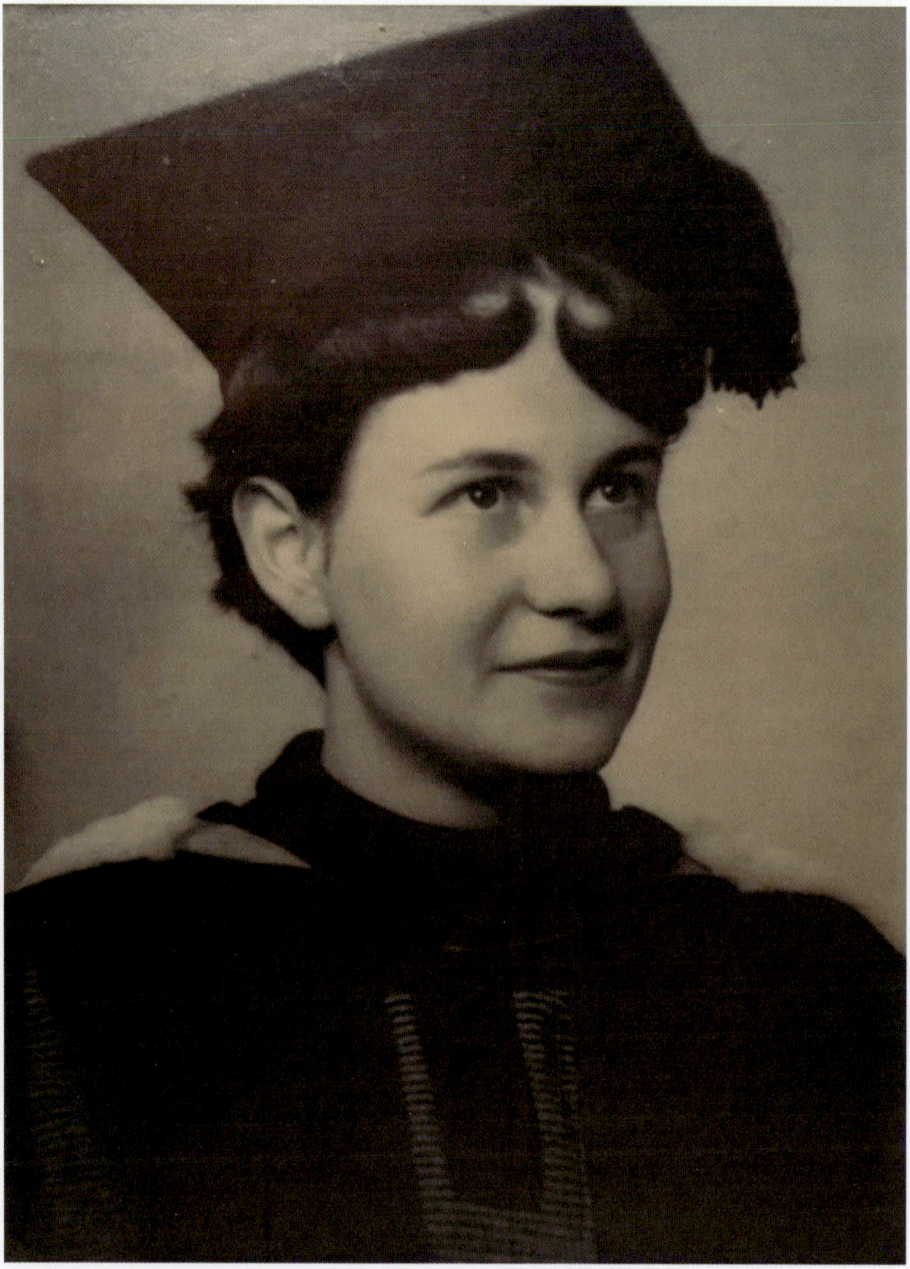

Hendrika Waal-Manning on her graduation day in 1957. *Courtesy Hendrika Waal-Manning*

In 1946, at the conclusion of the war, the Waal family was released from prison, but they were not yet out of danger. Over the five years of their occupation in Indonesia, the Japanese had encouraged the Indonesians to rebel against their colonial governors, the Dutch. At the end of the war, the Indonesians declared independence and ended up fighting against the Dutch. Not long after the family had been released, a group of nationalists came and murdered several Dutch people in Bandung. 'My parents decided that we couldn't stay. And we were offered New Zealand, Australia or Canada. The first ship was departing to New Zealand, so that's where we went.'

When the Waal family landed in New Zealand late in 1946, they were directed to the Miramar Transit Camp in Wellington for a medical examination. It was a big adjustment period for all. Her mother had to learn housekeeping skills, now that they had no housekeeper, and none of them could speak English. Waal-Manning attended Wellington East Girls' College, and as her English improved, she got good enough grades to be accepted to the medical intermediate course at Victora University College. She took one year to complete the course and was then offered a place at Otago Medical School.

Waal-Manning travelled to Dunedin at the start of 1952, but had been there only five days when the matron of St Margaret's College came to tell her that her father had died suddenly. She immediately went to Wellington to support her mother and sister, then returned to Dunedin shortly after and resumed her studies. She continued to struggle with English but found that she learned more readily from books than from her lecturers — perhaps because, in books, she could read and reread passages. She graduated in 1957 having never failed a class.

After graduation, Waal-Manning was offered a house surgeon position in general medicine at Dunedin Hospital. She was a member of the Christian Missionary Society (CMS) and, in 1958, she went on a CMS weekend camp to Quarantine Island (Kamau Taurua) in the Otago Harbour, where she met Jolyon Manning, an accountant. The couple married in 1958 at Old St Paul's in Wellington, near where she had first lived after arriving in New Zealand.

Waal-Manning became a medical research officer in the medical school's hypertension clinic which was run by Horace Smirk. She dedicated her career to this clinic and published over 50 papers, including in the *Lancet* and *Circulation*, largely focused on beta-blockers and various treatments for hypertension. In 1973 she also published an article in the *New Zealand Medical Journal* titled 'Women in Medicine in New Zealand', which she co-authored with two of her Otago colleagues, Ngaire Walsh (née McKerrow; 1956) and Barbara Heslop (1948). She gained an MD by thesis in 1972: she was by then working full-time as well as bringing up three children, and only found time to work on her thesis 'in the smaller hours of the morning'.

Waal-Manning worked through all her three pregnancies and because there was no such thing as maternity leave she used her annual leave to have a few weeks off around the birth of each baby, bringing them to work with her in a carrycot when they were 10 days old. She never had any doubts about her choice to carry on working. After later retraining in general practice, in 2004 she retired to Alexandra, where she and Jolyon developed a reserve in the hills above the town which was named Jolendale Park. Now run by a trust, it is open to the public and protected from development by a QEII covenant.

Hendrika Waal-Manning died in June 2022; at the time of her death, she was taking an online course in epigenetics. The interview she gave to the EMWoNZ project was the first and only interview in which she discussed her childhood.[67]

VIOLA CORNELIA PALMER (NÉE HEINE)

1959 graduate

Viola Palmer was born in 1936 in Hamburg, Germany.[68] In 1939 her parents, who were political dissidents, made the decision to leave Germany. They were 'persecuted and uncomfortable so they decided to migrate. They were fortunate enough to be allowed to come to New Zealand, being accepted here as immigrants.' The family arrived in New Zealand early in 1940; however, her father was only in the country for a short while before he returned to Germany to look after his parents. He stayed there for the duration of the war.

Palmer's mother had been a housewife in Germany, but in New Zealand she had to join the workforce, so she found a job as a housekeeper. She had no money to support her four children, so the three older ones were sent to board with different foster families around New Zealand; Palmer, who was only three, stayed with her mother. Later in life, Palmer discussed this time with her mother, who described the experience of leaving her children behind as horrible.

In those early years, her mother was regarded as a spy and was constantly being interviewed by the police: 'Every time she shifted, she had to let them know where she was and that was ongoing and she didn't get put on Somes Island, but only narrowly averted that.'[69] Palmer believes her mother only avoided incarceration on the island in Wellington Harbour because she had four young children. Palmer's father returned to New Zealand in 1947, where he got a job doing scientific research in the laboratory at the Crown Lynn pottery in Auckland.

Palmer attended Avondale College in the second year of the college's academic stream. Her first choice for her university studies was veterinary science but that subject was only available in Australia and her family could not afford for her to go there. Her second option was social work, but students had to be 21 years old to enrol in the programme. So she enrolled in her third choice: medicine.

Palmer studied for her medical intermediate year in Dunedin rather than staying in Auckland. She has fond memories of Agnes Blackie, who taught physics in the intermediate year and who helped the women with physics because many of them were struggling, as most New Zealand girls' schools did not offer the subject at the time.

+++

Palmer had a bursary, but even so finances were tight. She worked every holiday break as a childminder, waitress or hotel maid, or as a nurse in one of the psychiatric institutions, and one summer she worked at Paul's Book Arcade on High Street, Auckland. Outside of her studies, she was a member of the university tramping club, where she met her future husband, Phil Palmer, who was a year behind her at medical school. On an expedition in Arthur's Pass, they were partnered up and roped together for support: 'We fell down a mountain together and managed to survive.'

They were married in Christchurch at the end of Palmer's fifth year. After she graduated along with nine other women in 1959, she and Phil were fortunate to gain house surgeon positions at Kew Hospital in Invercargill together: 'The part I remember best was the emergency room, where one was called upon to do all sorts of things which were totally strange and out of our range of knowledge.' Palmer said she felt that medical school had not adequately prepared her to be a junior doctor.

She worked at Kew for a year before becoming pregnant with her first child, Anne. Two years later, the Palmers moved to England for Phil to pursue further study in pathology. Since she had become interested in anaesthesia at Kew Hospital, where the registrar had begun training some of the house surgeons, Viola Palmer also decided to do some further study and enrolled in the one-year Diploma in Anaesthetics.

After she became pregnant with their second child, Roger, the Palmers returned to New Zealand and settled in Auckland, where Phil took up a microbiology position at Auckland Hospital. Viola worked part-time at Auckland Hospital as an anaesthetist, working only a few sessions each week so that she could be home to look after the family. The family remained in Auckland for only a short while, as Phil was offered a position in Christchurch. Two years later they moved to Tauranga, where Phil became a partner in a private laboratory. During their time in Auckland, Christchurch and Tauranga, they had four more children — Harry, Joyce, Sue and Mark.

In Tauranga, Viola Palmer retrained and worked as a part-time GP for 10 years. 'After having done anaesthesia, I really wanted to be working with people who are awake,' she said. She retired to Waikanae at the age of 70 but found retirement too quiet after a long career in medicine, so continued working for two local clinics.

MIRIAM FRANK

1960 graduate

Miriam Frank was born in a small village near Barcelona, Spain, in March 1936, only four months before the Spanish Civil War broke out. Her mother and father were not married but maintained a close relationship during her early years. In 1941, Frank and her mother, Käte Lichtenstein, spent a year in Marseilles as refugees. Eventually they were able to board a boat full of refugees that took them to Mexico via North Africa. In Mexico City, Frank attended the Spanish Colegio Madrid.

In 1944 Frank's father, Lou, came to live with them — the first time they had all lived together as a family. The arrangement did not last long, and when they separated, Käte decided to move closer to her family. Her sister Lotte had

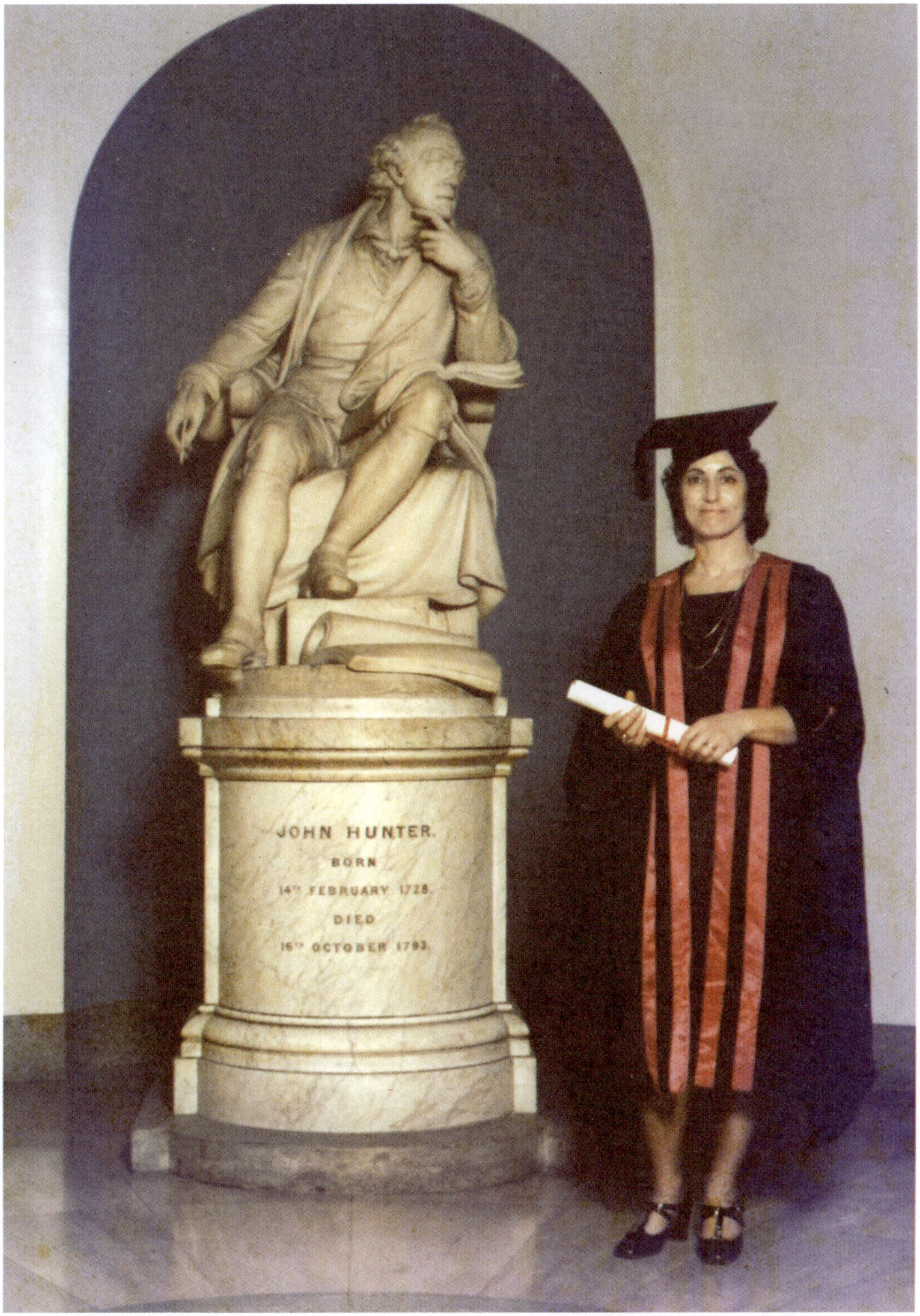

Miriam Frank after being admitted as a Fellow of the Royal College of Anaesthetists in London, 1975. *Courtesy Miriam Frank*

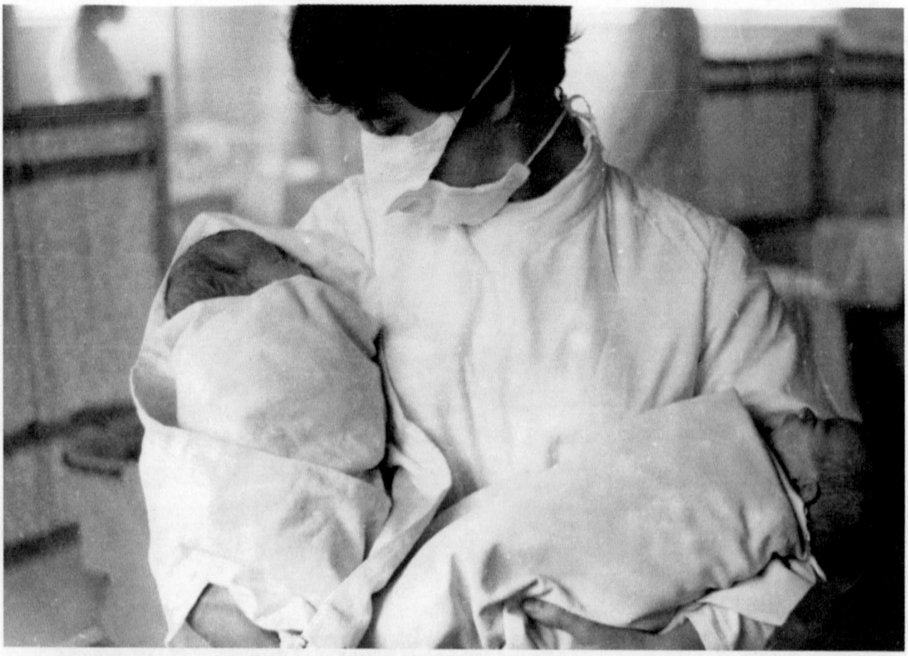

Miriam Frank at Queen Mary maternity hospital in Dunedin when she was a fourth-year medical student, 1957. The babies are her first two deliveries. *Courtesy Miriam Frank*

immigrated to New Zealand and 'encouraged her with letters full of glowing praise for her adopted country and its education and health systems'.[70] In 1948, Käte and Miriam landed in Auckland on the US Navy ship *Marine Phoenix*, then made their way down to Christchurch, where they arrived in 1948.

Miriam Frank entered medical school in 1955 along with 12 other women, including Viola Palmer, Rosalie Sneyd (née McPherson; 1959) and Norma Restieaux (1960). For the first year and a half in Dunedin she lived at St Margaret's College; later she moved to a bedsit just down the street, where she had independence and the freedom to set her own schedule. She remembers that the women generally sat in the front row of the lecture theatres, not because it was a requirement, but because the women tended to keep together. 'I do remember the Professor of Obstetrics and Gynaecology always starting his lectures with "Well, chaps", looking across and above the first row where we the women were sitting and addressing himself straight at all the men sitting behind us. It was a way of saying, "What are all you women doing here? I shall opt to ignore you."'[71]

Frank remembers her clinical experience well. In their third year, the students would cross 'the road in our short white coats and our stethoscopes dangling prominently from our necks to take part in ward rounds, learn to take histories and examine patients, and watch operations'.[72] Alongside this, they were taught some nursing skills, such as bed-making, intramuscular injections and catheterising.

In the fourth year, the requirement of delivering 20 babies was added. Frank remembers thinking the Plunket system was beneficial in that it had reduced infant mortality, but bad in that it ignored the value of bonding between mother and baby. In the fifth year, they studied public health and medical jurisprudence. Their sixth year was spent in a hospital in any of the four main New Zealand cities: Auckland, Wellington, Christchurch or Dunedin. Frank spent her house surgeon years in Auckland, where she worked between three hospitals in the Auckland Hospital group — Middlemore, Greenlane and Auckland. Frank completed her two years of registration and then decided it was time to leave New Zealand.

+ + +

By the end of 1962 she was in Israel, where she wanted to connect with her Jewish heritage. She accepted a year-long position as an anaesthetist at Hadassah University Medical Centre in Jerusalem. In 1964 she finally made her way to London, but her plan for postgraduate study was sidetracked when she met the eccentric German artist Rudolf Kortokraks (Kraks), who had trained under Oskar Kokoschka. They married in Salzburg in 1965.

After the wedding, the couple moved to wherever Kraks was commissioned to paint, getting by on very little. Eventually Frank's funds ran out and the couple decided to return to London. At first, she did a few locums around London, then she joined an Islington–Highgate medical practice as a full-time junior partner. After her first child, Rebekah, was born in 1966, Frank transitioned to part-time work.

This time in her life was very difficult. Kraks was suffering from frequent emotional episodes and an alcohol addiction, and so was often unable to care for Rebekah; instead, Frank would bring her daughter to the surgery, where the receptionist would look after her. At one point, Frank became so ill from overworking that she was confined to bed. She returned to work before she had properly recovered and was eventually diagnosed with chronic fatigue syndrome (ME/CFS; at that point just called myalgic encephalomyelitis).

After three years at the Islington–Highgate practice, Frank resigned to take up a part-time position in anaesthesia at Royal Northern Hospital. After this, she obtained a position as an anaesthetist at the prestigious Great Ormond Street Hospital for Sick Children for her senior registrar rotation — 'the last step before qualifying for a consultant post'.[73] In this placement, she covered the emergency department and the cardiac and respiratory intensive care wards.

Near the end of her rotation at Great Ormond Street, Frank was awarded the position of senior lecturer in anaesthesia at London Hospital Medical College. For this part of her career, she worked at Royal London and Newham hospitals in London's East End. She played a vital role in developing anaesthesia for epidurals and caesareans — specifically so that mothers could be awake, and husbands could remain in the room for the birth, which meant the mother and baby could instantly be with each other after the birth.

Throughout her studies and career, Frank did not feel that she was discriminated against; instead, she 'felt recognised and appreciated for what I offered. I was twice presented with prizes for what was described as my dedication above what was expected from my position, and I also received a Merit Award for Clinical Excellence. My being a woman never interfered with my work, and both male and female doctors doing their postgraduate training remarked on finding my teaching helpful.'[74]

Frank retired in 1993 and has spent the years since living between her homes in Duncan Terrace, Wellington, and in London, Greece and Italy. She has written two autobiographies and translated many books from Spanish into English. She is currently writing a third autobiography. Her advice to women seeking a career in medicine is to 'Go ahead! With enthusiasm and without fear . . . Your achievement will be your reward.'[75]

MIRDZA PALMER (NÉE ROBINS)

1961 graduate

Mirdza Palmer (née Robins) was born on 21 January 1930 in Ligatne, Latvia.[76] Her parents' farm was situated 60 kilometres from the capital city, Riga, in rolling hill country with a large forested area. In 1940, when Mirdza was 10 years old, the Russian army invaded Latvia from the east. The farm was confiscated, and communal farming was to be established; but in the interim, the family was able to continue living and working there. In 1941, the German invasion drove the Russians out of Latvia. As the war progressed, food and other goods became scarce and were rationed. Towards the end of 1944, as the progress of the war shifted and the German army was retreating westward out of Russia, the front line was just 40 kilometres from the farm, so the family decided to escape. From Latvia they caught a boat to Lubeck, in Germany, and then moved to a family friend's home in Austria, where they waited out the war. From there, the family was transferred to a displaced persons camp, where they obtained permits to leave Europe.

Palmer and her mother arrived in New Zealand when they were 21 and 49 years old. They had one US dollar between them, each had a suitcase and, importantly, Palmer had in her pocket the high school certificate she had gained by studying in a displaced persons camp in Germany.

The main stipulation of their visa was that they both had to work for two years before they had the freedom to move wherever they desired. They were placed in the kitchen of a local hospital in Pahiatua. When the two years were up, they moved to Wellington, where Palmer worked for the Wellington Gas Company as a junior office clerk, and her mother worked as a cook at Ewart Hospital. Eighteen months later Palmer started at Victoria University College, hoping to study medicine.

In 1946 Palmer's father died after three months in the displacement camp hospital. Palmer remembers his final message to her: 'We have lost our country, our home and farm, but remember whatever knowledge you acquire in your head you will never lose.' Palmer always remembered that and applied herself to her school work.

She had two attempts at the medical intermediate in Wellington before being successful, and she entered Otago Medical School in 1957, one of six women students. Her mother took a job as first cook at Wakari Hospital so they could make the move to Dunedin together. At first Palmer had difficulty understanding scientific terminology in English, and although she did not fail her first year, her grades were not high enough to earn her a place at the medical school. She continued to experience language difficulties, but over time her grades improved. In her final pathology exam, her professor advised her to explain her circumstances to the external examiner, particularly where she had come from and why her

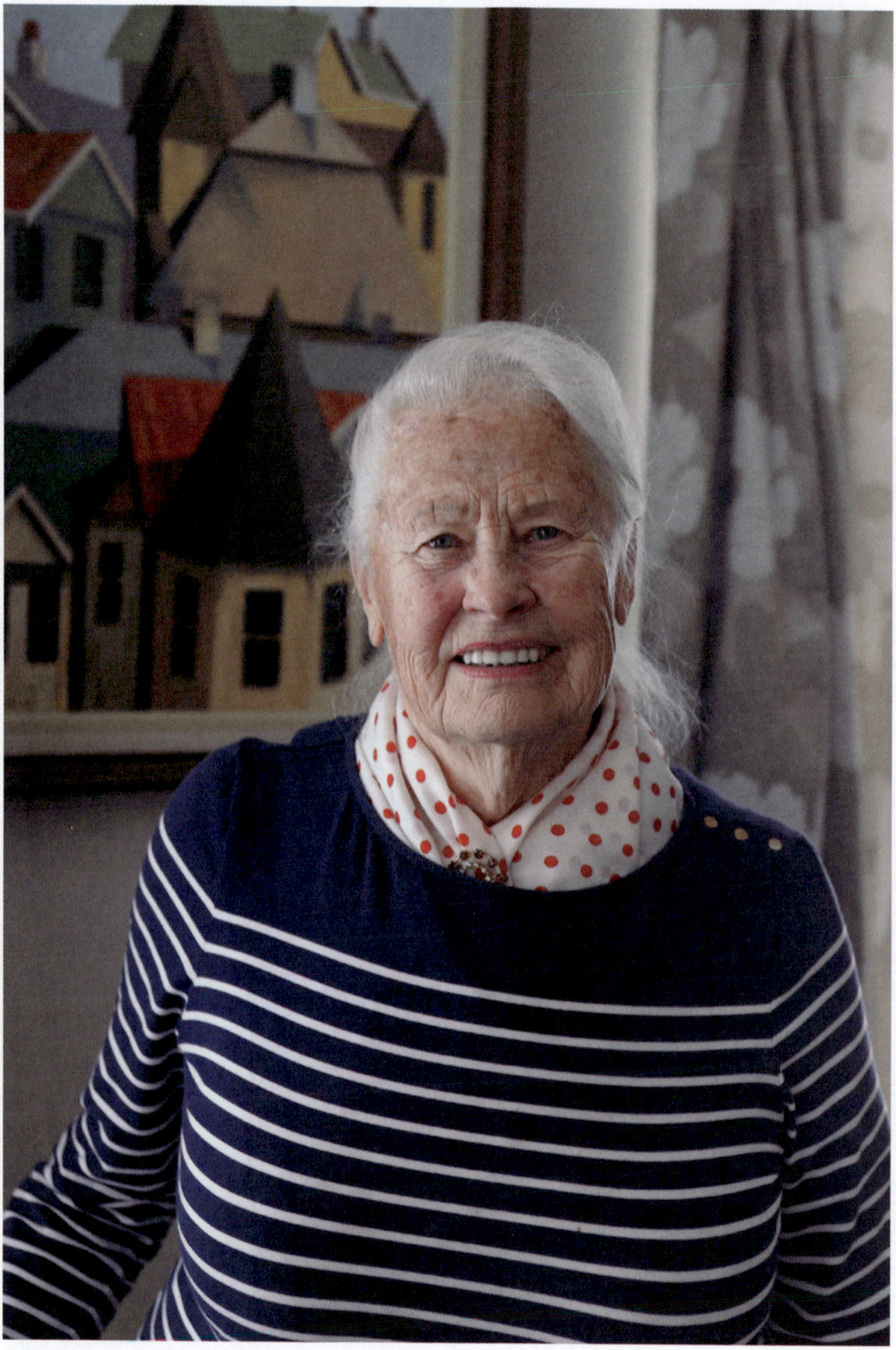

Mirdza Palmer in 2017. *Summerset Scene Summer Edition*

handwriting was so bad. To the second question, she replied that she had spent six years in the barracks in a displaced persons camp, doing her homework in the top bunk where she could not sit up.

Palmer graduated in 1961, 10 years after she had arrived in New Zealand. She felt that she had achieved her father's wish, but she also acknowledged that without her mother's help she would not have succeeded to this point. After graduation, Palmer progressed through the usual steps of junior house surgeon, then senior house surgeon, junior and then senior registrar at Dunedin Hospital: patients told her that she was the first female doctor they had ever had. She was awarded a grant to visit hospitals in America, including the Mayo Clinic, as well as hospitals in Berkeley, Sacramento, Seattle, New York and Washington DC.

By now she had met David Palmer, a rheumatologist at Dunedin Hospital and later professor in medicine. They married a few months after she returned to New Zealand and went on to have three sons. While she was raising the family, Palmer worked part-time in the audiovisual department for student teaching at the medical school, and in a part-time position as clinical assistant in rheumatology that was created for her and involved outpatient clinics and student teaching. She retired in 1990.

The third-year Otago Medical School class of 1959. The women students (front row, from left), are: Cecily Anne Cowie (née McNulty; 1962), Maureen Joan Peskett (née Lester; 1962), M. L. Harvey (did not graduate), Dorothy Jean Kral (1962), Ngaire Jean Jeffreys (née Twose; 1963), Jocelyn MacKnight (1963), Helen Robyn Hewland (1962), Mary Victoria Miller (née Cameron; 1962). Second row, from left: Meon Carolyn Shand (1962), Dorothy Haydn Cameron (née Bell; 1962). *Otago Medical School Archives*

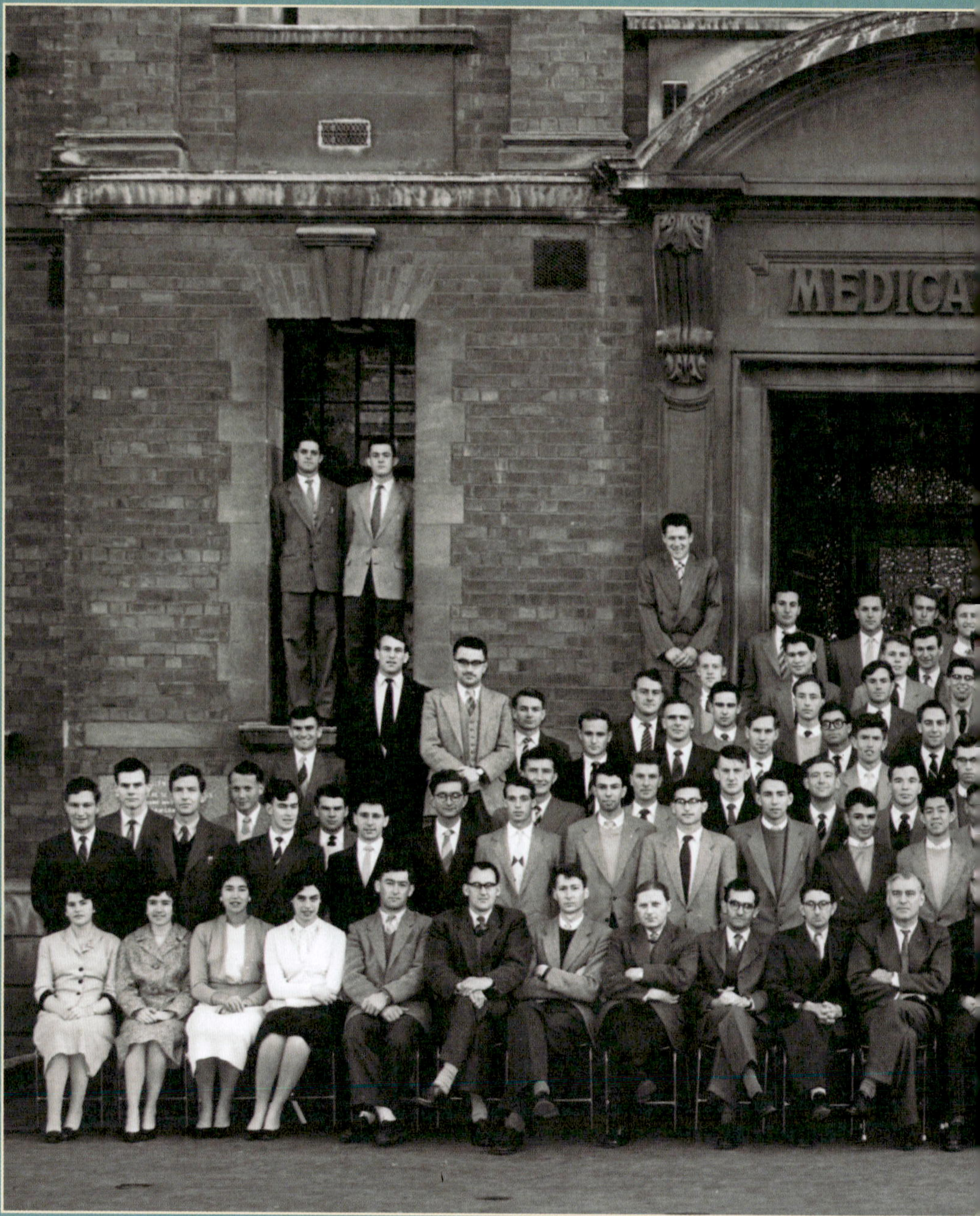

6. Agents of change 1948–1967

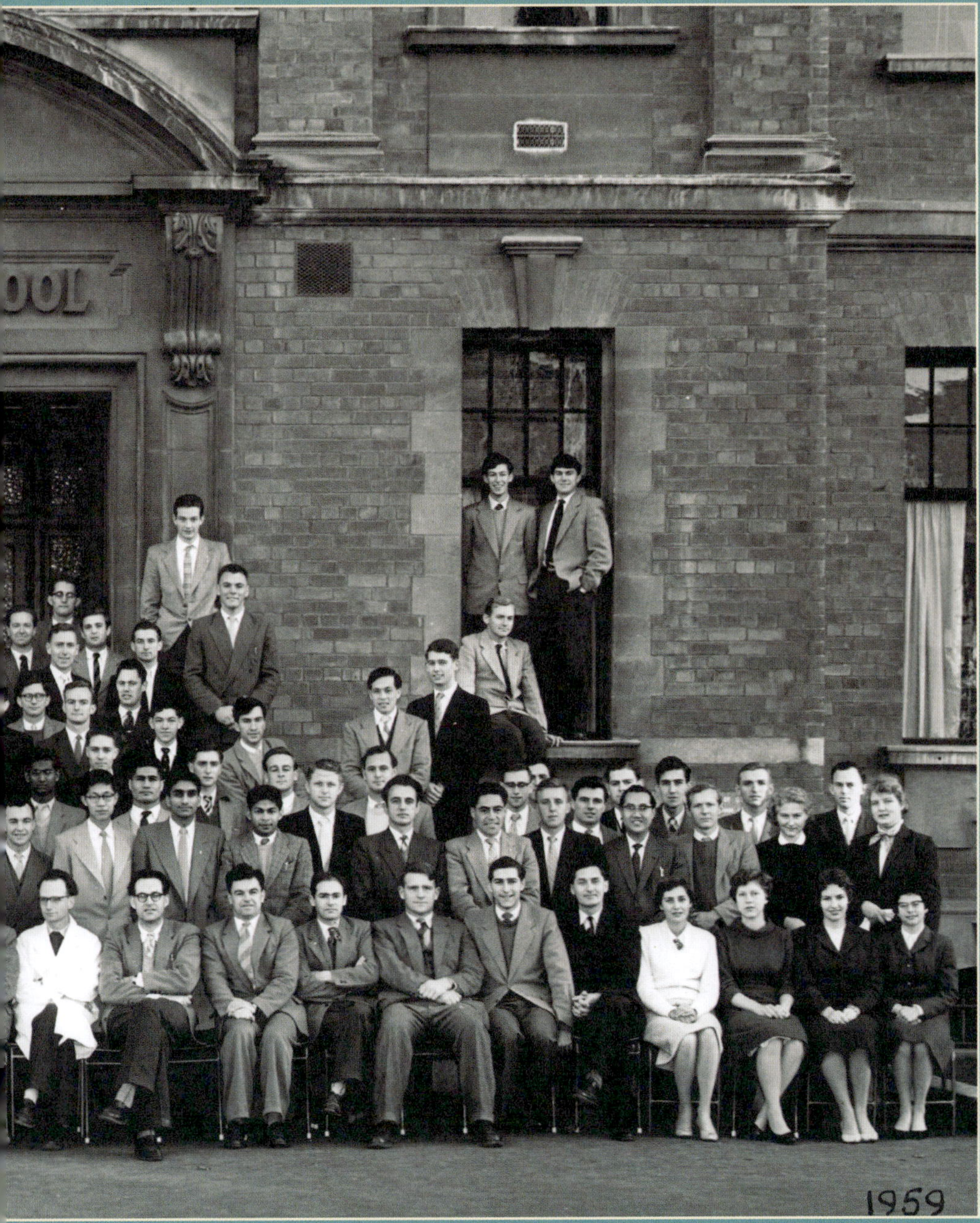

There were marked improvements for the lives of women after the end of the Second World War: the baby boom brought a renewed focus on the health of women and children; with the sexual revolution came a recognition of the need for better sex education; and the rise of second-wave feminism spurred a reconsideration of women's place in society and challenged patriarchal practices in the professions. Sexual health courses were more readily available, as was oral contraception or 'the pill', which gave women greater control over their own bodies.

Within six years of its introduction in New Zealand in 1961, 20 per cent of women of reproductive age were taking the pill — 12 per cent more than in the United States and 17 per cent more than in Britain — and by 1975, 35 per cent of women were using oral contraceptives. The introduction of the pill was ground-breaking for women, whether in the workforce or not, single or married. Families could manage the number of children they had, and this, in turn, improved their financial situations, with fewer mouths to feed. Women could plan their careers, earn more and demand better equality in the workplace.[1]

The women doctors who graduated from Otago Medical School from the 1940s to the 1960s were increasingly advocating for better conditions for society's disadvantaged. There were important changes to outdated antenatal and postnatal care practices as well as to the care of children and the aged, and for those who had experienced sexual abuse and mental health crises. These changes were occurring not only nationally but also on an international level, as women sought to bring adequate medical training and care to isolated or disadvantaged communities.

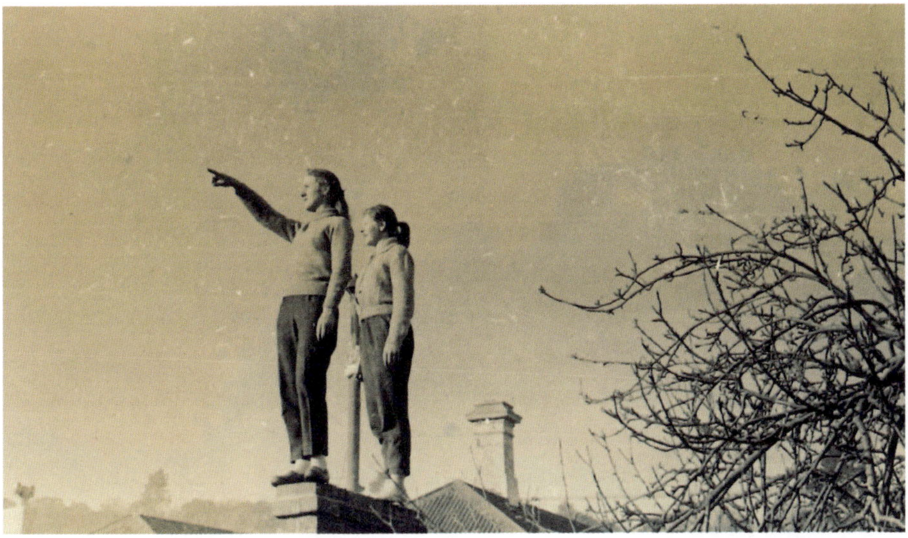

Heather Leslie (née Macallan; 1960) and Judith Barfoot (née Radcliffe; 1960) standing on the roof of their Castle Street flat, Dunedin, 1958. *Courtesy Judith Barfoot*

Graduates during this period typically worked long hours on unsociable rosters, and in lengthy training programmes — conditions that were unsustainable. In many instances, those with children struggled to balance their work with the needs of a young family. Joan Shirley Chapple (1957) worked in Australia, Britain, Russia, India and the United States as a specialist in hand surgery, then, in 1961, she was appointed to a full-time post in the plastic surgery unit at Middlemore Hospital, working under William Manchester. She was the only woman surgeon on staff, and she never felt welcome in the Auckland surgical fraternity. It was understood that she would not attend regular meetings at the men-only Northern Club. In 1972, she gave birth to a daughter, Raven. She requested just five months' maternity leave, but this was denied and her job was terminated. Her family believed this was because she was unmarried, rather than due to her competence in her job — reflecting the continued misogyny embedded in the medical system. At that time it resulted in considerable controversy in the medical and wider community.

Margaret Clare Gibberd (née Sidey; 1954) was met with a similar response when she announced she was pregnant while working in a chest clinic in London. According to Gibberd, the reason she was dismissed by the head of her clinic was simply: '"You would embarrass the patients." That was the attitude in those days, that people would have been embarrassed by being looked after by a pregnant woman. Pregnancy was not flaunted in any way.'[2] She returned to work in 1963 at a radioisotope laboratory set up by Lewisham Hospital.

In England in 1967, Ailsa Morrison-Galt (née Smith; 1960) qualified as a radiology registrar while she was pregnant, and felt she was unemployable. When she did get a job, she took her two-month-old son with her and was breastfeeding while she worked, with limited success; she later said that, in retrospect, she would have approached it differently.[3]

Wendy Hadden (née Fitzwilliam; 1968) also chose to specialise in radiology, largely because it did not involve night shifts and the hours were better than surgery or intensive care — specialties her supervisor had suggested she investigate. Hadden pushed hard for the Royal Australian and New Zealand College of Radiologists to allow her to train part-time so she could more easily balance her work and childcare responsibilities. After six months, the college allowed her to work seven-tenths in a training position that spanned all Auckland hospitals.

One of the reasons Miriam Frank switched from general practice to anaesthetics was because it enabled her to work part-time while raising children. Her supervisor granted her one day of leave a week on full pay to attend a three- to four-month course that worked towards the Fellowship of the Royal College of Anaesthetists. These women later went on to spearhead clinical developments in their respective specialties.

As noted in the preface, when Meredyth Gunn discovered she was pregnant just before returning for her fourth year she delayed telling her parents until she returned to Dunedin in March 1947. Within a week of arriving back, she had married fellow student Bryce Gunn and they told both sets of parents. Gunn feared telling her parents, but she knew she had to continue the course as her mother was a school teacher and very much wanted her daughter to graduate as a doctor. This was also at a time when women students who married (with or without children) were generally expected to leave the course; by this point this pressure came not so much from their teachers, but more from their families and other students.

Six weeks after Gunn gave birth, her mother-in-law took the baby back to Wellington so that Gunn could sit her exams. The baby stayed in Wellington while she went back to Dunedin to do her fifth year. In her sixth year Gunn was at Wellington Hospital but failed her exams and had to repeat the year. She passed the following year, while pregnant, and finally graduated in 1952. While Gunn would never have considered herself an agent of change, she was one of just a few women to continue their training after having children. She was very grateful to her extended family for their support.

For women who were not given the option to work or study part-time, the solution was often to hire a nanny — or to delay their studies. Diana Mason's nanny came from Monday to Friday so she could study towards her membership to the Royal College of Physicians and Surgeons.[4] Joan Walton (1945) hired a nanny while she was studying towards the Royal College of Physicians examinations, even though money was tight and rationing was still present in London.[5] Helen Bichan (née Simpson; 1958), on the other hand, had her five children while continuing to work part-time as a medical officer at Porirua Hospital; it was only later that she decided to pursue postgraduate training in psychiatry and work towards her Fellowship of the Royal Australian and New Zealand College of Psychiatrists.[6] Katharine Bowden (née Thomson; 1954) also followed this route: she trained for the Royal New Zealand College of General Practitioners after a specialty change, more than 20 years after she had completed her original degree; by this point, her six children were old enough not to need full-time care.[7]

From the 1940s to the 1970s, medical women in New Zealand were also campaigning for better sex education, better access to contraception and abortion, and better care for people who reported sexual assault. They also set up and ran clinics and community courses in family planning. Alice Bush, for example, gave lectures on topics such as 'Men and Women's Relationships in Wartime', which included detailed discussions on the physiology of the sex organs, sexual intercourse and the prevention and treatment of sexually transmitted diseases.[8] Early in her career, Margaret Sparrow (née Muir; 1963) worked alongside education officer Grace Taylor to develop a comprehensive sex education course in New Plymouth: the venue was so overcrowded that it risked breaching fire regulations. Not long after, Sparrow began work on a venereal disease education programme for the Department of Health.[9]

Along with discussions on sex education came those surrounding abortion. Many of the women medical graduates who entered general practice found that women came to them with questions about family planning, menopause and

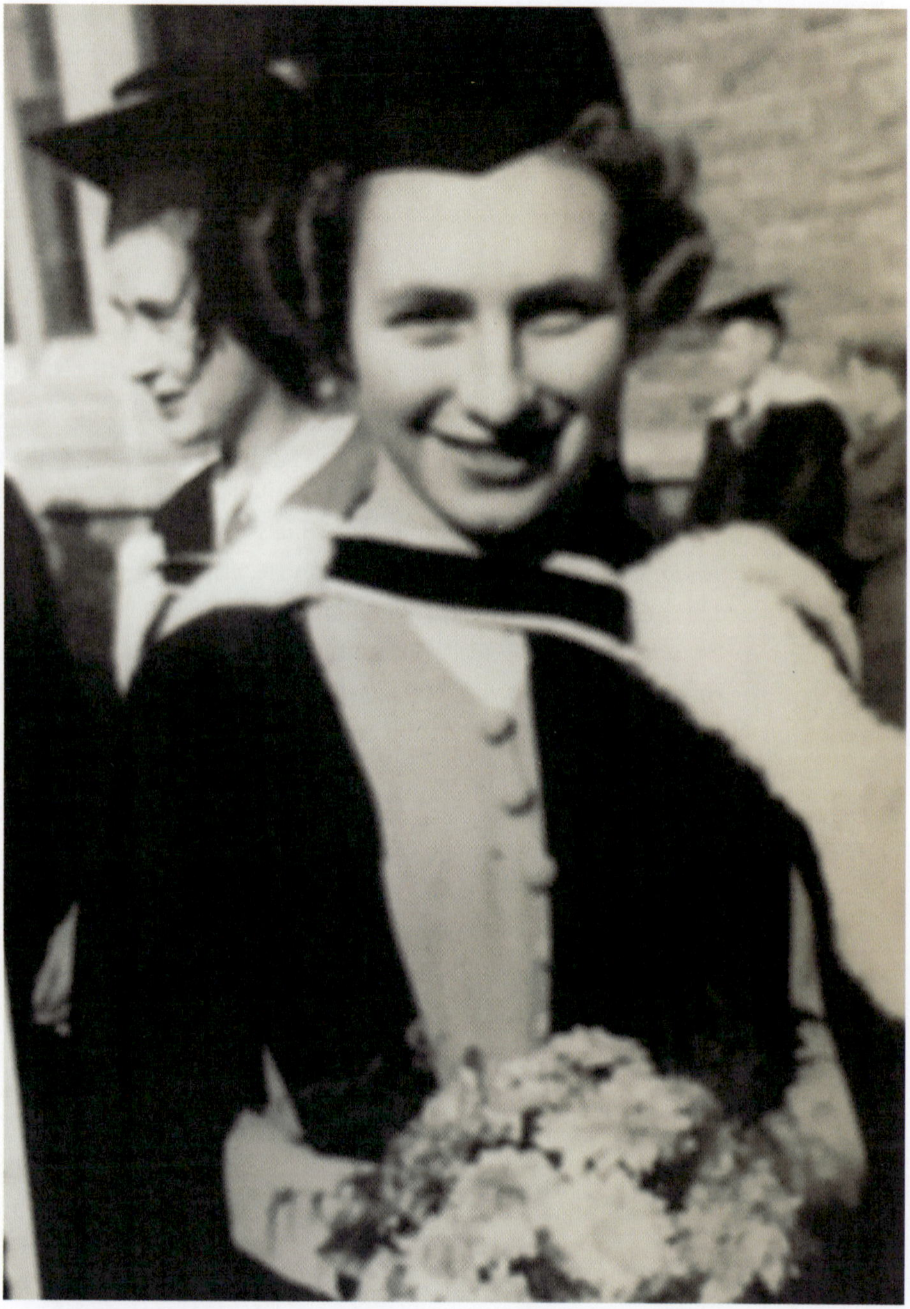

Mary Litster O'Halloran on her graduation from Otago Medical School in 1950. *Family collection*

sexual assault — subjects they often felt uncomfortable discussing with their male GPs.[10] When Margaret Sparrow became student health officer at Victoria University of Wellington in 1969, students would come to her for help and advice on contraception or unwanted pregnancies. She was reluctant at first: abortion was still illegal in New Zealand, and students who were refused help in their hometowns would opt to travel to Australian clinics that were often untested or monitored.[11]

Sparrow's approach changed radically when a pregnant student phoned her from Melbourne to say that she had turned up at one of the addresses she had been given, but it did not exist. Sparrow decided she needed to get involved, and she turned to the Family Planning Association (FPA) for help. The FPA had been established in 1936 and, during the 1940s, was primarily involved in providing contraception by mail. Over time, the association established clinics in cities throughout the country. Carol Shand (1962) and her husband, Erich Geiringer, were instrumental in establishing the clinic in Wellington, where they gave students contraception and advice free of charge.

Through the association, Sparrow met other people who were working to improve access to abortion by ensuring that women who went to Australia for an abortion had an official letter and a verified address for the clinic. This was made easier from the late 1960s, when judges in two court cases in Australia had ruled that abortion was lawful in certain circumstances.[12] As a result, doctors in New Zealand were now able to write legitimate referrals to clinics in Melbourne and Sydney. Sparrow became a de facto medical travel agent, organising addresses and travel and writing referral letters.[13]

In 1974, the Auckland Medical Aid Centre (AMAC), New Zealand's first abortion clinic, opened in Auckland. After only five months of operation, AMAC was raided by the police and the head operating doctor, Jim Woolnough, was arrested and charged along with other referring doctors, including Margaret Sparrow.[14] A young student whom she had referred for an abortion was selected as the key witness by the prosecution, so Sparrow and her patient had to travel to Auckland for the depositions in the magistrate's court and then two trials in the high court.[15] The first trial ended in a hung jury. In the second trial, Woolnough was acquitted, and that decision was confirmed following an appeal. Finally New Zealand was moving in the same direction as Australia.

In 1977, the Contraception, Sterilisation and Abortion Act was passed into law in New Zealand. As a consequence, in 1980 Margaret Sparrow and Carol Shand, along with Leigh Minnitt and Winifred Kennedy (née Fisher; 1964), opened Parkview Clinic, Wellington's first abortion clinic. The clinic performed abortions on women who were in their first trimesters of pregnancy. It was a constant site of protest throughout the 1980s and 1990s, including a bomb threat in 1998.[16] Not only was this clinic a site for family planning care, but the doctors also conducted research on the patients they saw there. In an article published in the *New Zealand Medical Journal* in 1982, Sparrow reported that of 1000 cases from Parkview Clinic, 50 per cent of women seeking abortions had been using contraception when they became pregnant. She used this article to recommend improvements in contraception practice.[17] Kennedy found that contemporary family planning services were not as accessible as they should be and many women could not afford them. Remedying this was one her motivations for working at Parkview.[18]

In 1999, Shand, Sparrow, Diana Edwards (née Montgomery; 1948), John Tait and Peter Stone established the not-for-profit pharmaceutical company Istar in order to import the French-made abortion pill Mifegyne (mifepristone), which no established pharmaceutical firm would touch.

There were also improvements in medical assessment services for women and children reporting cases of sexual abuse and assault. In 1985, Carol Shand helped establish and became a trustee and rostered doctor for Wellington Sexual Assault HELP (now called Wellington Sexual Abuse HELP), which provided medical assessment and counselling to women after sexual assault. Working closely with the police and support services, she was one of a small group of on-call women doctors who examined and treated any complainant of a sexual assault in the Wellington area. She was also a founding member and later president of Doctors for Sexual Abuse Care, now Medical Sexual Assault Clinicians Aotearoa (MEDSAC), which organises training for those providing medical care to men, women and children who have reported sexual abuse or assault. Shand helped develop training manuals for doctors working in this area and worked closely with the police to improve their response.[19]

Robyn Hewland (1962), who specialised in psychiatry, focused her efforts on improving support for men, women and children who had been sexually abused and were seeking assessment and therapy from mental health services. She lobbied hard to improve the Accident Compensation Act to include claims for trauma related to sexual abuse.

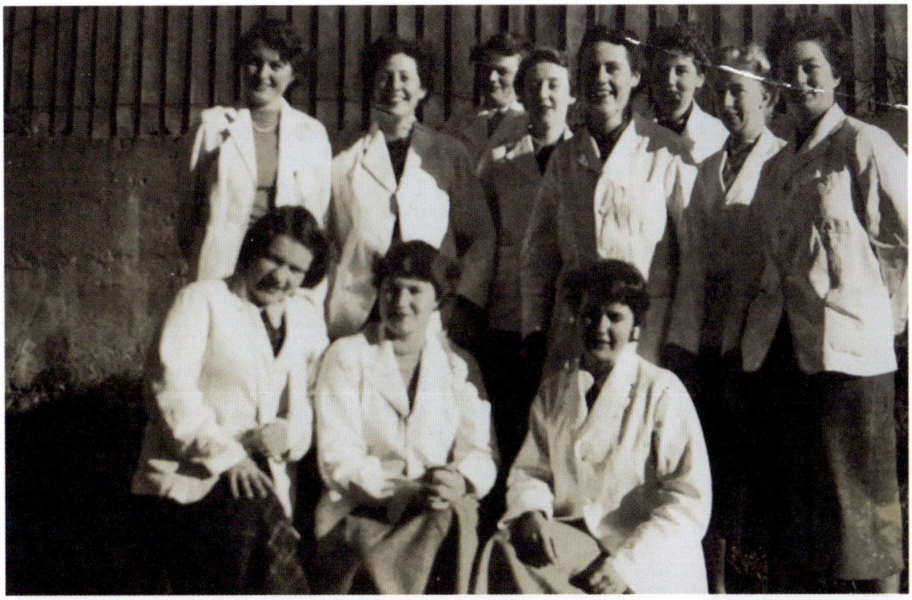

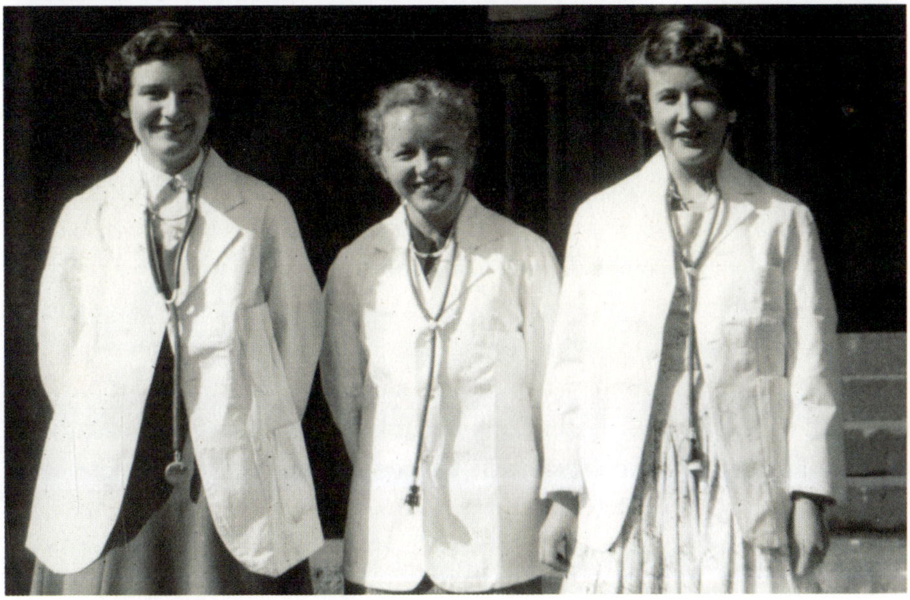

ABOVE: Otago Medical School graduates in 1954. Back row, from left: Margaret Belton (née Hart), Bronwyn Robinson (née Broomfield), Patricia Bassett, unknown, unknown, Kathleen Bradford (née Johnstone), Elizabeth Naylor (née Beauchamp), Katharine Bowden (née Thomson). Front row: Margaret Gibberd (née Sidey), Ann Weston (née Coates), Gwen Allison (née Hookings). *Courtesy Ann Weston*

BELOW: Otago Medical School graduates from 1960 (from left): Patricia Houghton, Rachel Maule (née Senn) and Elaine O'Brien (née Tutchen). *Family collection*

Alongside increasing awareness and improving practice in sex education, abortion and care for sexual assault complainants, women doctors enacted change for vulnerable populations in New Zealand and overseas. Robyn Hewland was appointed as a psychiatrist for the New Zealand Mental Health Review Tribunal, where she assessed appeals by patients who disputed their committal under the Mental Health Act. She discovered that the Act failed to cover many mental health issues, meaning some patients could be released without support. Hewland argued that committal under the Act should be based on a risk assessment rather than the presence of psychosis, and she lobbied for an amendment, which was finally addressed several years later.[20]

Margaret Guthrie (née Hoodless; 1951) led change in gerontology, helping facilitate mental wellbeing in the elderly. She became medical superintendent at Burwood Hospital in Christchurch in 1973 and later worked to improve facilities at rest homes, establishing bereavement counselling and social activities for older people to alleviate feelings of loneliness, in addition to providing training for specialised geriatric physicians.[21]

Cecily Pickerill (née Clarkson; 1925), Mercia Barnes (1955) and Margaret Liley (née Hunt; 1953) all worked to improve care for babies and children. In the late 1930s and early 1940s, Pickerill, a highly skilled plastic surgeon, pioneered plastic surgery for harelips and cleft palates alongside her husband, Henry Pickerill.[22] She was the first to specialise in child plastic surgery in New Zealand, but because of suspicion and mistrust about the competence of women doctors, parents were often not told that she had been the one to operate on their children until after the surgery. Her advocacy work, however, extended beyond her pioneering surgery practice.

She advocated strongly for a new system of postnatal care that would prevent the spread of infection: her method of 'insulation, not isolation' meant that each mother and baby had a room to themselves, which was sanitised before they arrived. Contact between the baby and anyone other than its mother was kept to a minimum. Not only did this reduce anxiety in the babies, but it also stopped the spread of infection — something that was very important in pre-penicillin days. After an operation to repair a baby's cleft palate or a harelip, Pickerill would show the mother how to massage the lip to prevent scarring and would ensure the mother was successfully nursing her baby.

Mercia Barnes spent 30 years as Hamilton's only woman gynaecologist, working in the obstetrics and gynaecology department at Waikato Hospital. She helped establish the Royal New Zealand College of Obstetricians and Gynaecologists (RNZCOG) in 1982; she was the first secretary, and in 1990 she became the first woman president of the organisation.[23] Barnes was a dedicated doctor, working tirelessly for her patients and her much-loved specialty of obstetrics and gynaecology. She died in 1994 only a few weeks after completing her presidency, aged 61.

Margaret Liley was involved in a complete overhaul of obstetric practices at National Women's Hospital in Auckland in 1957, led by Harvey Carey, who set up a trial 'rooming-in' ward where babies slept with their mothers in the same room rather than in a separate nursery, so that the mothers had greater access to their babies and could become familiar with managing 'demand feeding'.[24] From 1957, Liley ran antenatal classes for pregnant women and their husbands or other support person, to teach them what to expect and how to deal with childbirth. They encouraged fathers to be present for the birth. Liley kept records, including a baby's weight at birth and at discharge, breastfeeding, night crying, and the staphylococcal carrier status of nurses present at the birth.[25] She then compared the data from the trial ward with that from other wards. As a result of the findings, the hospital was redesigned for rooming-in, and this practice was eventually adopted nationwide.

There was a marked increase in women graduates making careers for themselves overseas in this period, especially in specialties or positions that were not available to women in New Zealand, or in providing aid to communities in need. Anaesthesiologists Miriam Frank and Patricia Mackay (née Wilson; 1948) and radiologist Ailsa Morrison-Galt implemented vital changes in their fields. Frank studied anaesthesiology in London from 1970, and in 1975 she became senior lecturer in anaesthesia at London Hospital Medical College, where she taught, researched and consulted on the subject. She played a vital role in improving the use of anaesthetics in epidurals and caesareans — specifically so that mothers could be awake during the birth and mother and baby could instantly bond after the birth.

During her tenure as anaesthetist at the Royal Melbourne Hospital, Mackay established an acute pain service and introduced a new and improved anaesthetic chart used to record data during anaesthesia, for future use. She was at the forefront of developing a quality assurance programme in her department, which

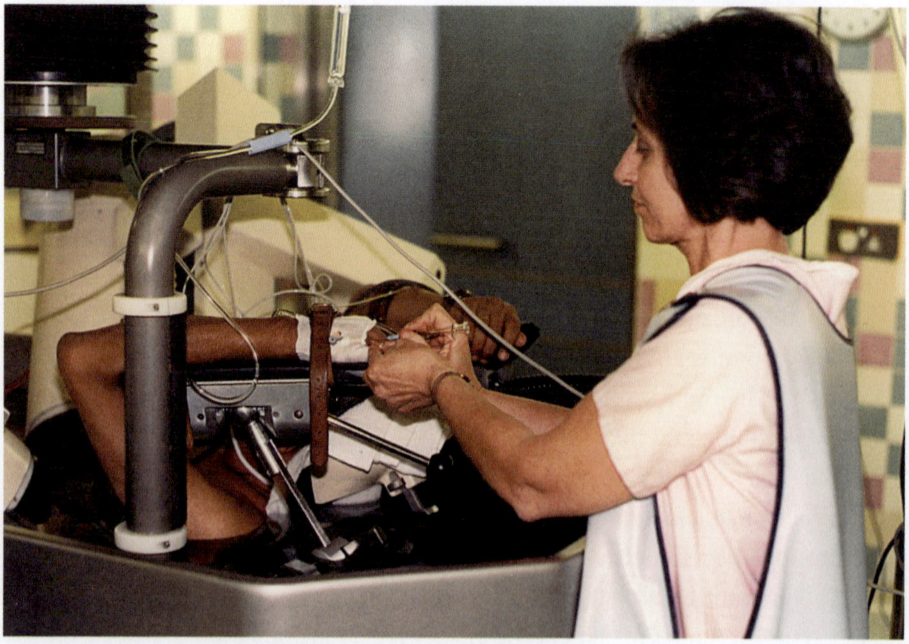

Miriam Frank working as an anaesthetist, c.1970. *Courtesy Miriam Frank*

eventually grew into an independent body, the Victorian Consultative Council of Anaesthetic Mortality and Morbidity, in 1976. The council received and reviewed voluntary reports of possible anaesthesia-related cases of mortality and morbidity in Victoria, with the goal of continuing to identify opportunities to improve the quality and safety of anaesthetic care.

Ailsa Morrison-Galt became a prominent radiologist who advocated for mammography, CT scanning and bone density studies throughout her time as a partner at the South Coast Radiology group for 20 years.

Some medical graduates from Otago went to work in remote areas in developing countries, especially after the Second World War. Linnie Calvert (née Tombleson; 1948) and her husband, Peter, also an Otago graduate, worked for the London Missionary Society (LMS) after completing their house surgeon years. They attended an eight-month course in tropical medicine at Sydney Medical School and then, in 1954, they went to work at a mission hospital

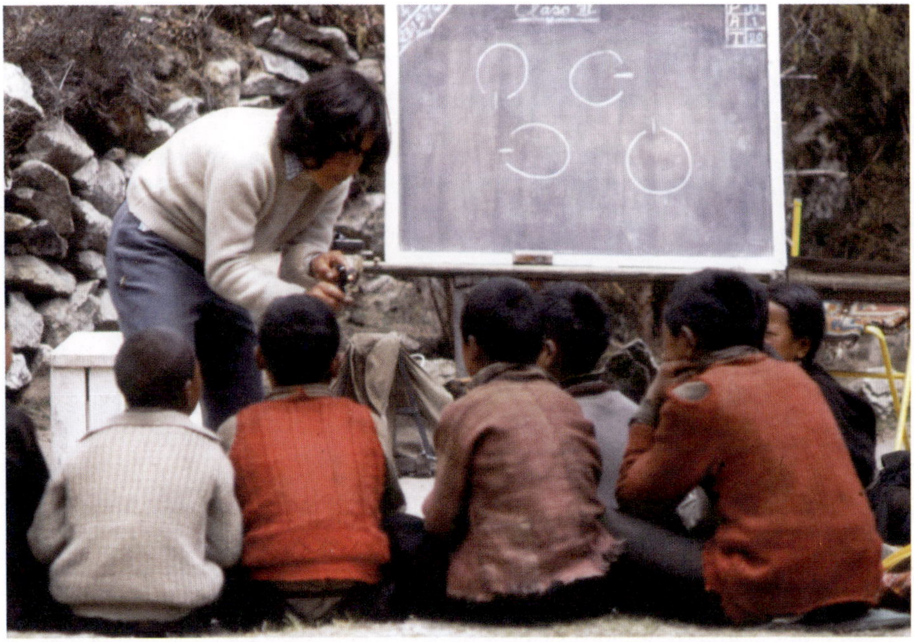

Ann Lang teaching in Nepal, c.1970. *Family collection*

in Kapuna, a remote village in the Gulf of Papua that is accessible only by boat. Through their time at Kapuna Hospital, they served more than 45,000 people. Phyllis Charlton (née Taylor; 1961), a daughter of missionaries in China, returned to China after graduating to work as a doctor with the Leprosy Mission.[26] Ailsa Barker (1967) moved to Indonesia in 1974 to work as a lecturer at Universitas Methodist Indonesia; she returned to New Zealand in the 1980s to complete a BA in theology, then returned to Indonesia for the rest of her career.[27]

Ann Lang (née Philipp; 1967) and her husband, fellow Otago graduate Selwyn Lang, went to work at Kunde Hospital in Nepal for two years. During the monsoon season in 1970 they visited every home in Khumbu to conduct a health and demographic survey; at the same time they vaccinated locals against smallpox and tuberculosis and administered iodine injections to prevent and treat goitre.[28]

Beryl Howie (1949) radically upended the local medical training system in Punjab, India, which had always lost postgraduate doctors to hospitals in Bombay, Britain or North America. As head of the obstetrics and gynaecology department at the Christian Medical College and Hospital (CMC) at Ludhiana, she supervised postgraduate and doctoral students, many of whom were working on research topics that addressed local needs. She was then able to offer them permanent positions when international doctors left or retired. She managed to get international recognition for the postgraduate programme at CMC so that, by the time she left, the majority of the locally trained staff were internationally qualified.

Patricia Hill (née Cruickshank; 1967) worked as a doctor for the Salvation Army. She was initially sent to work in Zambia from 1969 to 1970 and, after some additional training in tropical medicine in London in 1971, she was sent to Rhodesia (now Zimbabwe), where a civil war raged. She worked in the hospital there, mostly in obstetrics, for the next 10 years. She considers one of her main career achievements to have trained up the workforce in the maternity department to cope without a resident doctor.

Back in New Zealand, Hill continued working for the Salvation Army and eventually worked full-time in the Te Aro Health Centre (TAHC) in Wellington. The centre, established in 1985, had grown out of the early work of a group of retired doctors. They ran a first-aid post helping young and old homeless people with a range of problems, including addictions. Hill loved this work, and continued it until she retired in 2007.

In 1964, Papali'i Viopapa Annandale-Atherton (née Annandale; 1964) graduated as Otago Medical School's first Pacific Island student, and the first Samoan woman to become a doctor.[29] She is the only woman of Pacific heritage in this cohort of early medical graduates. She went on to establish and head a World Health Organization (WHO) clinic in Sāmoa for maternal and child health and family planning, and established the Soifua Manuia Clinic in Apia. She travelled to many developing countries to assist and advise on their family planning programmes, advocate for women's rights and fight for the vulnerable.[30] She was awarded an honorary doctorate by the University of Otago in 2019.

CECILY MARY AROHA WISE PICKERILL (NÉE CLARKSON)

1925 graduate — first woman plastic surgeon in New Zealand; first plastic surgeon to specialise in paediatrics; New Zealand's first medical dame

Cecily Pickerill was born on 9 February 1903 at Ruanui Maternity Hospital, Taihape.[31] She and her four siblings attended Taihape School until the family moved to Auckland in 1914, after which she boarded at Diocesan School, where she was a diligent student and focused on becoming a doctor. Entry into medical school at the time was based on exam results in English, Latin and French. Diocesan allowed her to study only two languages, but as three were required for entry to the medical school, she got up early in the mornings and taught herself French before school. Her perseverance paid off: she passed the exams and began her medical studies in 1920.

As the daughter of a minister, Pickerill was awarded a clergy scholarship that covered her university fees, but her parents had to pay for her board at St Margaret's College. Medical school was a stark contrast to her sheltered childhood — after just one anatomy class involving the dissection of a cadaver, she was ready to go home. She struggled with chemistry and physics, which she had not studied in school, and even had nightmares about them. Throughout medical school, she was often the only woman in a group of eight men. But she prevailed and graduated in 1925 at the age of 22.

Her first house surgeon position, in 1926, was with a former lecturer, Henry Percy Pickerill (affectionately known as 'Professor Pick'), who was New Zealand's first plastic surgeon and the first director of the Dunedin Dental School. In 1927, she did a short stint in California while visiting her family who were living there. She arrived with three references: one from R. Faulkner, the medical superintendent of Dunedin Hospital, one from Charles Hercus, dean of the medical faculty, and the third from Henry Pickerill, who praised her as the 'best house surgeon I have had for some years'. She secured a psychiatric residency but soon realised it was not to her liking. By this point, Henry Pickerill was working in Australia and offered her a position as his student, understudy and assistant; they worked part-time at St Luke's Hospital and Royal North Shore Hospital. In December 1934, they married in a small, private ceremony.

In 1935 the couple moved to Wellington, where they worked at Wellington Hospital with injured returned soldiers — Henry as a plastic surgeon and Cecily as an anaesthetist. Henry taught Cecily his methods of plastic surgery as they worked together and allowed her to perform some operations. In 1938, they established specialist plastic surgery consulting rooms in Kelvin Chambers on The Terrace; they conducted the operations at Lewisham Hospital in Newtown. Between 1941 and 1951, they also operated on a small number of patients, primarily with cleft lips and palates, at the Home of Compassion in Island Bay.

+++

In 1940, Cecily Pickerill secured a position as assistant plastic surgeon at Wellington Hospital. In 1945 she was appointed acting senior plastic surgeon. When she asked for the position to be made permanent, however, she was turned down, most likely because she had no formal postgraduate training. As her biographer Beryl Harris wrote, 'She was criticised for not being qualified, but in fact, there were no qualifications available for women until 1947 and she started in the field in 1935. In fact, she had the best apprenticeship possible, working alongside Henry Pickerill for 25 years.'

In 1939 the Pickerills established the private Lower Hutt hospital Bassam, initially as a hostel for mothers and babies who were undergoing operations at Wellington hospitals. By 1942 it had become a plastic surgery clinic for children with congenital disorders such as a cleft palates or harelips. Although it was privately run, Bassam did not charge mothers: it received support from the Crippled Children's Society, and supplemental income came from private cosmetic surgeries performed by the Pickerills on Wednesdays. From 1945, Cecily Pickerill took over all of the surgeries at Bassam as Henry's health began to fail. He died in 1956, aged 77, and she continued working at the Bassam for the next 10 years.

Cecily Pickerill was the first plastic surgeon in New Zealand to specialise in operating on children. But despite her success, it was not always easy. Working in the private sector meant she was isolated from her peers, and she never felt completely accepted by others in the profession. In 1958 she was made an Officer of the Order of the British Empire (OBE), and in 1977 she was made a Dame Commander (DBE) for services to medicine, especially in the field of plastic surgery. She was New Zealand's first medical dame. She retired in 1968: it was better to stop while she

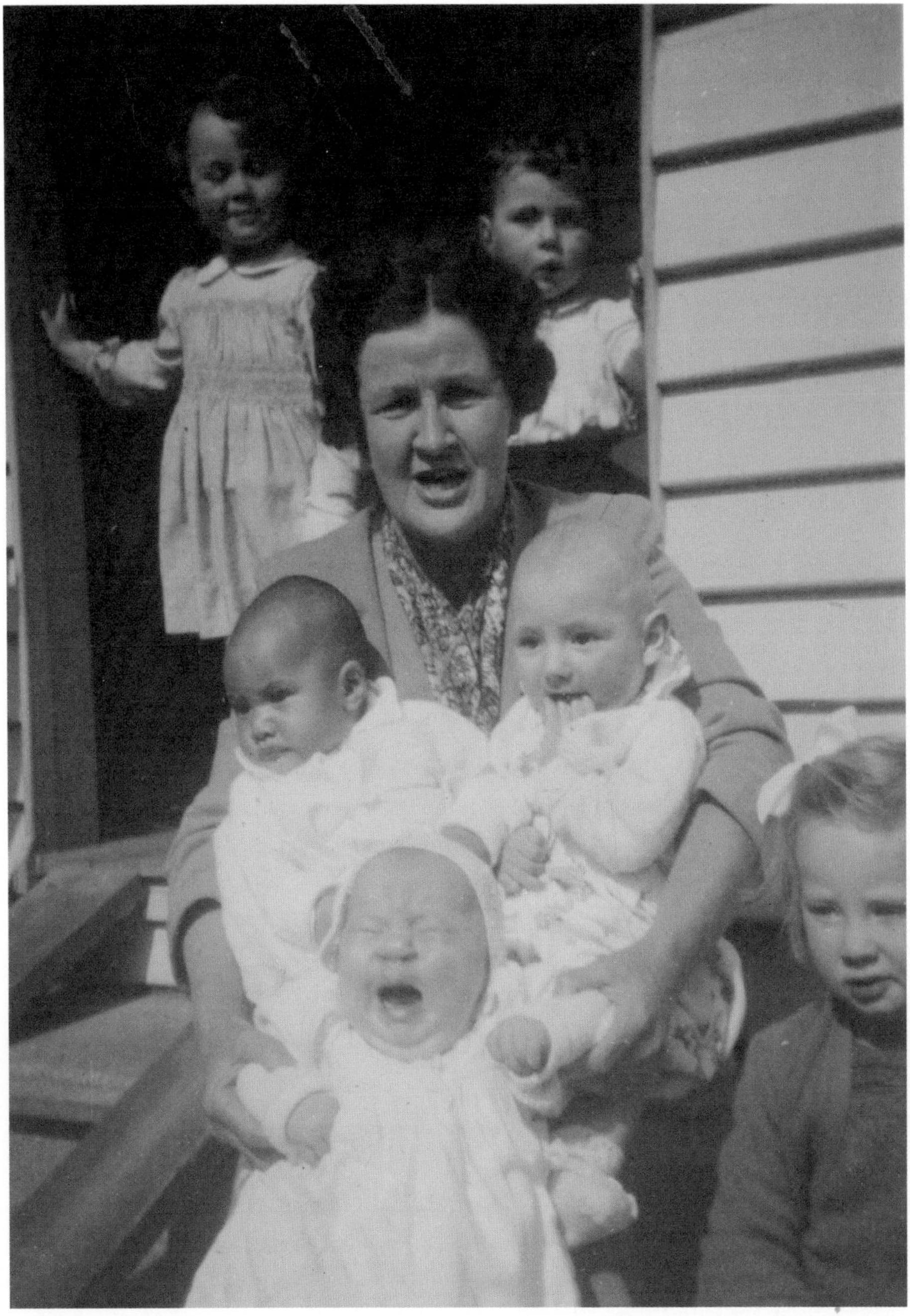

Cecily Pickerill and child patients at Bassam Hospital, 1967. *Hocken Collections Uare Taoka o Hākena, C.M.W. and H.P. Pickerill papers, MS-3066/044/001*

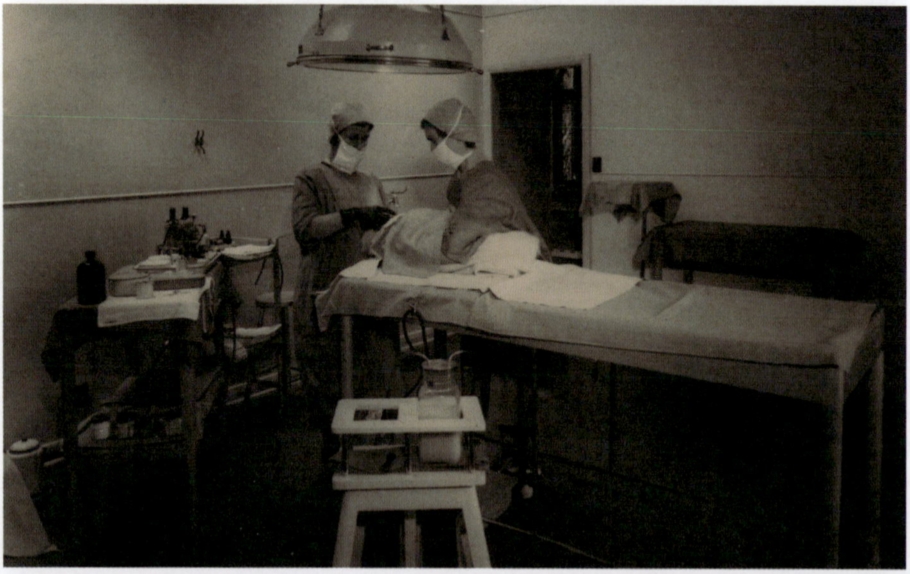

An operating theatre at Bassam Hospital (date unknown). *Hocken Collections Uare Taoka o Hākena, C.M.W. and H.P. Pickerill papers, MS-3066/040/001*

was still enjoying her work rather than wait until she was not, she said. When the plastic surgery clinic at Bassam closed in 1969, the site was turned into a rest home. Pickerill moved there in 1986 and died two years later, in the same building where she had worked with dedication for so many years.

MARGARET ISOBEL ERSKINE NEAVE

1943 graduate

Margaret Neave graduated from Otago Medical School in 1943. She worked first as a junior doctor in Wellington, then trained as a paediatrician in Britain. She spent most of her career outside New Zealand, working with children in developing countries such as Tokelau, Sāmoa, New Guinea, Vanuatu, Vietnam and the refugee camps in Hong Kong, with Volunteer Service Abroad and Save the Children. In Sāmoa in 1965, she developed a paediatric service within the village clinics. Her

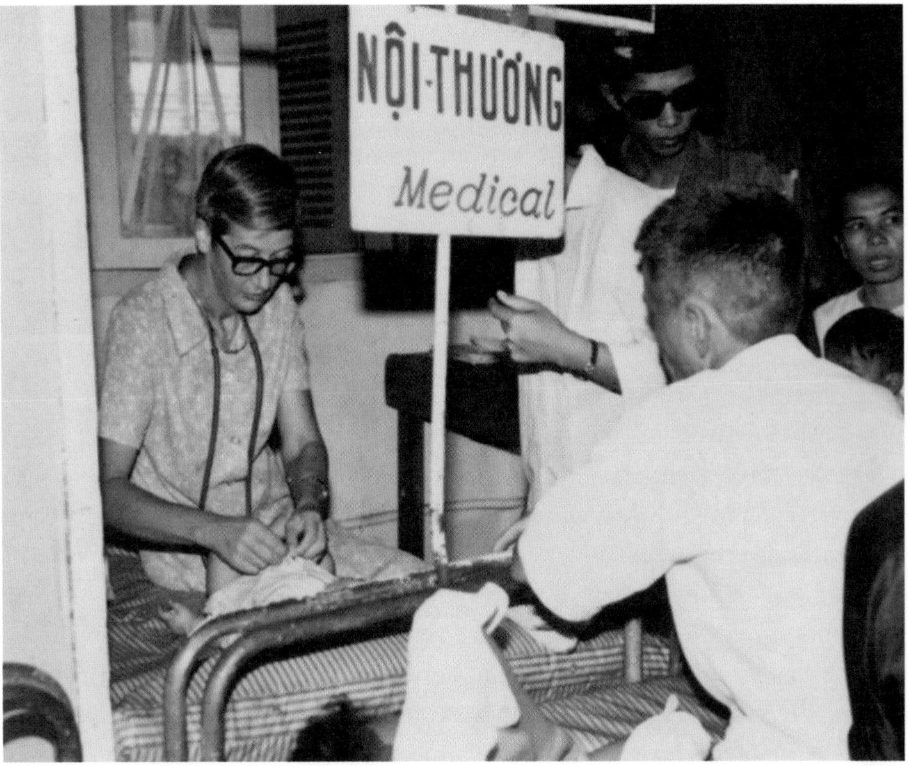

Margaret Neave working in Vietnam during the war, 1972. *Courtesy David Morris*

work philosophy was progressive and holistic, and she worked closely with local doctors, nurses and midwives to spread this approach.

She spent nearly seven years in Vietnam from 1969 to 1975, providing healthcare to local people in the Binh Dinh Province at Qui Nhon Provincial Hospital as part of the New Zealand specialist team, alongside civilian volunteer surgeons such as Al Grant, David Morris and Bill Sugrue. The team were there to support the local hospital staff and provide healthcare to civilians with war injuries as well as a range of other conditions.

The Viet Cong (VC) headquarters were also in the Binh Dinh Province. Al Grant recalled that Neave was not overly worried about her personal safety — she would cross the front lines if she needed to get somewhere for her patients. She was famous, where children were concerned, for refusing to make any distinction between VC and government-run villages: she would get in a Jeep and drive into 'enemy' territory if necessary. The American generals had nightmares about her crossing the lines; the VC simply waved her through. She left Saigon on one of the last New Zealand evacuation flights.

After Vietnam, Neave spent three years working in Papua New Guinea and then six years working in Vietnamese refugee camps in Hong Kong. The British Commission at the time tried to give her an honour for all she achieved there, but she refused it.

+++

When Neave arrived in Vanuatu in 1988 as a volunteer doctor she was welcomed by the New Zealand high commissioner, Tony Browne, with a small reception; both the president and the prime minister turned up to meet her. After she left, a chief from the island remarked, 'When Dr Margaret was with us our people didn't die.'

She was nominated to be honoured by the New Zealand government for her work but turned it down. In the *Evening Post* that year, the government responded to criticism that in one honours list, no woman had been made a dame, while four men had received knighthoods. Don McKinnon explained that they had had an excellent candidate, but she had refused to accept the honour. Had Margaret Neave accepted, she would have been the third dame in our New Zealand medical women, following in the footsteps of Cecily Pickerill and Margaret Sparrow. Margaret Neave died in Wellington in 2007.

PATRICIA MACKAY (NÉE WILSON)

1948 graduate

Patricia Mackay was adopted in 1926 in Balclutha, South Otago.[32] She told her children very little about her early life and parentage and never learned who her biological parents were. At 16, she became one of the youngest students to qualify for a bursary to attend Otago Medical School. She began her studies there in early 1943 and graduated five years later, in 1948.[33] She then spent two years as a house surgeon and a year as a registrar at Dunedin Hospital.

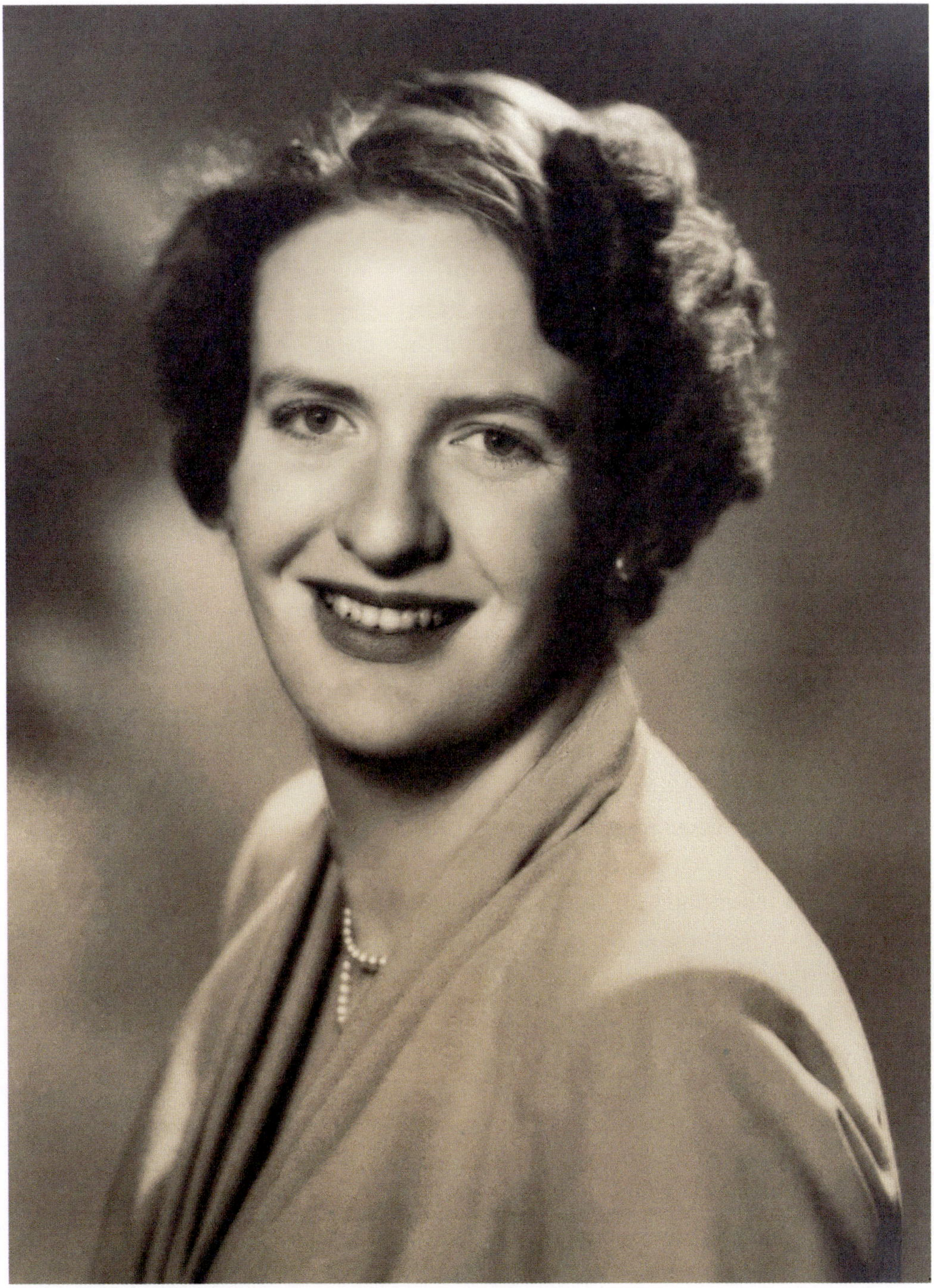

Patricia Mackay (date unknown). *Family collection*

During this time Mackay was drawn to the field of anaesthesiology. As a junior doctor and with little training, she was often called on to take on the role of anaesthetist — and found she enjoyed it. She later recounted how she was asked to administer the anaesthetic for a caesarean section; the surgeon said he thought the baby was dead, but Mackay was able to ensure the baby was born alive and healthy. It was at this point that she decided to be an anaesthetist.[34]

In 1952 Mackay moved to Melbourne, where she trained at the Austin, Alfred and Royal Melbourne hospitals and obtained her Diploma in Anaesthetics (DA) at the end of the year. She then spent a year at Oxford and gained her British DA in 1953. She enjoyed the academic atmosphere at Oxford, where she was taught by the well-known New Zealand-born anaesthetist Robert Reynolds Macintosh. Mackay returned to New Zealand at the end of 1953 and spent six months as a junior anaesthetic specialist at Dunedin Hospital, as well as lecturing in anaesthesia at Otago Medical School. In 1954 she was elected to membership of the Faculty of Anaesthetists of the Royal College of Surgeons.[35]

While she was in Melbourne, Mackay had worked with Norman James, the first director of anaesthesia at the Royal Melbourne Hospital. In 1954, he offered her a position there as a specialist anaesthetist and assistant director of anaesthesia, which, she recalled, was an offer too good to refuse, especially as she already had a romantic interest there — Ian Mackay.[36] They married in Melbourne in 1958.

They had five children over the next five years, and the family became her main focus until the children were independent. She had part-time home help for eight hours a day from a Mrs Stead: 'Steady', as they called her, was an integral part of the family for 20 years and was like another mother figure to her children. When Mrs Stead went home at the end of the day, the children would sometimes accompany their mother on the drive to the hospital so she could do her pre-operative rounds for the following day.

+++

When the children were old enough, Mackay worked as a visiting anaesthetist at the Royal Melbourne Hospital, and this eventually became a full-time position. Her main focus was on neurosurgery anaesthesia. For many years, the role of the anaesthetist had not been considered especially important — they were only there to administer anaesthetics. Mackay and her colleagues were able to establish that anaesthesia was an essential service in the hospital, and they advocated for better education for their registrars.[37] Mackay was chair of the anaesthetics department at Royal Melbourne from 1984 to 1991, and after she stepped down in 1992 she remained on as a consultant anaesthetist.[38]

Mackay was also involved in establishing the Australian Patient Safety Foundation in 1988 to advance patient safety in anaesthesia care. This was achieved in part by creating systems that track and review incidents involving patient safety: the goal was to find weak spots in the system and fix them rather than merely counting the number of incidents.[39]

Patricia Mackay achieved many awards throughout her career. In an interview for the *Otago Daily Times* in 1991, she said one of the disappointments of her working life was that she never became president of the International Association of Anaesthetists, but she did achieve most of what she wanted to, as well as raising five children.[40] The award that gave her the most gratification, she said, was the 2008 Order of Australia, as it was based not only on her anaesthetic career but also on her community involvement.[41]

Mackay died in September 2015, aged 89. The Patricia Mackay Memorial Australian and New Zealand College of Anaesthetists (ANZCA) Research Award was established with a generous donation from her daughter, Indi Mackay, to improve the quality and safety of patient care.

BERYL OVERTON HOWIE

1949 graduate

Beryl Howie was born in Invercargill in 1924, and the family moved to Auckland soon after for her father's work.[42] She attended Maungawhau and Epsom Normal primary schools, then went to Epsom Girls' Grammar, where she did well academically and was appointed a prefect. Two of her uncles worked as missionary doctors in China, and they influenced her choice of career. She enrolled at Auckland University College to do her medical intermediate in 1943 and began studying medicine at Otago Medical School in 1945. While in Dunedin, she lived at St Margaret's College, and in 1947 she became president of the college's students association.[43]

Howie graduated in December 1949, then completed the required two years as a house surgeon at Tīmaru Public Hospital. In 1952 she went to Oxford for postgraduate studies in obstetrics and gynaecology. After qualifying, she worked and taught at Oxford until she obtained a position at the Christian Medical College and Hospital (CMC) at Ludhiana in the Punjab, India, where she arrived in December 1959.

Arriving at Ludhiana was overwhelming. The London office of the Ludhiana British Fellowship had appointed her as head of the obstetrics and gynaecology department but had neglected to tell the interim head, a newly qualified O&G specialist who had been doing the job very well before her arrival. This oversight was eventually sorted but the initial atmosphere was uncomfortable. It took three years for Howie to receive academic recognition from the University of Punjab: she was promoted to full professor on the basis of her postgraduate degree and teaching experience at Oxford.

During her first term, one of her MD students carried out a research project on the care of women and babies in one of the slums serviced by CMC. He found the care given by local dais (midwives), who had little or no formal training, to be inadequate. Howie and the student refined his recommendations for a new concept of maternal and child healthcare centred on home-based care. The study was an overwhelming success and in December 1979, at a WHO workshop in New Delhi, Howie presented results showing that lay urban health workers were an achievable solution for improving the health of mothers and babies, especially in immunisation and family planning, on which India was focusing. In addition, the method was economically feasible.

The population of Ludhiana doubled during Howie's time there, and the O&G building had become increasingly inadequate. Space was set aside for a new O&G block when the CMC hospital was built several years earlier, but the years went by without any progress. In 1973 the London-based RCOG officially recognised the CMC obstetrics and gynaecology department for training for their membership exam. In the latter part of her career in India, Howie raised funds and oversaw the construction of the new building. It was opened on 9 October 1982, and on 12 December, the six-floor wing bearing her name was dedicated by the moderator of the Presbyterian Church of New Zealand.

+++

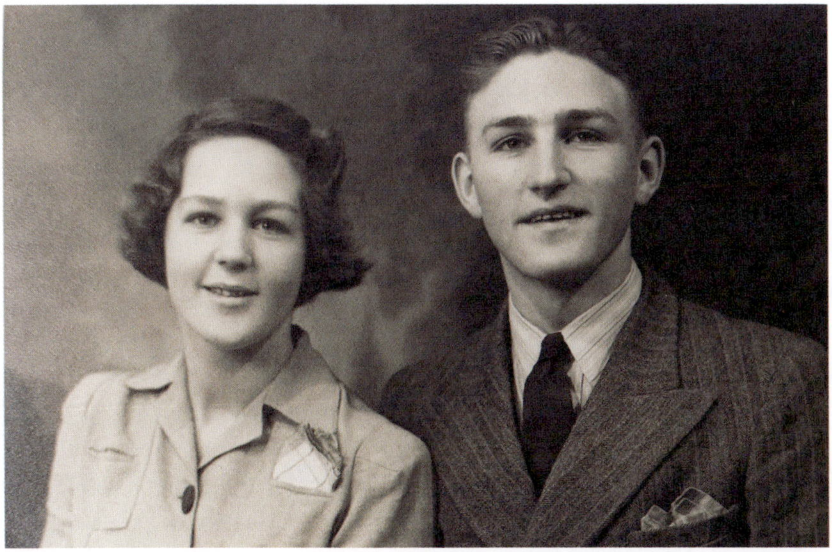

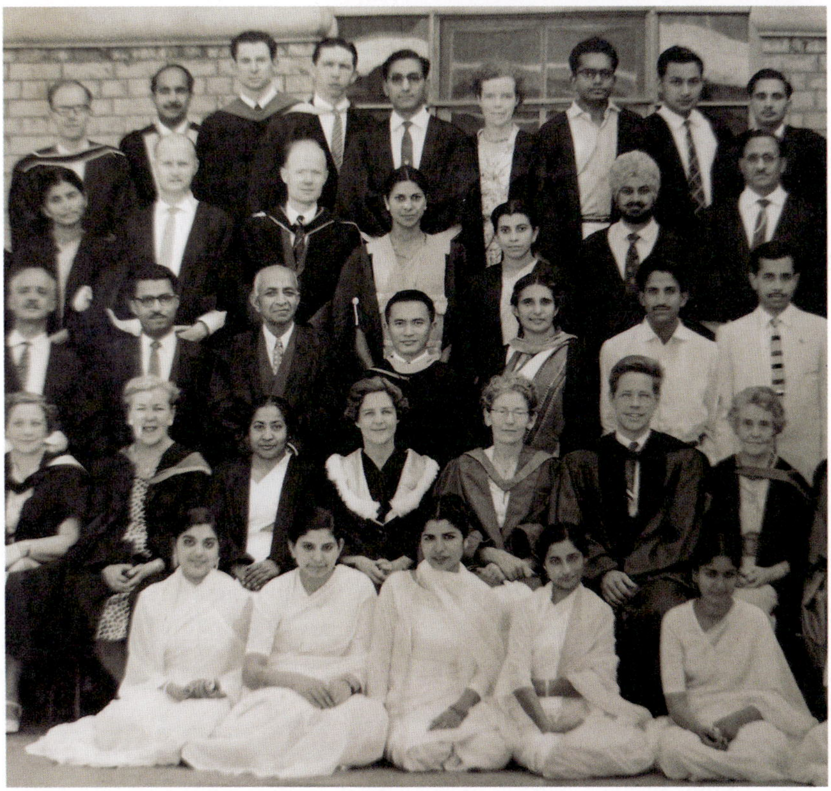

ABOVE: Beryl Howie and her brother John, c.1945. *Family collection*

BELOW: Beryl Howie (centre, second row) and her students at the Christian Medical College graduation in Ludhiana, India, in 1961. *Family collection*

Howie resigned in 1981 after more than 22 years in India. Some of the babies she had delivered in her early days were now returning as medical students; 84 per cent of the diploma students and 29 of her MD postgraduates were using their skills in India rather than working overseas. She had trained the head professor of the O&G department and five of the lecturers. After she left Ludhiana, she wrote a handbook for obstetric trainees, *High Risk Obstetrics*, that focused on the needs of women and babies in developing countries.

Howie settled in Auckland after her retirement. This was a time of major adjustment after leading a busy, structured life, but she found herself in demand as a speaker, and, with her wisdom and knowledge of international missions, she became a valued contributor on some mission boards as well as in organisations such as the Tertiary Student Christian Fellowship, Christian Medical Fellowship and the Missions Interlink council. When she died in December 2012, her obituary in the *New Zealand Medical Journal* noted that 200 people attended her memorial service in Ludhiana.[44] Former students, residents and registrars sent messages recalling her competence, compassion and determination, and the Ludhiana CMC board in the United States raised money to purchase a laparoscopic set for the obstetrics and gynaecology department that had been founded in her memory.[45]

MARGARET WINN GUTHRIE (NÉE HOODLESS)

1951 graduate — first female medical superintendent of a hospital of over 100 beds in New Zealand

Margaret Winn Guthrie was born in the 1920s in Suva, Fiji, to New Zealand parents.[46] After completing her primary school years in Suva, she attended Epsom Girls' Grammar in Auckland as a boarder. In 1941, she sat the Cambridge International examination — one of only two candidates in New Zealand. Her intention had been to travel to Britain for medical school; however, her family decided that because of the Second World War it would be safer for her to stay in New Zealand.

She struggled during her medical intermediate year but was offered a spot at the medical school. Even so, she felt that she needed more time to prepare, and she also felt she was still quite young to be a doctor, so she enrolled for a BSc instead.

When she finally entered Otago Medical School in 1946, Guthrie was one of 10 women among 120 admissions. The women were told that they were expected to sit in the front row 'under the immediate supervisory gaze of the lecturer to presumably protect precious males from the risks of female proximity'.[47] She refused to sit in the centre of the row; instead, she sat at the end closest to the door.

Most of the students in Guthrie's class were returned servicemen — including her future husband, Johnnie Wray, who was repeating his second year of medical school. They were married in 1947. Guthrie was criticised for being a married woman at medical school, and one of the professors told the class that he did not think she would complete the full degree. Even some of the other women medical students asked her, 'How can you be a woman doctor and a lady?'[48]

Guthrie became pregnant a few months after she finished her training. The couple went to live in Havelock North, where they established a general practice while they decided what to do next. Guthrie delayed her radiotherapy studies so she could work part-time as a GP with Johnnie while raising the children; she returned to work after their second daughter was born in August 1953. Their third child, a son, was born in July 1958. In March 1960 the couple sold their practice and travelled with the family to Britain. Wray died suddenly in 1963 while they were in England, and Guthrie returned to New Zealand later that year.

Her first job was as medical officer at RNZAF Base Woodbourne, near Blenheim, where she worked for three years until 1966, giving talks on sexual health and looking after the health and wellbeing of the young male recruits, many of whom suffered from homesickness. She met and developed a close relationship with Walter Guthrie, a sergeant who was considered professionally beneath her by her fellow staff. The relationship caused such a controversy that it landed on the desk of the air commodore at Woodbourne and of the secretary of defence, who summoned her to Wellington. She stood her ground, and a few days later, she received notification that her job was not, in fact, in peril: her contract would continue if she chose to marry Walter Guthrie, but they would need to live off-base. They were married on 28 March 1964.

+++

In 1973 Guthrie applied for the role of medical superintendent at Burwood Hospital. At her interview, a circle of men questioned her about her capacity to work,

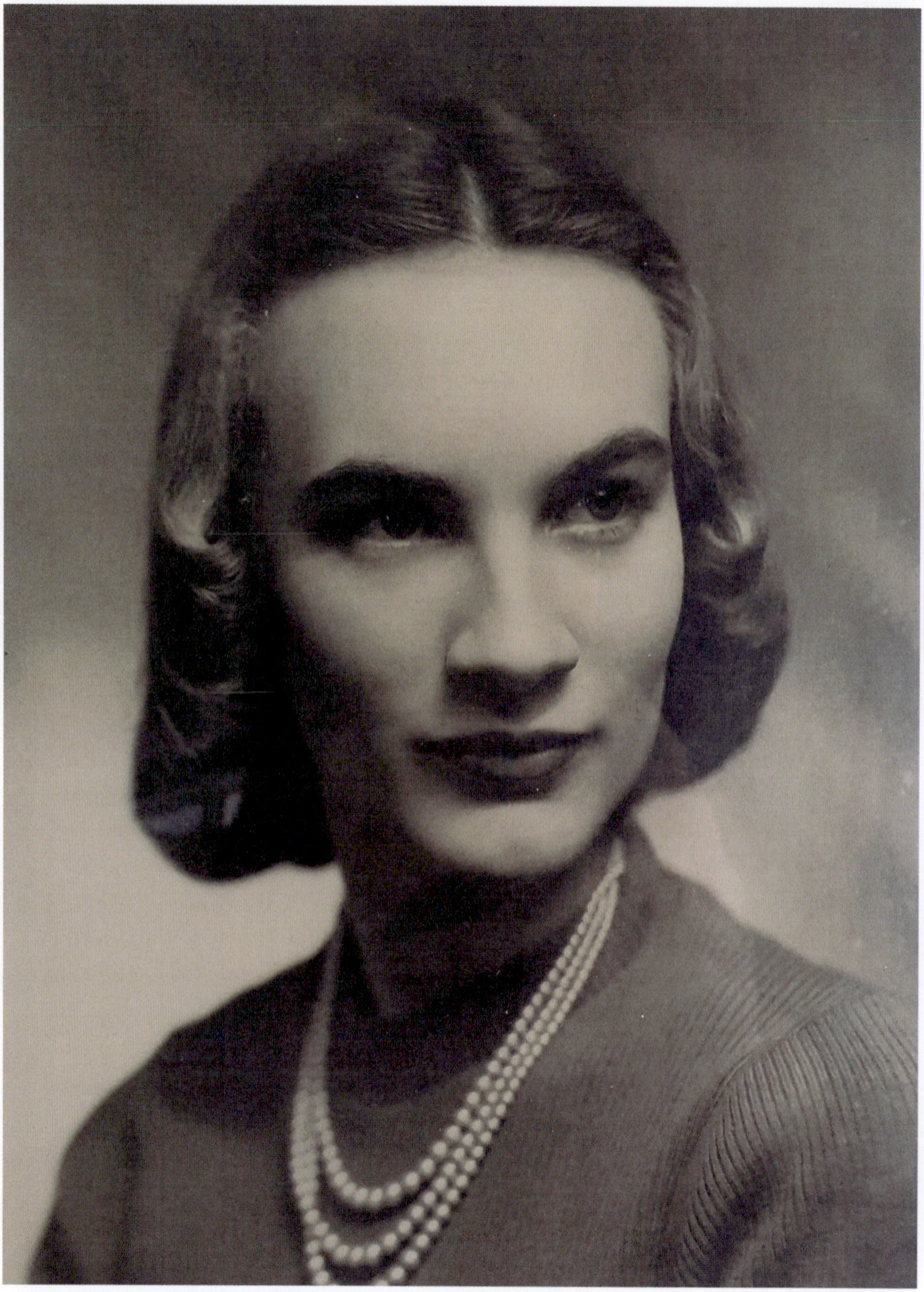

Margaret Guthrie, aged 21, in 1945. *Courtesy Margaret Guthrie*

considering she had three children: what impact would this have on her ability to be a good mother? Her answer must have been satisfactory because she was offered the position — making her the first female medical superintendent of a hospital of over 100 beds in the country.

Over the years at Burwood she developed an interest in gerontology, fired by her concern that many people were surviving into older age but were not receiving adequate care. In 1979 the Guthrie family moved to Wellington, where she was employed by the Department of Health to develop policy to improve and maintain the functioning and wellbeing of older people. As part of this role, she was an active member of the New Zealand Geriatric Society and the New Zealand Association of Gerontology. In August 1986 she was appointed manager of the elderly, disabled and handicapped (EDH) division of the Department of Health, where she became involved in a number of geriatric health education initiatives to combat the view that older people were either disabled or handicapped. This included a public education aspect, with a radio series and educational pamphlets written in English and te reo Māori.

In 1990 Guthrie reduced her workload and became an advisor to the Health of Older People Programme (HOPP), with which she had been heavily involved in the late 1980s. She was also involved in the Christchurch-based Nurse Maude Foundation, which provides hospice and palliative care to patients and their families. She was made a Companion of the New Zealand Order of Merit in 1997, and in 2001 she received an Epsom Girls' Grammar School Founders Award for services to medicine.

HELEN MARGARET IRWIN LILEY (NÉE HUNT)

1953 graduate

Margaret Liley was born on a farm near Te Kūiti in 1928 to William Irwin Hunt and Helen Maclaurin.[49] She attended a rural primary school in Te Kūiti before going to Waikato Diocesan School in Hamilton. Though she was academically ahead of her classmates, the school would not allow her to be placed in a higher year level, so she remembers misbehaving out of boredom. By her last year of high school, Liley

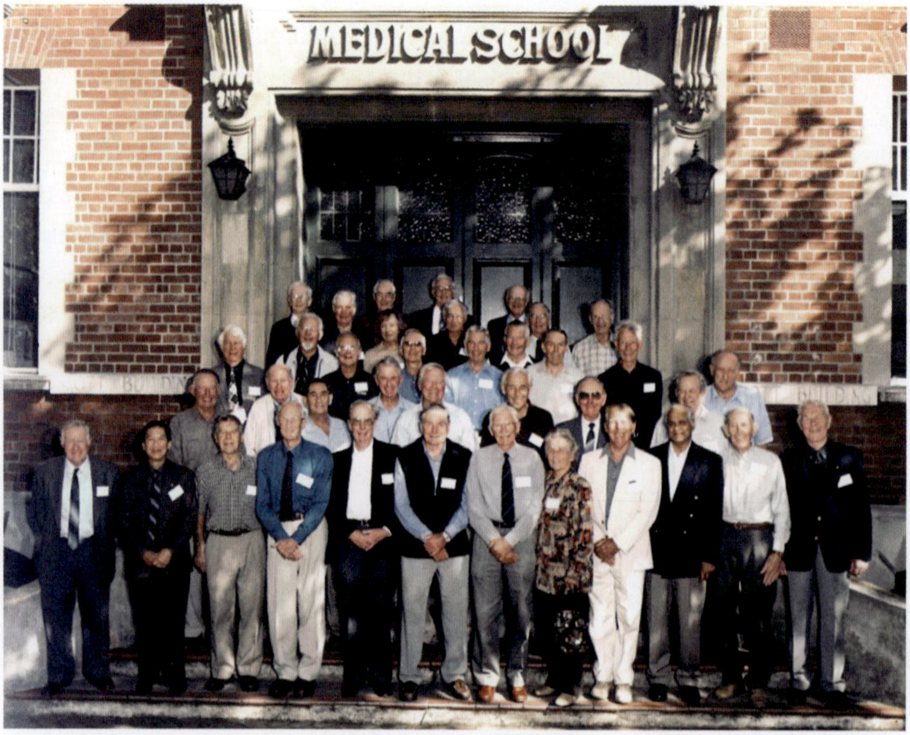

Margaret Liley (front row) with her graduating class from 1953 at a reunion in Dunedin in 2003. *Family collection*

had decided that she wanted to work on the family farm, but when her parents suggested this might be too physically demanding, she settled on medicine instead. She transferred to Epsom Girls' Grammar School to prepare for university. In 1946 she completed the medical intermediate year at the University of Otago and then decided to do a BSc before progressing to a medical degree. By 1949, she was a first-year medical student.

She met fellow student Bill Liley while at medical school, and they married in 1953. For their sixth year, the students were divided among the four university centres. Margaret was assigned to Auckland, where she worked as an intern, while Bill, who had taken a year out of his medical studies to complete a BMedSc, stayed in Dunedin. In January 1955 the couple moved to Canberra, Australia, where Margaret Liley was offered a position as assistant to the obstetrician and gynaecologist Moya Blackwell.

By 1957 the Lileys had two children, and they decided to move back to Auckland. Bill Liley had obtained a research position at National Women's Hospital (NWH), and Margaret Liley took on the newly created post of physician in charge of antenatal education, a role she held, working part-time, until 1984. While there, she worked on introducing a fresh approach to the ways in which unborn and newborn babies were viewed and cared for within the hospital and by their mothers, fathers and the wider family.

In 1964 Bill Liley took a sabbatical, and the family travelled to New York. Margaret Liley was paid 40 per cent of her salary from NWH for six months' work, during which she turned the material from her investigations at NWH into two books and many magazine articles. She wrote *Modern Motherhood* while the older children were at school. The book was revolutionary as it discussed pregnancy from the perspective not only of the mother but also of the baby, pre- and postnatal. After they returned to New Zealand, she continued to work part-time at NWH, teaching antenatal and postnatal care. She also worked part-time as an assistant to Neil Begg, the Dunedin-based medical director of the Plunket Society.

+++

Liley never completely gave up on farming. In 1973 she saw an advertisement in the *Herald* for a 900-hectare farm at Retaruke in the Ruapehu district; the Lileys bought the property the following year, and set about an extensive tree-planting project. Bill Liley died in 1983, and in 1985 Margaret Liley moved to Taumarunui, where she ran her own general practice for 17 years while managing the farm and other land and forestry interests. She retired from medical practice in 2004, aged 75, and only stopped working on the farm in 2019 when she was 91.

MARGARET DAWN MAXWELL (NÉE PARSONAGE)

1955 graduate

Margaret Maxwell was born in 1931 in Christchurch. She was an only child, and both her parents were teachers.[50] When she was about six, the family moved to

Nuku'alofa in Tonga, where her father was director of education for the next three years. Maxwell did most of her secondary school education at Wellington Girls' College, and by her final year she knew that she wanted to study medicine and become a doctor. She recalls that as a girl she often had tonsillitis, and when the doctor, Elsie Burnett, visited Maxwell she thought her job sounded interesting: 'I thought, well, I can have a go at it.'

In 1948 Maxwell studied her medical intermediate at Auckland University College, where she found that she lacked knowledge of the sciences compared to the male students, whose secondary school education had better prepared them for university. As she expected, she failed several subjects in her first year of medical intermediate, including physics and chemistry. Undeterred, she repeated the year, this time with more success.

'I was fortunate in finding that one of the guys who had been in the airforce was very knowledgeable in the physics/chemistry sphere, and without any other attachments, he agreed to give me a bit of coaching, which was probably largely instrumental in me getting the hang of the subjects and being able to follow on with them.' This time, she passed with a high enough grade to get into medical school, even with just 45 per cent in her least favourite subject — physics.

+ + +

Maxwell was one of 15 women in the 1950 intake at the medical school. The highlight of the first day was a surprise visit by Emily Siedeberg, the first New Zealand woman to graduate from medicine. She got used to sitting in the front row of the tiered lecture theatre with the other women, and although she herself found the teaching staff approachable, she could see how some of the women faced opposition from their male peers: 'I think they thought that it was a bit stupid that women were doing it — it was higher ranking than women should take on. Of course, we resented that, and so we carried on with perhaps an increased awareness of the importance of the group of women being in the classes.' Only the male students were offered sex education; there was nothing in the curriculum designed for women.

Maxwell moved to Auckland in her sixth year to complete her practical training at Auckland Hospital. She graduated in 1955, one of nine of the original 15 women from her intake year. During her sixth year, she met Roger Maxwell, who was working as a house surgeon at Greenlane Hospital; they married after she

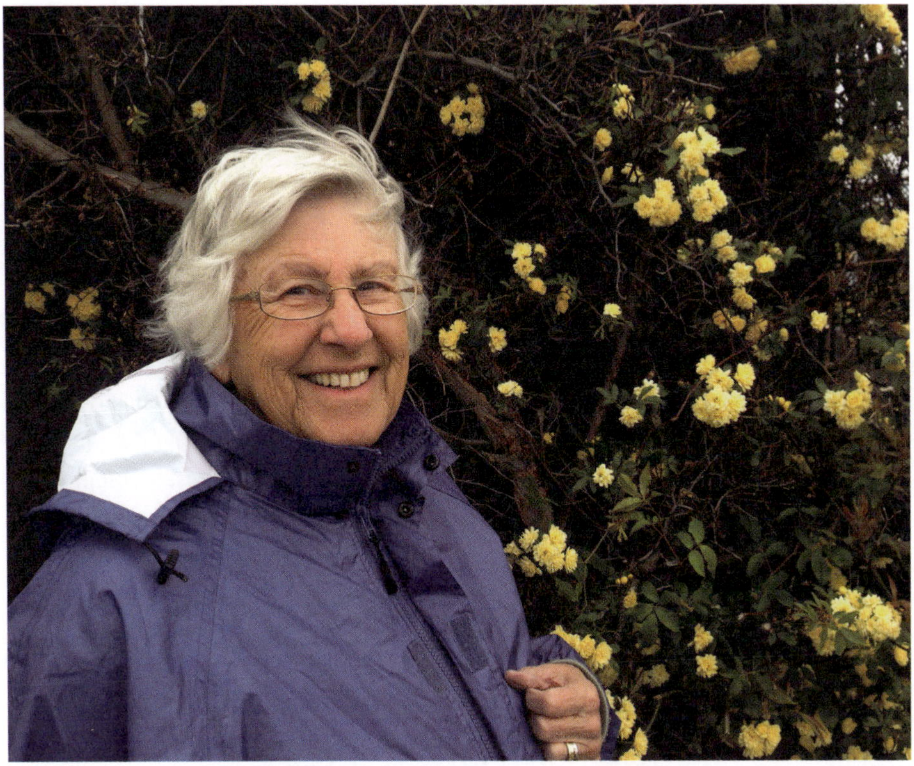

Margaret Maxwell in 2015. *Courtesy Margaret Maxwell*

graduated. Maxwell spent her first year as a house surgeon in the ear, nose and throat department of Auckland Hospital, first as a resident doctor and then as registrar. This gave her valuable experience in the procedures she would need for her future career in general practice. Maxwell and the other junior doctors lived in two houses on Park Road, near the hospital. There were no direct phone lines into the doctors' rooms, so an orderly would come and collect the female doctors if they were required to be in the hospital late at night.

After she completed her training at Auckland Hospital, she and Roger moved to London, where they lived for three and a half years. Maxwell worked part-time as a locum GP and as a medical officer for the Ealing Area Health Office (now the Ealing Park Health Centre).

They moved back to New Zealand with their three children in 1962, and in 1970 Maxwell opened her own practice in Takapuna on the North Shore in Auckland. As the sole GP, her schedule did not allow her to work part-time, and her neighbours often looked after the youngest child. She also wrote articles for *New Zealand Family Doctor* magazine and, later, for *Thursday* magazine under the pseudonym Margaret Greenford, in which she answered questions from readers on medical matters.

Throughout her career, Maxwell was involved with the NZMWA, and in 1971, she became the national corresponding secretary. The group met regularly to discuss feminist issues, write research papers and submissions to Parliament, and provide support for women who wanted to undergo further training. In 1990, Maxwell published *Women Doctors in New Zealand: An Historical Perspective, 1921–1986* — a book that collates historical records from the NZMWA over its lifespan, describes the life experiences of several prominent early women in medicine, and comments on the challenges that women in medicine have faced.

She worked for several years as a medical officer supervising the care of patients in a large geriatric hospital near her home until her retirement.

HELEN BEAUMONT ANGUS

1958 graduate

Helen Angus was born in Hastings in 1934 and grew up in various places on the east coast of the North Island.[51] She was dux in her final year at Gisborne High School and was accepted into Otago Medical School in 1954, one of fewer than 10 women. She lived at St Margaret's College with other young women who were doing a degree in the arts rather than medicine, and they remained lifelong friends. She graduated from Otago Medical School in 1958, alongside four other women.

Midway through her second year as a house surgeon, Angus decided that pathology appealed to her, and in 1967 she passed the examination to become a Fellow of the Royal College of Pathologists of Australasia and subsequently became a consultant anatomical pathologist with the Canterbury Area Health Board. She was well known for her diagnostic skills and sometimes acted as a consultant for other laboratories, including the Godfrey Laboratory — the forerunner of MedLab. In the 1970s, she was awarded a Cancer Society travelling fellowship, which funded her travel to North America for a course on malignant lymphomas — an area of interest for her — and when she returned, she passed on the information she had gleaned to New Zealand pathologists.

Although her main clinical work was spent in the laboratory, Angus also applied her specialist skills to the wider field of pathology. In the 1980s she acted as examiner for the College of Pathologists of Australasia and occasionally was asked to audit the work of colleagues in other centres. She was also a clinical lecturer at Otago Medical School's Christchurch campus, teaching medical students in pathology.

Helen Angus was never aware of any gender discrimination against her personally during her medical career. However, compared to her early years of training in Auckland, she noticed that the medical staff at Christchurch Hospital in the 1960s were almost exclusively male. She retired when she was 63 and, like many women doctors, had to adapt to no longer feeling needed and turning instead to other interests.

MEON CAROLYN (CAROL) SHAND

1962 graduate

Meon Carolyn (Carol) Shand was born in Wellington on 21 September 1939, just three weeks after war was declared.[52] Her mother, Claudia Shand (née Weston; 1936), was a doctor, and seeing her mother care for the community inspired Shand to follow in her footsteps and pursue medicine.

She studied for her medical intermediate year at Victoria University, as it was close to family. She achieved good results at school but only just scraped in to medical school — she lays the blame partly on the 'social rubbish' she was expected to attend outside of her university study, such as balls. After she was called into the dean's office and warned that she needed to focus on her studies, Shand turned her grades around: she passed the year and entered medical school in 1958.

There were only 10 women in the 1958 intake. 'Our [male] classmates were seldom unpleasant to us, in any way,' Shand remembers. 'We had their full support. But some of the lecturers were extremely offensive — remarks like "Why are you

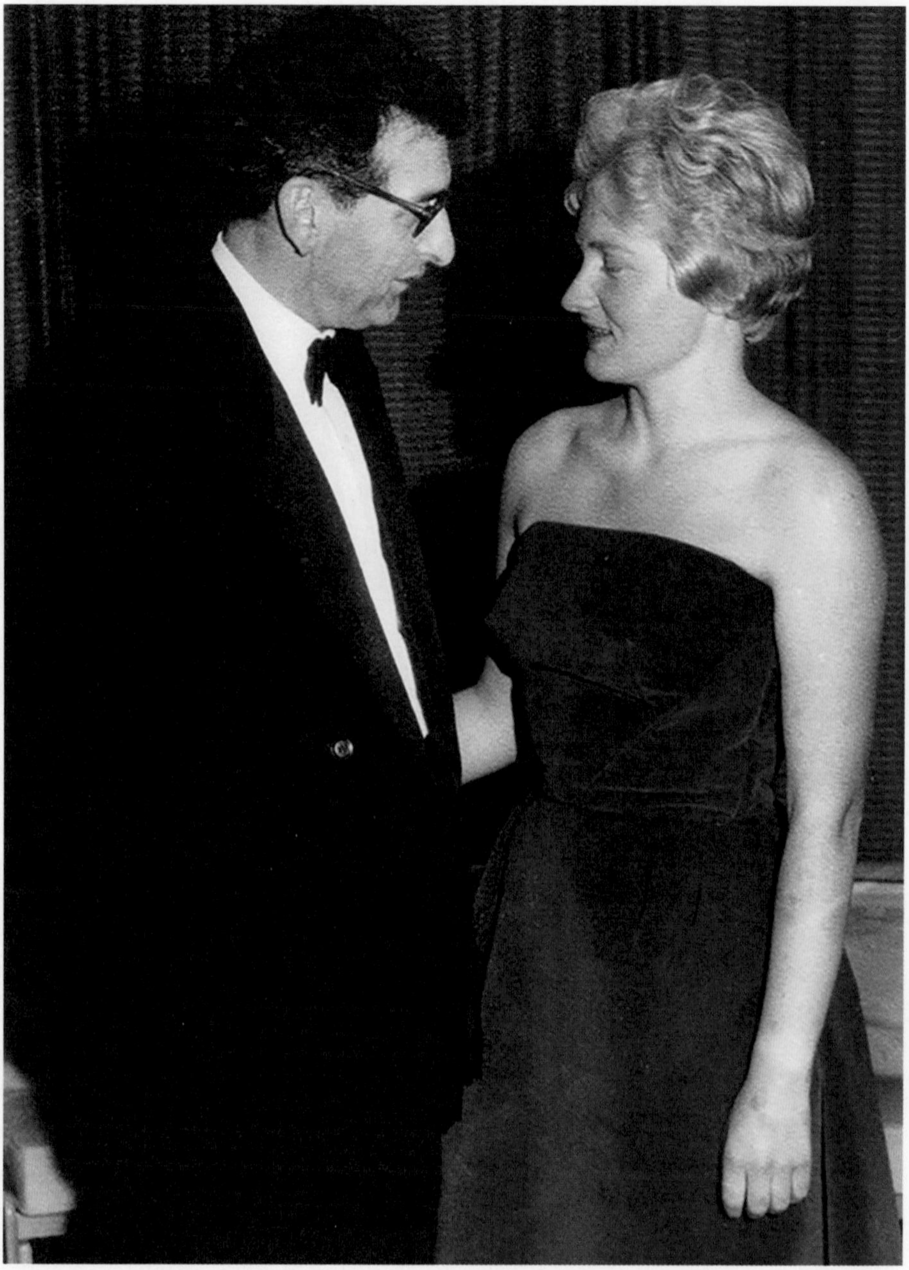

Carol Shand with Erich Geiringer at her graduation, 1962. *Courtesy Carol Shand*

taking up the place of a man who can be a proper doctor?"' In her fifth year, she and her fellow women students were not allowed to attend the traditional end-of-year dinner. Women had been barred from this event since its inception, but this was the first year they protested.

> And it was the big, end of term social event; the women were not allowed to attend the dinner. So, in our year, I organised that the women, and some partners of the men students, would come. It was in a hotel, and we got a room on the same floor nearby where we all sat and talked and drank. There was an open area at the end of the lecture theatre, and I sat beside it and listened to the speakers. Well, the reason they couldn't have the women come was because the lecturers liked to tell dirty jokes, and they couldn't tell them in front of the women. That was the last year that women were excluded; we made so much fuss.

Shand remembers that they learned very little about contraception or women's health in class. 'We had one annual condom lecture given by the dean of the O&G department. It was an open lecture, all the art students turned up, and at some point, he brought a condom up and stretched it. It was a useless lecture, really.'

Oral contraception was just becoming available as Shand graduated. She herself took Anovlar, one of the first contraceptive pills to be used in New Zealand. It was quite a big dose of oestrogen, and it caused her to feel premenstrual and nauseous all month. While she was a student, she recalled that 'some of us managed to get a diaphragm fitted. It was a humiliating experience to find a GP who would be helpful. There was something creepy about it.'

After graduating in 1962, Shand worked as a house surgeon at Wellington and Hutt hospitals. She registered as a doctor at the end of 1963 and did a few locums in general practice, but 'It was hard for women to get general practice locum in '63 . . . they didn't want you. Most practices didn't know what to do with a woman locum in general practice; they'd never had one. Their excuses were that there were no facilities or there was no accommodation.' Shand believes that the practices thought women could not manage the workload.

When she set up her own GP practice in 1964, there were only three or four women in general practice in Wellington. However, she quickly learned that there was a need for more women doctors: she often treated women patients for issues they did not feel comfortable discussing with male GPs, in particular contraception, unwanted pregnancies from failed contraception, menopause and sexual assault.

+++

In 1964 Shand married Erich Geiringer, her partner since her fourth year of medical school. From early in their relationship, when she was a final-year student, they had shared a keen interest in medical politics. Both spoke at public meetings, wrote articles and participated in TV discussions about the medical issues of the time, including abortion, contraception, sex education and the shortage of doctors.

As a GP, Shand was outspoken about women's health issues, starting with contraception for the unmarried and later extending this to abortion services in the 1980s after the 1977 Contraception, Sterilisation and Abortion Act became law. Before that, abortion had been illegal in New Zealand; the only exceptions were in case law, which interpreted abortion as legal to save the life of the mother. She had had to refer her patients to clinics in Australia for an abortion. A survey of GPs carried out by the NZMA showed that most were in support of liberalising abortion. Shand was employed as an operating doctor in the abortion service at Wellington Hospital from 1980 to 2016.

In 1985, Shand helped establish and became a trustee and rostered doctor for the Wellington Sexual Assault HELP Foundation, set up to provide medical assistance and counselling to people who have experienced sexual assault. She was named Companion of the New Zealand Order of Merit in the Queen's Birthday Honours in 2008.

MARGARET JUNE SPARROW (NÉE MUIR)

1963 graduate

Margaret Sparrow was born in 1935 in Inglewood, Taranaki.[53] After high school, she enrolled to do a BSc at Victoria University of Wellington, studying botany, zoology, chemistry and psychology. At the start of her third year she met Peter Sparrow, who was working as a carpenter but was considering taking a medical degree. He encouraged her to also consider doing a medical degree, so she enrolled in the physics course she would need for entry. Despite having no background knowledge in physics, she passed.

The couple married in January 1956 and moved to Dunedin later that year, where Margaret took a research position at Otago Medical School while Peter began his medical studies. She then discovered she was pregnant, despite having been fitted with a diaphragm. It was a difficult decision, but she made up her mind to have an abortion, as she was the breadwinner and needed to prioritise her career. Abortion was illegal, and arranging one was a dangerous and often traumatising experience. Sparrow met George Bettle, a well-known chemist in Christchurch, who gave her a large bottle full of a black mixture that she was instructed to take three times a day until it worked.

The following year, Sparrow began her medical studies. She felt distant from her fellow students as a married woman, and this feeling was exacerbated when she became pregnant again in her second year. She carried this pregnancy to full term, and when their son was born in October 1958, she took a week off and then organised a childcare schedule with fellow medical students in the same situation. After the birth of the Sparrows' second child, she took two years off her studies. The couple graduated together in 1963.

The year after graduation, they separated and Sparrow moved to Stratford, where she had been offered a position in the hospital. Two years later she took on a full-time position with the Department of Health in New Plymouth, where she worked alongside education officer Grace Taylor to develop a comprehensive public programme in sex education — something that had never been done before. Sparrow remembers bluffing her way through her first lecture on puberty, trying to make sure that she was using accessible language. She showed pictures and played a film on the topic. It got a great reception, and for months afterwards people in the street would ask her when the next one was going to be held.

+ + +

After four years in New Plymouth, Sparrow applied for a student health job at Victoria University, where she could continue her work in sex education. Many of the students she saw asked her about abortion.

From 1969, although abortion was illegal in New Zealand, doctors were able

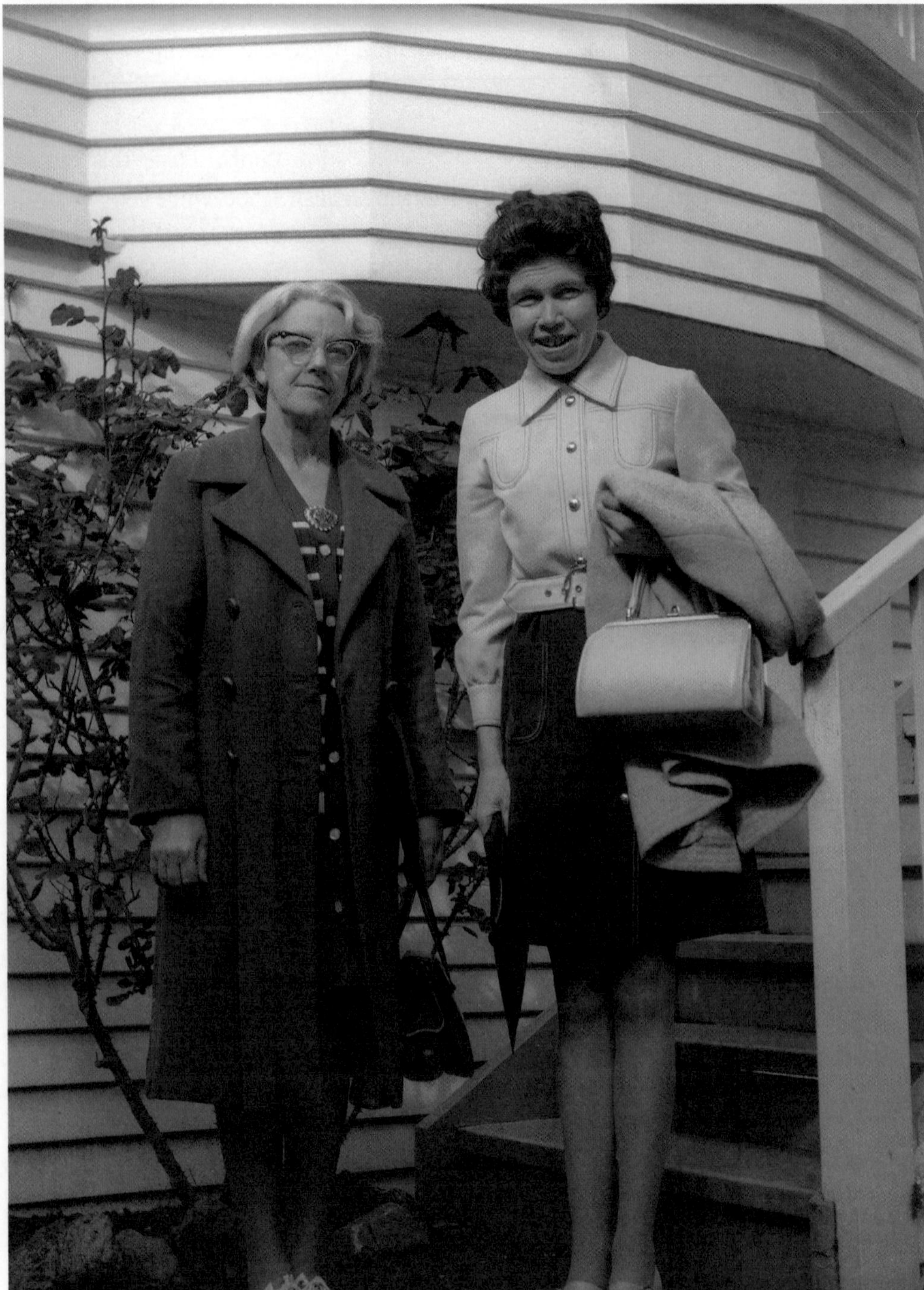

Otago Medical School graduates Alice Bush (left) and Margaret Sparrow in 1963. *Courtesy Margaret Sparrow*

to write legitimate referrals to clinics in Melbourne and Sydney. In 1973, Sparrow travelled to Australia for a student health conference, which erupted in applause when word came through that the landmark Roe v. Wade decision, upholding the constitutional right to have an abortion, had passed into law in the United States. After the conference, she visited as many abortion clinics as she could in Sydney and Melbourne to establish contacts for future referrals.

Around the same time as Australia was making some progress on bodily autonomy, the pro-life movement was emerging in New Zealand, and Sparrow was disturbed by much of the misinformation that was being disseminated. She decided it was time she took a public stand, and in 1972 she joined the Abortion Law Reform Association. In 1974 she was part of an all-women government delegation that represented New Zealand at the United Nations World Population Conference in Romania.

When she returned to New Zealand from a sabbatical in 1976, during which she had gained further training in venereology and performing vasectomies, Sparrow continued to work on abortion law reform. She began receiving hate mail, but this did not deter her. She was involved in setting up Parkview, an abortion clinic associated with Wellington Hospital, where she became an operating doctor. She also worked for the Family Planning Association in Wellington, ran a venereology clinic once a week, and was very involved in sexual health medicine, especially during the 1980s with the emergence of HIV/AIDS. She was the second woman in New Zealand to qualify in venereology, and the only woman venereologist in Wellington. She retired from her role with student health in 1981 so that she could juggle three part-time jobs at Family Planning, Parkview and the Sexual Health Clinic.

Margaret Sparrow was one of the first doctors to prescribe the emergency contraception pill in New Zealand, and her study of the emergency contraceptive pill was published in the *New Zealand Medical Journal*. Her pioneering work has been recognised with her appointment as a Member of the Order of the British Empire (MBE) in 1987; she was made a dame in the 2009 Queen's Birthday and Golden Jubilee Honours; and in 2012 she was honoured as a champion of public health by the Public Health Association. In 2020 she was named Senior New Zealander of the Year in the Kiwibank New Zealander of the Year Awards.

PAPALI'I VIOPAPA ANNANDALE-ATHERTON (NÉE ANNANDALE)

1964 graduate — first Pacific woman medical graduate and first Samoan woman doctor

Viopapa Annandale-Atherton was born at the Moto'otua National Hospital in Apia, Sāmoa, in 1940.[54] She came from prestigious origins: her paternal great-grandfather was Thomas Annandale (1838–1907), a well-known Scottish surgeon, and her maternal grandfather Ta'isi Olaf Frederick Nelson was a leader in Sāmoa's independence movement and was exiled twice by the New Zealand government.[55]

At the outbreak of the First World War, New Zealand annexed Sāmoa from Germany, and from then until the 1960s, relations between the two countries were tense as Sāmoa vied for independence. In 1935, the Labour government sought to improve the relationship by establishing a schooling system in Sāmoa that aligned with the New Zealand syllabus, and through a scholarship scheme that brought Samoans to New Zealand for high school and tertiary education.[56] Annandale-Atherton received one of these scholarships to attend Epsom Girls' Grammar in Auckland. She then won a university scholarship, and her mother encouraged her to set her sights high and become a doctor.

Annandale-Atherton arrived at the University of Otago in 1959 as a 19-year-old, not knowing anyone. She initially felt a bit lost, but the other young women at St Margaret's College were friendly, and she quickly settled into university life.[57] She recalls being treated 'in a rather special way' by her male colleagues and being the only 'sort of non-white student at the time'. She graduated in 1964 and spent her first year as a house surgeon in the surgical and medical wards at the Royal Infirmary in Edinburgh, where her grandfather had worked and where his portrait hung on the wall.

In Edinburgh she met John Atherton, who had also just graduated and was doing his internship. They married in 1965. After her first year as a house surgeon in Edinburgh, they moved to England, where Annandale-Atherton did various other jobs. The family spent several years travelling back and forth between Britain and Sāmoa.

From 1971 to 1974 they lived in Sāmoa, where they both worked at the Moto'otua

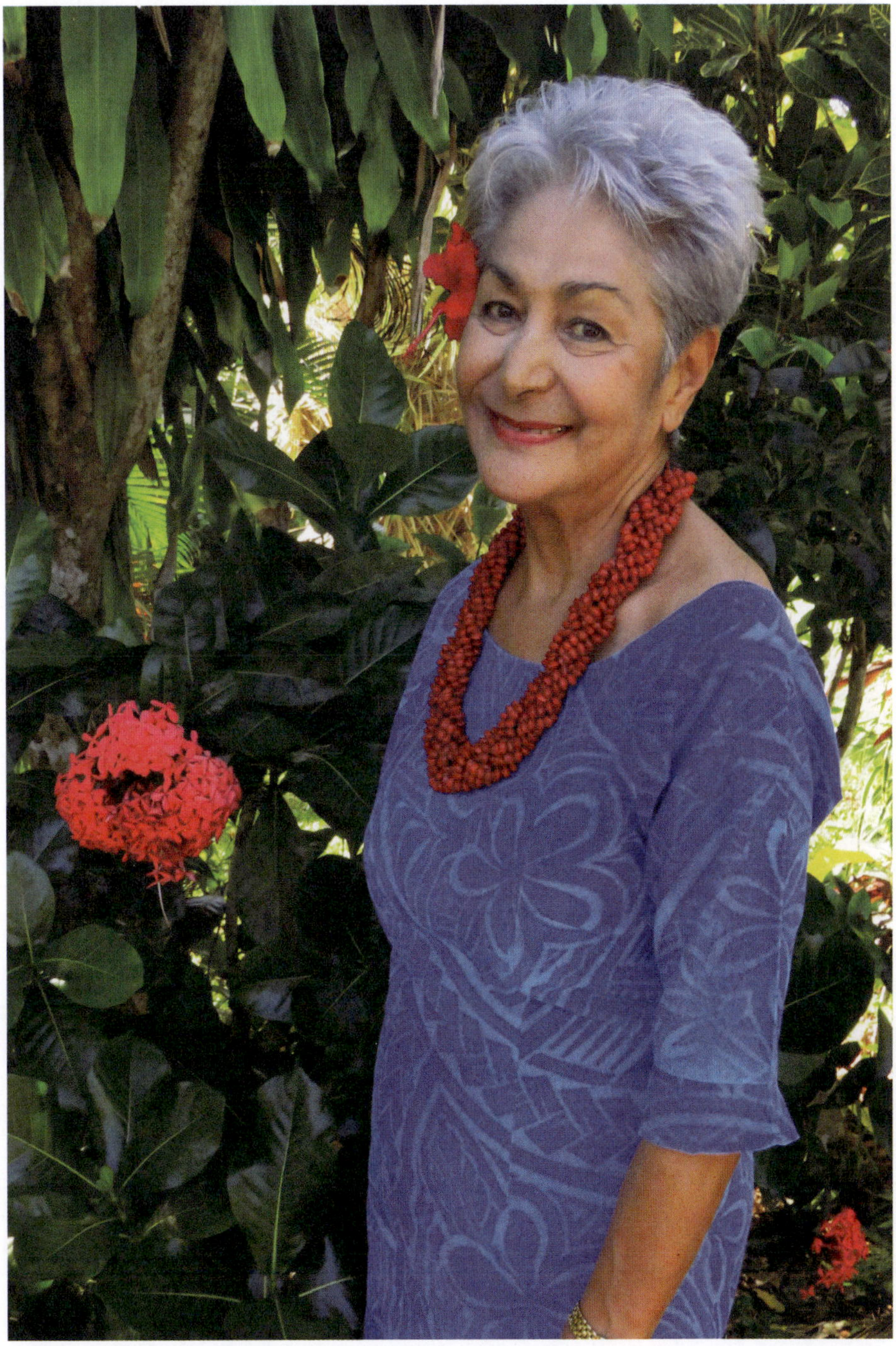

Viopapa Annandale-Atherton in 2019. *Courtesy James Atherton and University of Otago*

National Hospital in Apia. When they returned to Britain, Annandale-Atherton worked in family planning in Sutton, South London, as well as studying at the London School of Hygiene and Tropical Medicine, where she obtained a Diploma in Tropical Public Health in 1976. She was not overly drawn to clinical medicine; she particularly liked the social aspect of maternal–child health and family planning. In 1982, the family returned to Apia, where she worked with the Ministry of Health.[58] For a time, she was acting director of health. In 1979 she became a member of the Pan Pacific and South-East Asia Women's Association (PPSEAWA).

John Atherton's years as chief surgeon in Sāmoa were not recognised by the licensing body in Britain, so he made the decision to switch his career pathway to general practice. The family spent several years back in Britain, where he retrained and then worked in general practice in Norwich, and Annandale-Atherton headed the Family Planning and Well Women's Service.

In 1993 they settled in Sāmoa permanently. Believing primary care was important for the community, they set up the Soifua Manuia General Practice Matautu in Apia, where they both worked until it was sold in 2007. Annandale-Atherton retired from her clinical work at this time, but John Atherton continued to work in other general practices until his death in 2014.

Annandale-Atherton lived on the former pineapple plantation her mother managed during the 1970s and 1980s. The land was subdivided among various family members, and she was surrounded by her cousins, aunties and uncles. She continued with some advocacy work with the PPSEAWA.

In 2019, as one of four outstanding alumni, Viopapa Annandale-Atherton was awarded an honorary doctorate at the 150th anniversary celebrations of Otago University. When she was asked what the future held, she focused on the climate crisis challenges that Sāmoa and other Pacific nations faced: 'I am very proud of what our tiny nation and others in the Pacific are trying to do about reducing our carbon footprint, even though we contribute a minuscule compared to that of other nations. We must continue to speak out and defend and protect our blue Pacific.'[59]

Breaking barriers and creating opportunities for women and girls was the driving force of her life. As a result of her services to Sāmoa, she was awarded the chiefly title Papali'i from the village of Sapapali'i in Savai'i, which was conferred by the head of state, Malietoa Tanumafili II.[60] She died in Sāmoa on 4 November 2024.

WENDY HADDEN (NÉE FITZWILLIAM)

1968 graduate

Wendy Hadden was born in 1943 in Dunedin. She knew from a young age that she wanted to be a doctor, but her mother was not so keen — she told her, 'It'd be nice to marry a doctor, but I don't want you being one', and suggested she do something 'nice, like home science'.[61] Her father was enthusiastic about her choice, although he didn't think she would get into medical school. In the end, her mother was 'chuffed' that she did do medicine.

It was difficult to get through the intermediate year and into medical school. In her first physics exam Hadden got only 20 per cent, which shocked her. 'I needed to pick myself up. So I really tried hard. I got a C pass. Nearly a C plus. People didn't get As and Bs in our days, to get an A was almost unheard of, and B was pretty good.' Just before Christmas she received the letter with the news that she had been accepted, and she was ecstatic.

Hadden had grown up playing cricket. At the suggestion of her high school PE teacher, she joined the Young Women's Christian Association cricket club, and her talent secured her a place in the Otago team and, later, the New Zealand team. The team was chosen to play in the United Kingdom, which meant being overseas for several months. She was surprised when the dean of the medical school, Edward Sayers, gave her permission to go: 'Of course you must go,' he said. 'I let the men go to play their rugby, you must go and play your cricket.'[62]

When Hadden returned from overseas, she re-entered the fifth year of medicine in 1967. That same year, she was engaged to fellow medical student Bruce Hadden, who was by now a year ahead of her. They married at the end of her fifth year — just after his graduation. She was the only woman in her year group to marry before graduating. After she graduated in 1968, she spent two years working with one other house surgeon at the Mater Misericordiae (Mercy) Hospital in Auckland. No registrars were working there, so she was given more responsibility and learned a lot. While there, she applied to be a radiology registrar but pulled out after becoming pregnant; instead, she chose to work as a GP for the next three years.

Once Bruce Hadden had passed his fellowship exams, and now with two

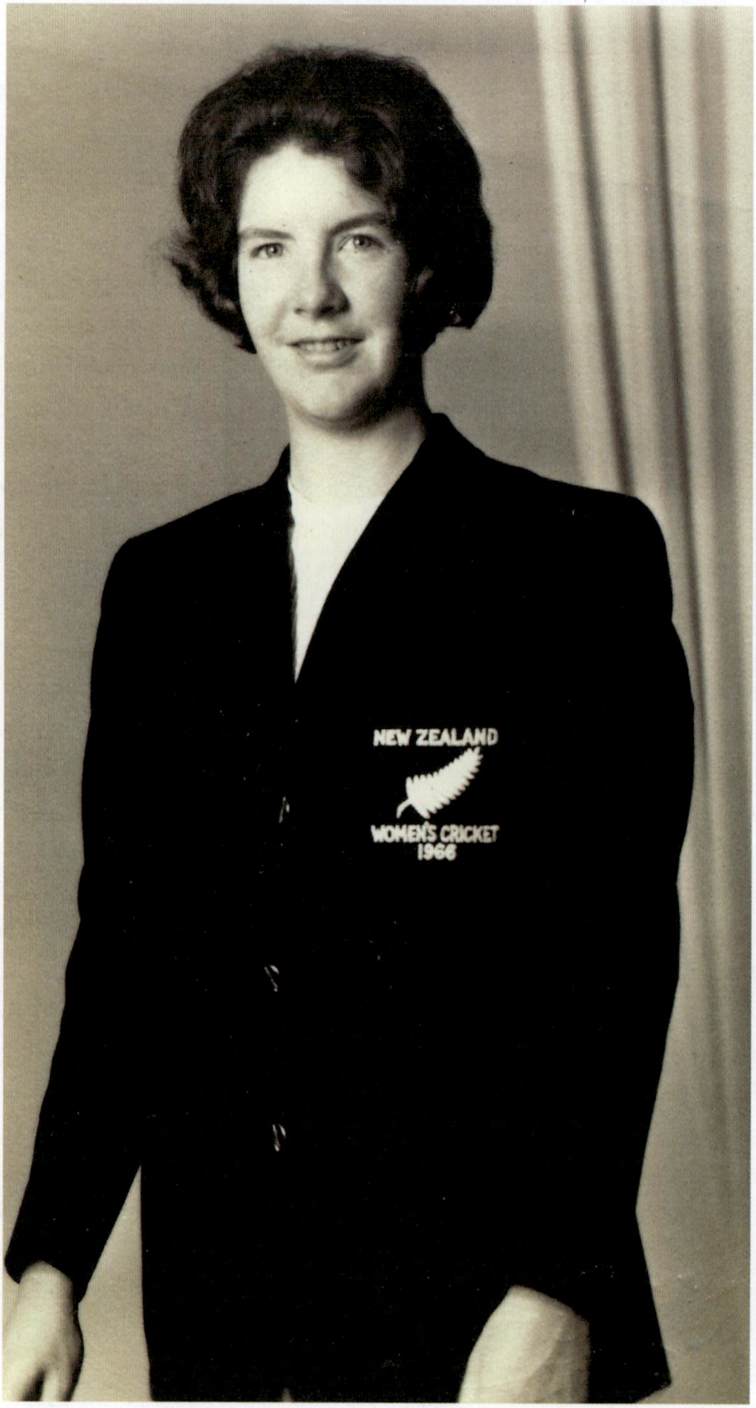

Wendy Hadden on the 1966 women's cricket tour. *Courtesy Wendy Hadden*

children, they moved to America for two years, where Hadden dedicated her time to being a mother. She then received a letter from Bryan Trenwith, director of radiology at Auckland Hospital, offering her a radiology registrar position. The family returned to Auckland, and she started as a radiology registrar at the end of 1974.

One of her radiology posts was at National Women's Hospital, which introduced her to obstetric work. During this time, the hospital introduced the first ultrasound scanners. Her assistant, whom the family called Auntie Howell, looked after the boys, and she would come home to find the ironing done and the meal cooked. 'Without her, I couldn't have managed. You need support. You can't do it alone.'[63] After her sons had grown up, Hadden increased her workload, working half-time at National Women's Hospital and half-time at Auckland Radiology. She retired on her seventieth birthday.

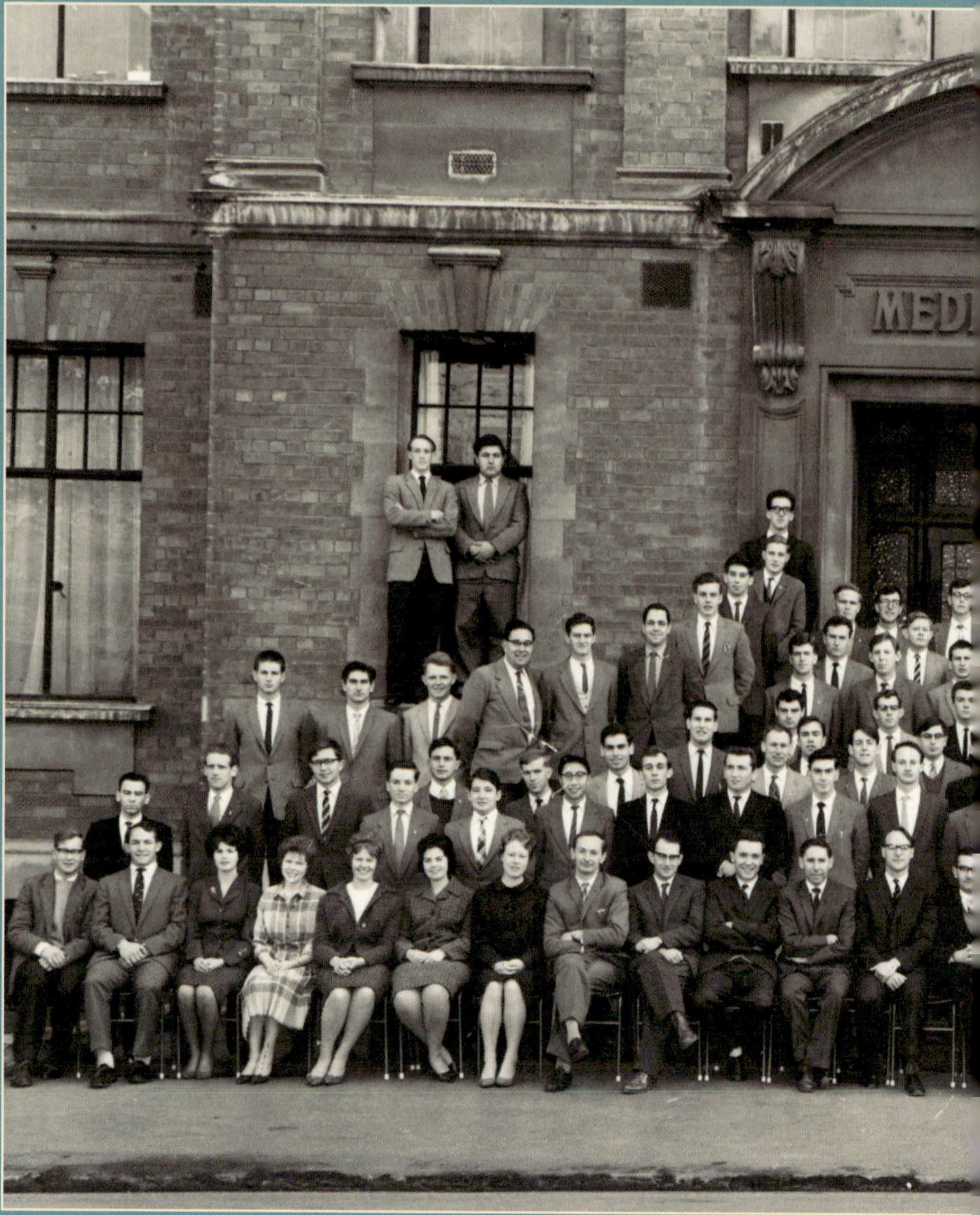

The third-year Otago Medical School class of 1962. Front row, from left: Dorothy Dowd (1965), Margaret Croxson (née Cunningham; 1965), Beth Synek (née MacGregor; 1965), Ann Steele (1965), M. A. Robertson, Noeline Butcher (1967), M. G. Jankovskis, L. V. Dwyer, Robin Briant (1965). Those for whom no dates are recorded either did not graduate or were members of staff. *Otago Medical School Archives*

7. Making their mark in research 1896–1967

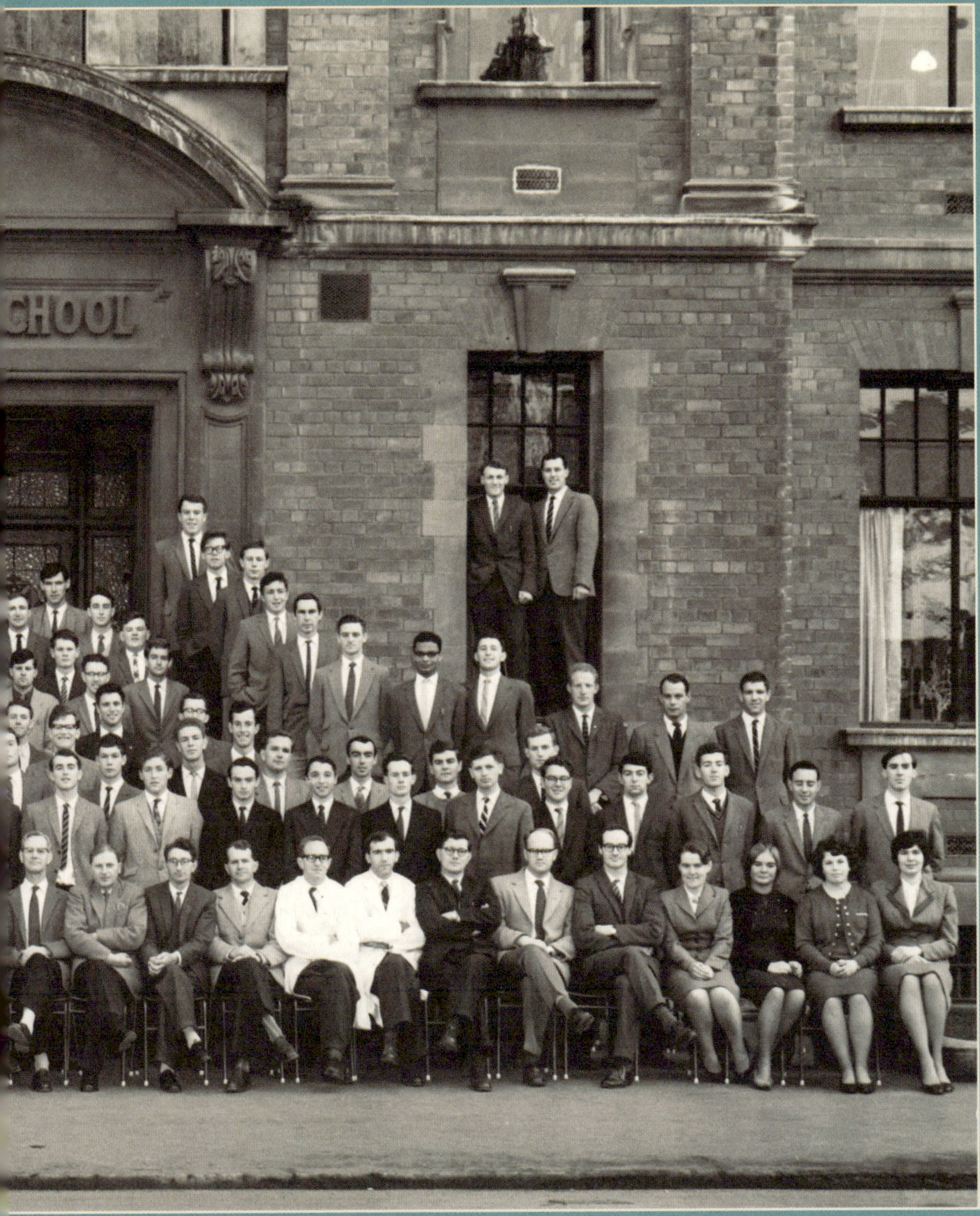

For Otago Medical School's 100th anniversary Gordon Parry was commissioned to write 'An Historical Sketch' of the school from 1875 to 1975. The monograph covers the foundation of the medical school and its expansion under the first three deans. The chapter dedicated to research at Otago Medical School focuses primarily on John Halliday Scott, Charles Hercus and Horace Smirk. In another chapter, 'Men Who Made Their Mark', Parry discusses how these same men 'championed' the state of medicine and paved the way for the future of research at the medical school. He concludes:

> Research. The word seemed for many years to be synonymous with Hercus; his encouragement was by example, and by the practical help of somehow finding money for projects . . The Dean's Fund, built up by Ferguson, was extensively used by Hercus, but what he gave most generously of all was his time and his understanding. His energy, skill, patience and leadership combined to make him one of the most important figures in the history of a School which has attracted and retained *so many men of distinction.*[1]

Parry neglected to mention the women who, during the same period, made their mark not only in the medical school but also beyond — even though, by the time he was writing his history, the first New Zealand-trained medical woman had achieved promotion to associate professorship at Otago Medical School. Many more had made their mark in New Zealand and had received a variety of accolades, including royal honours.

This chapter outlines how Otago Medical School produced women of distinction in research and academic medicine, and highlights some of the women who 'made their mark'. There was not enough room to include all the early medical women graduates who undertook research after graduation — in 1917, for example, Emily Siedeberg (1896) was appointed as anaesthetist to the dental school and lecturer on anaesthesia to dental students, and Shirley Tonkin (née Curtis; 1945) made substantial contributions to SUDI research. The focus here is on early women graduates who completed a postgraduate research thesis and were awarded an MD or PhD, and who worked in the research environment.

During the first three decades of Otago Medical School, teaching loads were heavy, salaries were low and most lecturers supplemented their wages with other work, usually in private practice. Moreover, staff numbers did not keep pace with the increase in student numbers, especially after the First World War. All this meant that staff had little time for research.[2]

There were, of course, exceptions. The staff member credited with making the largest difference to research at Otago Medical School was Charles Hercus,[3] who developed a programme of research and enlisted doctors to conduct field research. One of those was Eleanor McLaglan, who assisted Hercus with his early goitre research. McLaglan travelled around New Zealand to collect data for a survey, first throughout the South Island and then from districts as far away as Tauranga. The observations were conducted solely by McLaglan, to ensure the results remained as consistent and uniform as possible: she examined each child's neck while a teacher recorded one of four letters — L, M, S or O (large, medium, small or zero) — for the right, middle and left lobes of the thyroid. The result was a comprehensive map of incidences of goitre in New Zealand.

In 1937 the government established the Medical Research Council (MRC) in the Department of Health: its members included Hercus, Muriel Bell (1922) and John Malcolm. The department established committees to focus on various fields of research such as nutrition, cancer and obstetrics, and scholarships for students to conduct research and to bring 'stimulating visitors to the department'.[4] This increased funding meant more research could be undertaken and supported.

Hercus recognised the importance of introducing students to research during their medical training. In 1923 he added a new assignment to the curriculum for students in their fifth year at the medical school, in line with his stated policy: 'Unless the professor undertakes some research of his own, at the same time encouraging and stimulating his staff continually to do likewise, there will be no vitality in his department.'[5] In place of an examination on preventive medicine, students could complete a public health research project on a topic of their interest (although Hercus would sometimes assign topics based on his research requirements), and they could conduct their research in the summer break between the fourth and fifth year.[6]

Students wrote up their findings in a dissertation, which they then defended in front of the class. The research projects were extremely popular, and most students selected this option over the final examination. Many of these dissertations are still held in the University of Otago Medical School Library or Hocken Library Archives, and some were published in the *New Zealand Medical Journal*.[7]

These projects are remembered fondly by women medical graduates from this time, as it gave them their first experience in doing research. Helen Bichan, for example, used a holiday job in the casualty department at Dunedin Hospital to gather data for her dissertation — a project on wound healing, which later evolved into a larger project investigating how casualty departments operated nationwide. She was awarded a distinction in public health for her research.[8] Monica Lewis (née Moody; 1967) conducted research on burns in children; and Hendrika Waal-Manning researched the health camps designed for 'youngsters who have been deprived of fresh air and exercise and good nutrition'.[9] Meredyth Gunn and Marion Boock both undertook research on aspects of breastfeeding.

In 1926, Hercus also established a mid-degree research year that remains in place: the Bachelor of Medical Science (BMedSc).[10] Selected students could delay their medical studies by a year to focus on a research project under the supervision of one of the professors at the medical school. Some of the women who undertook this research year were Marianne Fillenz, Norma Restieaux, Hendrika Waal-Manning and Jocelyn MacKnight (1963). The success of the BMedSc led to the establishment of the MMedSc, which could lead to studying for a PhD or an MD.[11]

The MD was more popular, as it was tailored for a medical graduate and allowed for study and clinical work at the same time. In the early years of the programme, a candidate for an MD at the University of Otago was required to submit a thesis and pass written and oral examinations in one of the following subject groups: anatomy and physiology, surgery and anatomy, medicine and pathology, or public health and jurisprudence.

Seventeen of the early women graduates went on to complete an MD. For some, this was the beginning of a distinguished academic career; for others it was a requirement for specialty training. Margaret Cruickshank is the first graduate recorded as completing an MD, but there is no record of her thesis topic and her career was cut short by her early death. None of the women graduates from Otago Medical School completed a PhD at Otago in this period, but four completed PhDs overseas: Marianne Fillenz (Oxford University, 1955), Norma Kent (Cambridge University, 1955), Keitha Farmer (University of London, 1963) and Senga Whittingham (University of Melbourne, 1970).

At first there were no clear training routes for graduates who developed an interest in particular branches of medicine, as many of the specialty colleges had not been established. The Royal Australasian College of Physicians was founded in 1938; before that, New Zealand and Australian physicians had to seek membership in the Royal College of Physicians in Britain. Paediatricians in Britain did not have a separate college until 1996, when the Royal College of Paediatrics and Child Health was established; and the Australasian College of Physicians did not move to a separate paediatric identity from the Royal College of Physicians until 1998. The College of Pathologists of Australia was founded in 1956; before that, trainees in pathology were expected to do an MD as well as written papers.

SYLVIA GYTHA DE LANCEY CHAPMAN

1921 graduate

Sylvia Gytha de Lancey Chapman gained her MD in 1934 as part of her specialty training. Her research for her thesis on the subject of perinatal toxaemia laid the foundation for the discovery of the Rh factor.[12] She went on to have a distinguished career in New Zealand and Britain, including as part of a committee of inquiry into abortion in New Zealand (1936–37); offering advice that led to the establishment of the Family Planning Association (1936); being the first woman appointed to the senate of the University of New Zealand (1938); and fostering the establishment of the New Zealand Council of Organisations for Relief Service Overseas (1944). In Britain, she did clinical work and became the registrar of the newly formed College of General Practitioners. Sylvia Chapman died in 1995.

MURIEL EMMA BELL

1922 graduate

Muriel Emma Bell was the first of the women medical graduates to make their mark in research. She was born on 4 January 1898 on her parents' farm at Four Rivers Plain near Murchison, a pioneering environment where roads were scarce and rivers had to be forded on horseback. The Bells were a prominent family in the area. Nelson was a day-long journey away if there was a need for medical treatment, and accidents were often fatal. Bell's father, Thomas, taught himself medical and rudimentary surgical skills. He owned a set of surgical and dental tools and could set limbs, extract teeth and assist in emergency surgeries.[13]

Bell's brother, Leslie, was a medical student at the University of Otago when the First World War broke out. He interrupted his studies to serve with the New Zealand Medical Corps. When he heard that his sister had started university, he wrote to suggest that she study medicine. Bell wrote 'a very careful letter to her father asking what he thought of the idea. He was delighted and telegraphed his wholehearted approval.' In an interview later in life, she speculated that at the 'back of his ready consent was his own thwarted desire to be a doctor'.[14]

Muriel Bell graduated from Otago Medical School in 1922 and completed her MD in 1926: her thesis was titled 'Clinical Studies in Goitre Cases in New Zealand'. Her lab partner at medical school, Frances Preston, noted Bell's careful and particular approach to scientific method.[15] John Malcolm, professor of physiology, was a mentor and an inspiration to Bell, and she became interested in the nutritional research he established at Otago.

After she graduated, Malcolm offered Bell a position in his laboratory as assistant lecturer in physiology from 1923 until 1927.[16] At this stage in her career, as well as completing the MD she also published papers on metabolism and nutrition in some of the leading European journals of the time, including 'The Blood Sugar Level in Vitamin B(1) Deficiency', 'Cystine and Nephrotoxicity' and 'High-protein Diets and Acid-based Metabolism'.[17] After two stints overseas and some time working in pathology in Napier, Bell returned to Otago Medical School and continued with nutritional research as senior assistant in physiology and lecturer in experimental physiology from 1935 to 1940.

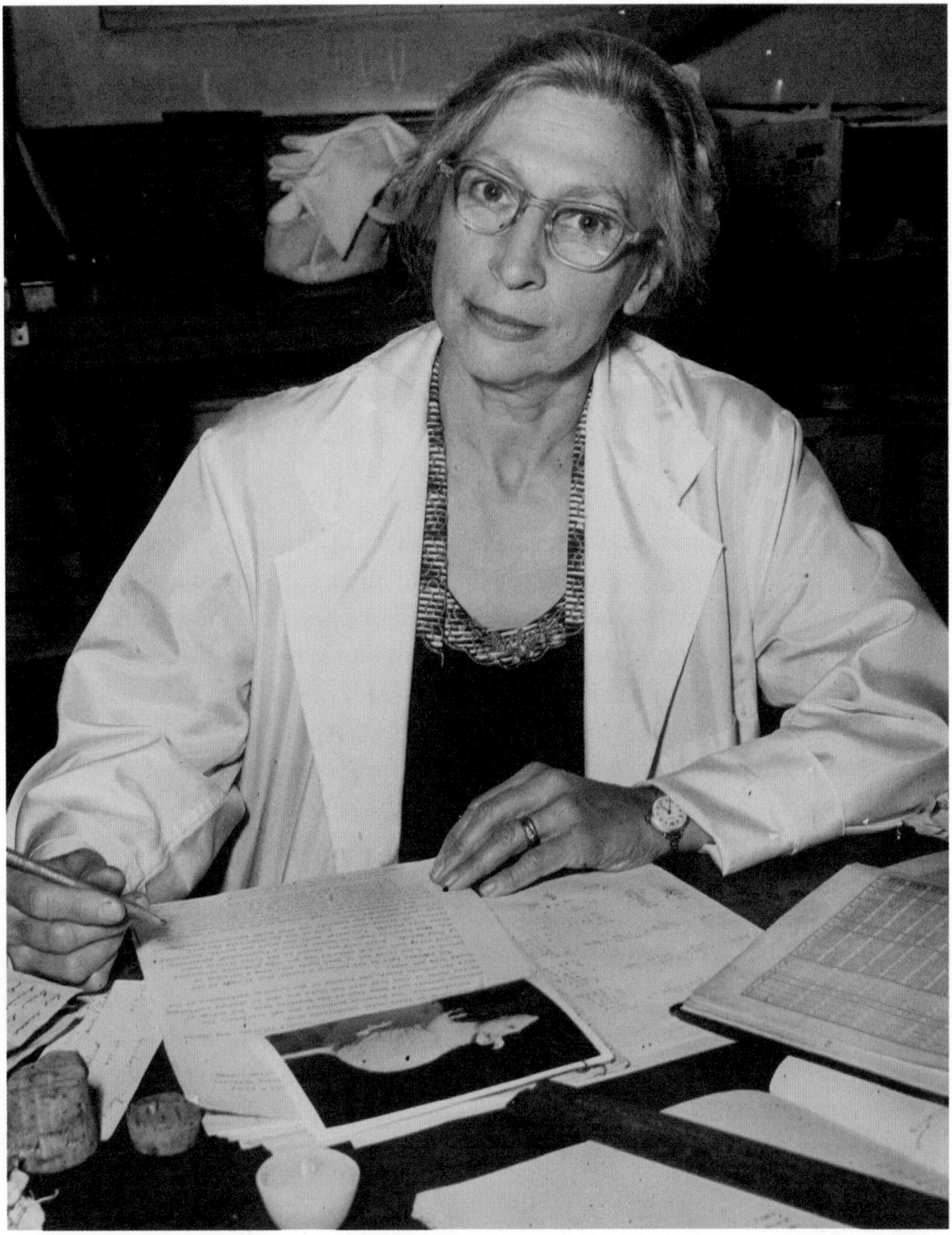

Muriel Bell, director of nutrition research, Otago Medical School, and state nutritionist, 1940–64. *Hocken Collections Uare Taoka o Hākena, MS-1078-111-003*

In 1938, Bell was appointed to the newly established Medical Research Council as a member of the nutrition research department, which was part of the Department of Health but based at Otago Medical School. In her role overseeing this department, Bell made major contributions to improving the health of New Zealanders, including implementing programmes such as the school milk scheme; making milk and butter affordable; and providing nutritional advice to Edmund Hillary's trans-Antarctic expedition. She also carried out nutrition surveys in Fiji and Sāmoa. In this role from 1940, she was listed in the university calendar as a research worker associated with the university but not listed as having an academic title.

+++

Towards the end of her career, Muriel Bell was the leading scientist advocating for fluoride to be added to town water supplies around the country. She was pivotal in educating the New Zealand public about nutrition through publications aimed at the general reader and in her regular columns in the *New Zealand Listener*. She edited *Good Nutrition Principles and Menus*, which was written for nurses, doctors and the general public. It included chapters on the scientific evidence for the nutritional advice provided by Otago home science graduates Elizabeth Gregory and Elizabeth Wilson, a chapter by John Malcolm on the digestion of food, as well as menus and recipes. It even gave recommended shopping lists.[18]

Bell married twice but had no children of her own. Her work was everything to her. She had an international reputation and travelled widely; she spent time on sabbatical at Harvard University as a research fellow in nutrition, and she visited the National Institute of Health Research institute in Bethesda, Maryland. She was the first medical woman graduate to receive an honorary degree from the University of Otago (DSc, 1968) and the first medical woman to be made a Fellow of the Royal Society (1952). She became a Fellow of the New Zealand Institute of Chemistry in 1941 and of the Royal Australasian College of Physicians in 1959, and that same year she was made Commander of the Order of the British Empire (CBE). The New Zealand Dental Association made her an honorary member for her work on fluoride.

Bell was a long-term member of the Nutrition Society of New Zealand, and each year, at their annual conference, a memorial public lecture is held in her name. The department of nutrition at the University of Otago awards the Muriel Bell

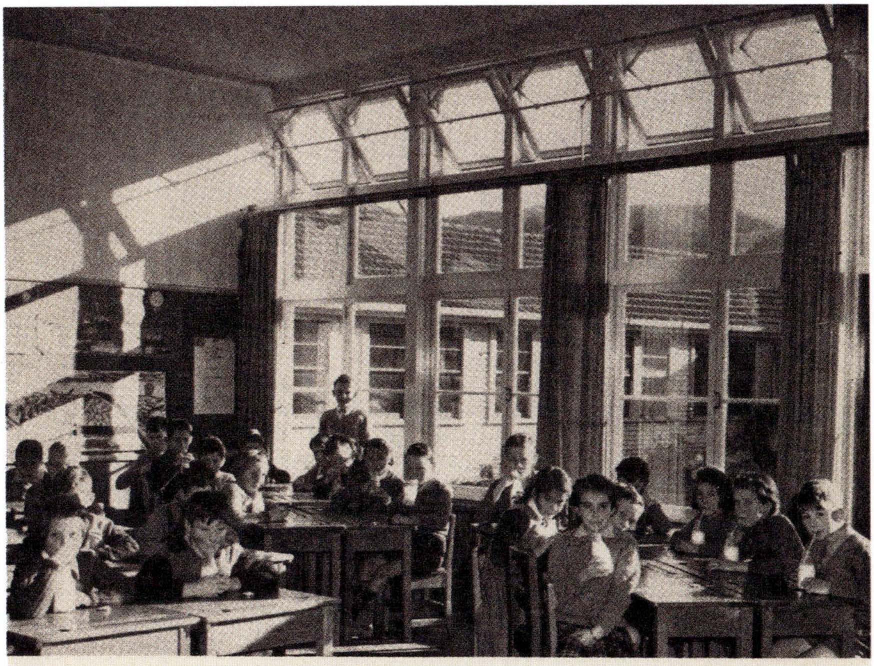

K. E. NIVEN PHOTO

MILK in Schools

ISSUED BY THE NEW ZEALAND MILK BOARD

'Milk in Schools', published by the New Zealand Milk Board, discussed the low levels of calcium in the New Zealand diet. Advocating for children's consumption of milk was a significant portion of Muriel Bell's role as state nutritionist. *Hocken Collections Uare Taoka o Hākena*

Memorial Prize annually to the 400-level undergraduate student who is 'judged to have achieved the highest standard of attainment in Human Nutrition'.[19] Muriel Bell died in May 1974.

HELEN DEEM (NÉE EASTERFIELD)

1924 graduate

In 1928, Helen Deem became the third woman graduate of Otago Medical School to be awarded an MD. Deem had science and research in her genes: her father, Thomas Easterfield, was the foundation professor of chemistry at Victoria University College and director of the Cawthron Institute in Nelson from 1919 to 1933.[20] Her sister Theodora Hall also studied medicine and graduated a year later. Deem initially worked as a house surgeon in Whanganui and Ōamaru. She was the first recipient of the Lady King Scholarship, set up to honour Isabella King, wife of Truby King, after her death in 1927.[21] She used the scholarship to study infant feeding and nutrition.

Her MD thesis, 'Observations on the Milk of New Zealand Women', was published in *Archives of Disease in Childhood* in 1931. While practising medicine in Whanganui she was appointed lecturer and honorary physician to the Stewart Karitane Home. In 1933 she became a member of the Plunket Society's newly formed medical advisory committee, which was set up to address concerns among paediatricians about some of the society's infant feeding recommendations.

After Deem's husband, John, died suddenly in 1933, she moved overseas for postgraduate studies in paediatrics. On her return to New Zealand, she worked initially as a school medical officer in the South Auckland Health District and as assistant to Harold Turbott in the Department of Health. She was appointed to the role of medical advisor of the Plunket Society in December 1938. At the time of her application for the role, she had testimonials from Turbott and from Michael Watt in the Department of Health, Dudley Carmalt-Jones of Otago Medical School, and Brian Corkill, a doctor who had been critical of Truby King's methods. Her Whanganui medical colleague Herbert Robertson also supported her application, saying she had a mind 'somewhat like her father, which was adapted to investigating and to research matters'.[22]

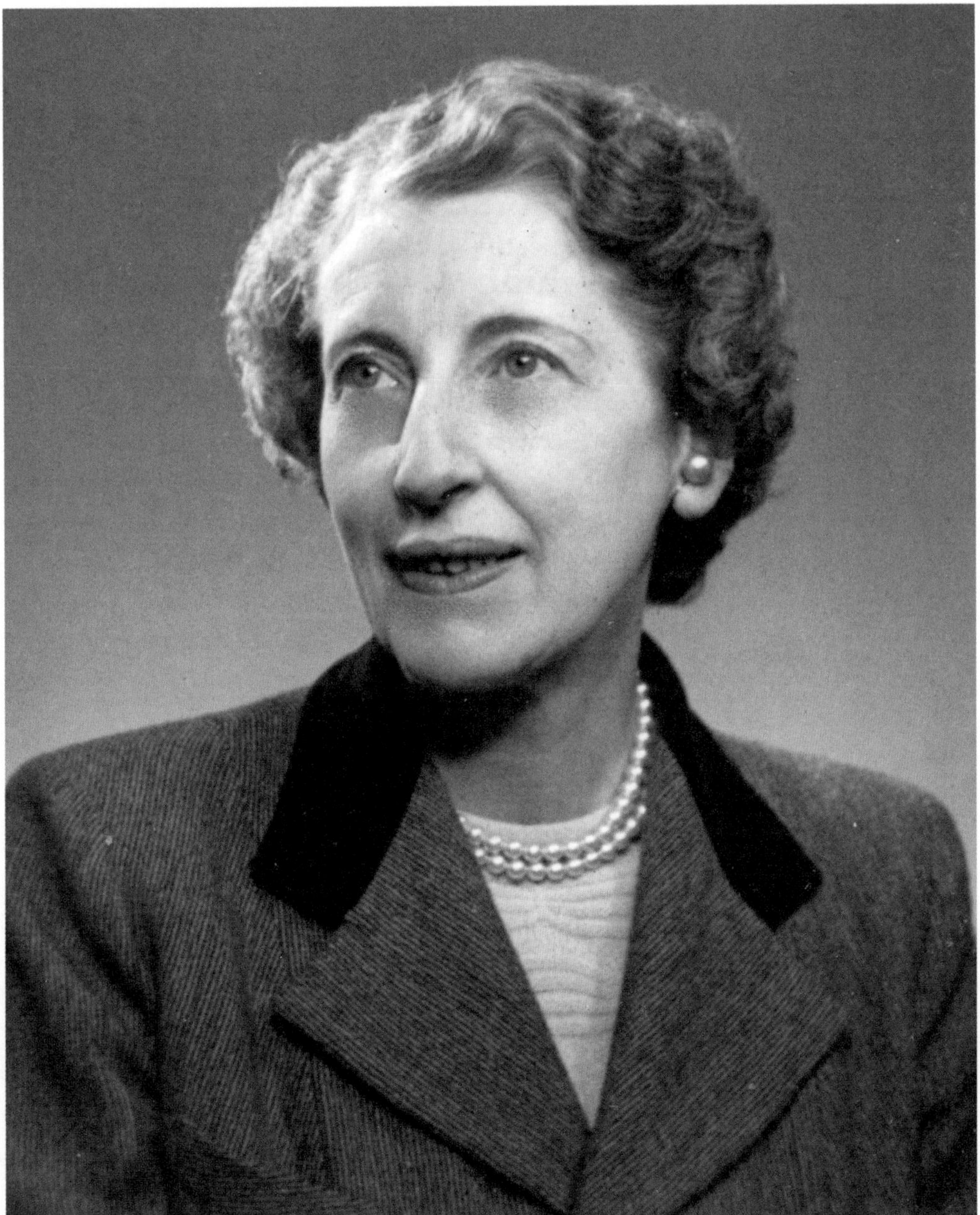

Helen Deem, doctor, medical officer, Plunket medical advisor and university lecturer, c.1950–55. *Alexander Turnbull Library, 1/2-190191-F*

Deem brought an evidence-based approach to the Plunket Society and an ability to work with paediatric colleagues who had become detractors of the society's work. Through her careful research, the growth of thousands of infants in Plunket care could be studied to determine what were described as 'satisfactory' growth curves. She wrote a new handbook for Plunket, *Modern Mothercraft: A Guide for Parents*, published in 1945, and a second edition in 1953. During her term at Plunket, Deem advocated for education for fathers, and she introduced antenatal classes. She later turned her attention to the preschool age group — she set up a preschool centre that opened in Dunedin in 1941 and still carries her name.

In 1946 she was appointed lecturer in preventive paediatrics at Otago Medical School, the first woman in a paediatric academic role. She introduced visits to Plunket centres for students as part of the medical curriculum so they could learn more about the care of infants. In 1952 Deem was appointed Officer of the Order of the British Empire (OBE) for services to child health. She died in 1955 at the age of 55 of lymphocytic leukaemia. Helen Deem has not remained as much of a household name as Truby King, but she can be credited with endeavouring to make the Plunket Society systems of the time evidence-based.

MARIE PAYNE BUCHLER (NÉE STRINGER)

1932 graduate

Marie Payne Buchler graduated from Otago Medical School in 1932. She was awarded the Lady King Fellowship by the University of Otago from 1935 to 1937 and used the award to carry out her MD research: the title of her thesis was 'An Analysis of 20,319 Obstetrical Case Records of the New Zealand Obstetrical and Gynaecological Society'. The study focused on stillbirths and neonatal deaths, as the Obstetrical and Gynaecological Society and the Plunket Society 'were anxious to know how much of this wastage of life was preventable'.[23]

This is a remarkable piece of audit research, done without modern methods of documentation to aid analysis. She advocated for postmortem diagnosis and examination of the placenta in these cases. Moreover, she advocated for the importance of determining the primary cause of death, for example, specifying pneumonia in a preterm infant rather than just putting it down to prematurity, which was a co-factor but not the reason for the death. These recommendations are still current for perinatal mortality review.

Marie married lawyer Arthur Buchler in 1934, and their first child was born in April 1936. With a small baby at home, Buchler resigned as honorary medical officer in Dunedin, and the family moved to New Plymouth, where two more daughters were born.[24] In 1941, Buchler joined the staff of the Department of Health in Wellington, and from then on she was based in Lower Hutt. Her main interest was child health, but she did some general practice and worked as a school medical officer in Petone. She was a vocal advocate for Montgomery Spencer's call for a review of the infant feeding recommendations of the day, espoused by the Plunket Society; she wrote three letters to Spencer in support of his stand.[25]

While she was working in the Department of Health, Buchler was involved in an important MRC-funded project on screening for tuberculosis: 2204 office and factory workers and secondary school children were screened using a chest X-ray. Buchler reported that the project found an incidence of active and inactive TB of 2.8 per cent: this showed that not all community cases of TB had been recognised clinically. The data collected from the project was published in the *New Zealand Medical Journal* in 1944.[26]

During her career, Buchler contributed her expertise and support to St John, the Speech Therapy Association and Plunket, but she did not further develop her research career. She seems to have had difficulty finding someone to help at home so she could continue with her work: she placed a number of advertisements seeking domestic help in the *Evening Post*, including one headed 'Wanted urgently!'.[27] Marie Buchler died in 1982.

MARY (MOLLY) JOYCE MARPLES

1944 graduate

Molly Marples completed her MD in 1951 on the topic 'Some Observations of the Distribution of the Fungi Pathogenic to Man'. She earned a BA and an MA in zoology at Oxford University before immigrating to New Zealand in 1937 with her husband, Brian, who had been appointed professor of zoology at the University of Otago. Marples had two young boys but was clearly ready for something new: she enrolled in Otago Medical School and graduated MB ChB in 1944. During her medical training, she completed a preventative medicine project on the topic 'A Survey of Ringworm in Dunedin'.

In 1946 Marples was appointed to the staff of the department of bacteriology and public health at Otago Medical School. This was the first appointment of a woman academic who was expected to teach and carry out research. Marples was greatly respected by her colleagues in what later became the department of microbiology at Otago.[28] She was involved in a major development in the department, whereby microbiology was taught to science students as well as medical students: the course, which Marples proposed and promoted, first became available to science students in 1949. She participated in several research expeditions to Western Sāmoa from 1950 to 1951 to research medical mycology; this was the basis of her MD thesis and her book, *The Ecology of the Human Skin* (1965). In 1969 she published an article on 'Life on the Human Skin' in *Scientific American.* Two articles co-written with her PhD student John (Sandy) Smith were published in *Nature.*

Unlike Muriel Bell, by the time Molly Marples was looking for an academic position after graduating, she was able to secure a position as assistant lecturer; she was promoted to associate professor in 1960 and retired in 1967. In 1981 Molly Marples was made an honorary member of the New Zealand Microbiology Society. Her wide influence is demonstrated in the April 2017 edition of the University of Otago alumni magazine cover story, which reports on the career of university alumnus Robert Webster, an international expert in avian flu. Webster, who initially was studying chemistry at Otago, reports that his early career path took an unexpected turn when Molly Marples spoke to the chemistry club in the microbiology department she was heading up: 'She talked about microbiology — micro-organisms, bacteria, viruses, yeasts — and captured me, as it were, to the idea of putting together chemistry, disease and animals. So, I moved my focus to microbiology.'[29] Molly Marples died in 1998.

HELEN RARITY MCCREANOR (NÉE YOUNG)

1947 graduate

Helen McCreanor graduated in 1947 with distinction in medicine and surgery. She worked as a house surgeon at Wellington Hospital until she married Jack McCreanor in 1949 — they had met at medical school.[30] They travelled to England, where she cared for their growing family.[31] When the family returned to New Zealand, McCreanor returned to work in the department of pathology at Wellington Hospital in 1966, where she was encouraged to establish a medical genetics unit. McCreanor completed her MD later in her career, in 1972, titled 'Studies in the Human Karyotype: A Contribution to the Study of Robertsonian Translocation in Man'.

She did not continue in research but spent the rest of her career focused on clinical work. She was greatly respected by her peers and was admitted as a Fellow of the Royal Australasian College of Physicians in 1977.[32] After her death in 1979 at the age of 55, Jack McCreanor endowed funds to the Royal Australasian College of Physicians to establish the Dr Helen Rarity McCreanor Travelling Fellowship to support postgraduate research and training in human genetics.

BARBARA FARNSWORTH HESLOP (NÉE CUPIT)

1948 graduate

Barbara Heslop graduated from Otago Medical School in 1948 and went on to have an impressive research and academic career.[33] From 1950 she was assistant lecturer in the University of Otago pathology department, and during this time she completed her MD (1954). She then moved to Britain with her husband, John, to pursue postgraduate studies: she held a research position in the paediatric pathology department at Great Ormond Street Hospital, and John did surgical training.[34] They arrived back in New Zealand in 1957 with a new baby.

With the support of her mother-in-law, Heslop took on a part-time role in the

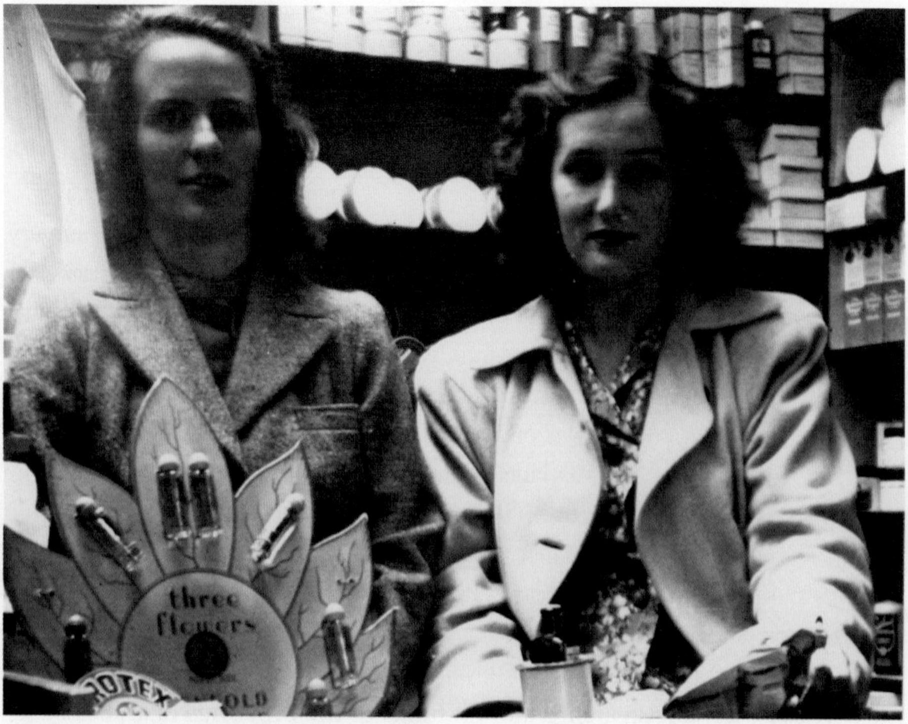

Barbara Heslop (right) and Patricia Mackay (née Wilson; 1948) in a Dunedin shop after completing their end-of-year exams, c.1947. *Courtesy Helen and Hilary Heslop*

---

pathology department at the University of Otago and, the following year, became a senior research officer in the department of surgery, working in the transplantation research group with Norman Nisbet. In 1964 she became head of the research group, and she remained in this role until her retirement in 1990. She was promoted to associate professor in 1972 and to professor in 1984 — the first medically qualified woman to achieve these milestones in the department of surgery.

While Heslop was well known for her research, which was funded by the MRC and widely published, she became somewhat of an icon in Australasian medical postgraduate circles by convening the postgraduate training programme for the Royal Australasian College of Surgeons (RACS), a role she took over in 1978 from John Borrie, who had started the course only a year earlier. Under her leadership, the course maintained a high reputation and was considered a 'must-do' for all surgical trainees; it is still running in the department of surgery to this day. In his survey of medical research at the Otago Medical School, Ted Nye argued that Barbara Heslop was 'without doubt the most influential non-surgeon investigator within the Department'.[35] She had an international reputation that resulted in her being flown around the world to give lectures, and she 'nurtured hundreds of aspiring young surgeons' through her courses.[36]

In 1975 she was made a Fellow of the Royal Australasian College of Surgeons for her contribution to surgical science. She was the second female medical graduate to be made a Fellow of the Royal Society of New Zealand (1990), and in 1991 she was appointed Commander of the Order of the British Empire (CBE) for services to medical education. In recognition of the work of both Barbara and John Heslop, the RACS has awarded the Heslop Medal since 2004 to 'a person who has made a long-term and outstanding contribution to the surgical science and clinical examinations committee and its subcommittees'.[37] Since 2014, the Barbara Heslop Memorial Scholarship has been available at Otago Medical School to assist students in undertaking one-year research degrees such as a BMedSc (Hons), BSc (Hons) and BBiomedSc (Hons) in the disciplines of pathology or immunology. Barbara Heslop died in 2013.

MARIANNE FILLENZ

1948 graduate

Marianne Fillenz was born in Romania in 1924 but came to New Zealand with her family in 1939. She graduated with a BMedSc from the University of Otago in 1946.[38] Her first paper, 'Acetylcholine and Neuro-muscular Transmission', was based on her BMedSc research and co-authored by her former classmate Mary Coldham (née Hanafin; 1948); it was published in 1947 in the *Journal of Neurophysiology*. Fillenz graduated in 1948, and in 1949 the *Press* announced that she was living in Christchurch and would be placing her name on the medical register.[39]

This may have just been until she received confirmation of being admitted to Oxford University for postgraduate study. John Eccles, a professor at Otago Medical School, had recognised her talent for science research and recommended that she go to Oxford to study for a DPhil. She arrived in Oxford in 1950 and soon after met her husband, John Clarke, an Australian Rhodes Scholar. They married in 1951.

For her DPhil, Fillenz studied receptors responding to stretch of the eye muscles; her thesis supervisors were Sybil Cooper and David Whitteridge.[40] She then spent nine years as a lecturer at St Hilda's College Oxford and a demonstrator in the physiology laboratory at Oxford University while she continued her research.[41] She was one of the first people to use and further develop the technique of voltammetry to measure the release of the neurotransmitter catecholamine deep in the brain. In 1963, she won a tutorial fellowship at St Anne's College, and she remained based there throughout her time at Oxford.

She had a remarkable career as a physiologist with a focus on the anatomy and physiology of the autonomic nervous system. In 1990, she published an important book, *Noradrenergic Neurons*, which examines the mechanisms regulating the release and synthesis of noradrenaline, a neurotransmitter important in the stress response. She was highly respected by students and colleagues alike and a role model for women students.

Marianne Fillenz was the first woman to be appointed as a university lecturer in physiology at Oxford. On her retirement from this position in 1992, she was made senior research fellow in recognition of her ongoing work. In 2000, she was awarded a DSc by the Faculty of Physiological Sciences for her research output. In 2003, she published *Neuroscience: Science of the Brain: An Introduction for Young Students*. On PubMed there are 141 publications in her name, including 33 as first author. The *Guardian* obituary for her husband, written by her children, highlighted his support of her career; this was noted as being different to other academic fathers.[42] It is fitting that her last published paper in 2012 in the *Journal of the History of Neurosciences* was titled 'Memories of John Eccles' — her first research mentor. She died later that year.

In January 2018, the inaugural Marianne Fillenz Memorial Lecture was hosted in the department of physiology, anatomy and genetics at the University of Oxford. The presenters since then have all been at the level of professor — a title of which Marianne Fillenz would have been more than worthy.

RUTH MITCHELL (NÉE ADAMS)

1949 graduate

Ruth Mitchell entered Otago Medical School in 1944, along with 10 other women. She earned her BMedSc in 1946 in the department of anatomy, and then returned to do fourth-year medicine. Her thesis involved a microscopic analysis of the connections in the midbrain of the tuatara. During her university years, Mitchell was interested in mountain climbing. In the summer of 1947, she was climbing in the Mount Cook region when she had a serious accident, falling 20 metres. She suffered head and facial injuries, multiple fractures of her left elbow and a lumbar spine fracture. For three nights, Edmund Hillary, who was a member of the hiking party, sat with her until a rescue could be organised. A dominant left-hander, she had to learn to write with her right hand.

Despite a disrupted year in 1947 as a consequence of this accident, she managed to pass her final examinations and completed her sixth year of training in Christchurch, graduating in 1949.[43] In 1950 she married Robert Mitchell, and in 1952 they travelled to England, where she completed a Diploma of Child Health at Great Ormond Street Hospital. Although Mitchell was contemplating further training in paediatrics, she felt that a career might not be compatible with her desire to be a mother. The family returned to Dunedin, where she was a lecturer in anatomy at the medical school. In 1959 they moved to Australia, and Mitchell became a lecturer in anatomy at the University of Queensland. Here she developed her interest in the electron microscope, studying skin pigmentation and the melanocyte.

In 1963, now with three children, the family moved to the United States, where Robert had been awarded a Carnegie Fellowship to study renal transplantation. Mitchell was awarded a fellowship and lectureship at Harvard University in the dermatology department at Massachusetts General Hospital, where she continued her study of melanocytes. The family returned to Queensland in 1965, then moved to Hobart in 1967. She continued her research there and completed her MD in 1968: her thesis was titled 'The Effect of Prolonged Solar Irradiation on the Human Skin'.

She was appointed lecturer in the pathology department at the University of Tasmania, and when the family moved to Sydney in 1977, she was appointed senior lecturer in pathology at the University of New South Wales and specialist pathologist at St George Hospital. Here she continued with general pathology and electron microscopy and designed the electron microscopy unit. She resigned from these positions because of ill health in 1989 and died in 1990. She leaves a record of 17 publications.

SENGA WHITTINGHAM

1953 graduate

Senga Whittingham went into a full-time career in research without an initial MD qualification; she later completed a PhD in Melbourne, Australia, in 1970.[44] In 1958, she moved to Melbourne to work for the Red Cross, which at that time had research laboratories. She worked under Rachel Jakobowitz, who had trained in Berlin as a scientist, and Whittingham acknowledges that this was where she learned about scientific methods. Her first project was in Rh disease, where she identified a case of autoagglutinin as well as pan-hemagglutinin.

This led her to a Diploma in Clinical Pathology in England. She worked at Hammersmith Hospital after her course and then returned to Melbourne, where she obtained a position as senior research fellow and honorary assistant physician to Ian Mackay, head of the Clinical Research Unit in Melbourne, a joint initiative between the Walter and Eliza Hall Institute of Medical Research and the Royal Melbourne Hospital. Between 1965 and 1991, with Mackay, Whittingham carried out important research in autoimmune diseases in a unit comprising research laboratories attached to a 27-bed ward at the Royal Melbourne Hospital.

During this time, she was also a committee member and international advisor for World Health Organization and the Royal College of Pathologists of Australasia (RPCA), chief examiner for Immunology RCPA and associate editor of the RCPA journal *Pathology*. Throughout her career, Whittingham published over 150 research papers.

TATIANA (TANIA) ROBERTA GUNN (NÉE TARULEVICZ)

1955 graduate

Tania Gunn graduated from Otago Medical School in 1955.[45] She completed her MD later in her career, in 1989, through the Auckland School of Medicine. She gained experience in research and teaching during her residency at Montreal Children's Hospital, which led to a position as lecturer in the department of pediatrics at McGill University, Montreal, as well as acting director of the Neonatal Follow-Up Clinic at the Montreal Children's Hospital.[46] While there, Gunn co-authored papers with renowned researchers such as Gordon Power and Percy Pease.[47] In 1975 she became a Fellow of the Royal College of Physicians and Surgeons of Canada, and she gained her American Board of Pediatrics certification and Neonatal–Perinatal certification.

One of Gunn's postdoctoral positions was with Jacob Aranda at McGill. Her research focus was on caffeine: she demonstrated that its use significantly decreased the need for and duration of mechanical ventilation in low-birthweight babies because it improved the regularity of their breathing. She published a paper on this research, titled 'Sequelae of Caffeine Treatment in Preterm Infants with Apnea', in the *Journal of Pediatrics* in 1979; Aranda acknowledged the contributions of three fellows at McGill, including Tania Gunn, to research on the use of caffeine citrate to treat apnoea of prematurity, which was recognised by the American Academy of Pediatrics Neonatal Landmark Award in 2022. Gunn also completed work on risk factors in retrolental fibroplasia (an eye disease related to prematurity), and she published a letter in the prestigious *Lancet* journal on the incidence of this condition.

Gunn returned to New Zealand and continued to carry out research while working at St Helens Hospital in Auckland. From 1979 to 1989, she was also honorary senior lecturer in the department of paediatrics at the University of Auckland, where she published with researchers such as Peter Gluckman and Shirley Tonkin in a range of areas. Her MD thesis was titled 'Responses of the Fetal Lamb to Alternations of the Thermal Environment in Utero'. In 1990, she retired from fulltime clinical work but continued with research, and she was made honorary associate professor in the department of paediatrics at the University of Auckland; this was upgraded to honorary professor in 1999.[48]

One of her most important research achievements came during this period

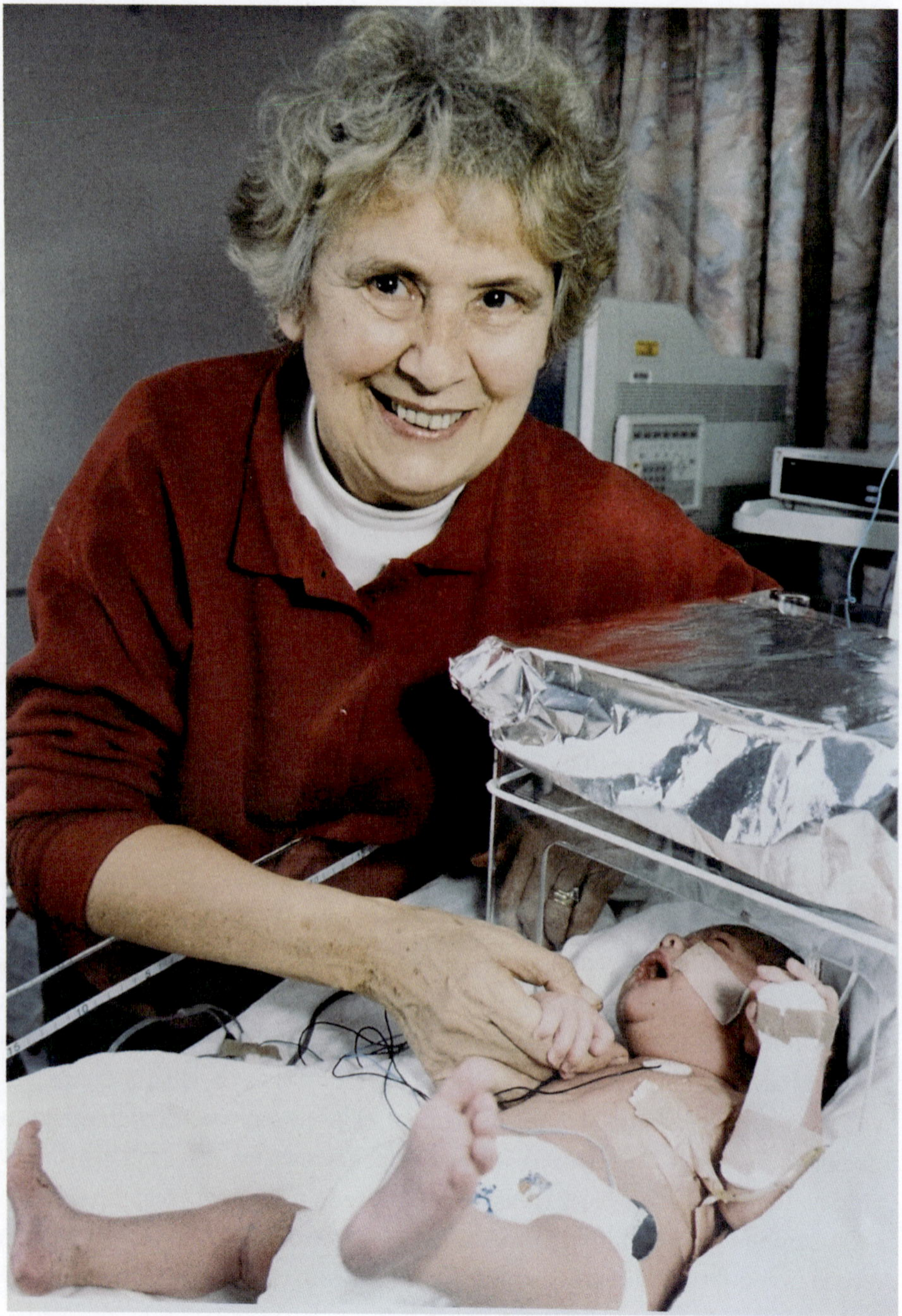

Tania Gunn with a young patient, c.1989. *Courtesy Alistair Gunn*

in collaboration with her son Alistair, also a paediatrician and professor of physiology at the Auckland School of Medicine. He had started to think about the effects of temperature on neonatal outcomes and discussed this with his mother, who had experience in cooling animals from her own research. Together, they developed this research idea in an animal model and later they conducted the first-ever randomised pilot study of head cooling for infants with birth asphyxia. Further research studies replicated positive findings for infant outcomes, and this management is now standard treatment worldwide for infants exposed to birth asphyxia. Tania Gunn died in 1999.

NGAIRE MARGARET WALSH (NÉE MCKERROW)

1956 graduate

Ngaire Walsh did well at medical school and was always among the top students.[49] She graduated first with a BSc in physiology in 1952, then MB ChB in 1956 and MD in 1963. She was awarded the Lady King Scholarship in 1959 and 1961 and used it to undertake data collection for her MD thesis, titled 'Nutritional State and Serum Cholesterol Levels in Relation to Normal Feeding Regimes in the First Year of Life'. Walsh married in 1963. In 1964–68, while she was looking after her two small children, she held various part-time and relieving clinical posts at Dunedin Hospital. She was president of the Dunedin branch of the Medical Women's Association, and during her tenure a working party under the leadership of Barbara Heslop documented the professional activity of medical women in New Zealand; the results were published in the *New Zealand Medical Journal* in 1973.[50]

This group contributed to the political discussion that resulted in the medical reserve scheme, which provided medical employment opportunities for a small number of women with family commitments. In 1970, Walsh was appointed part-time lecturer in anatomy and histology for medical and home science students at the University of Otago. In 1975 her health deteriorated and she resigned from this role as she required cardiac surgery. From then on, she worked more in a voluntary capacity and was involved in the natural family planning movement both in New Zealand and overseas. Ngaire Walsh died in 1982.

HENDRIKA JACOBA WAAL-MANNING

1957 graduate

In the late 1930s, Horace Smirk was appointed to the medical school and argued strongly for an increase in staff and an upgrade of laboratory facilities.[51] His specific focus was on hypertension research: he set up a clinic to further this research, which developed an international reputation.[52] Hendrika Waal-Manning was one of his long-term employees; she worked for the clinic until it closed in 1992. She had completed a BMedSc degree during her medical student years and, after graduation, wanted to work in pharmacology so she returned to the university to train with Fred Fastier and Gary Blackman. After this she joined Smirk's team as a medical research officer.

Her research into beta blockers and various treatments for hypertension was published widely and in 1972 she submitted her MD thesis on her research work undertaken in the clinic.[53] The thesis runs to 137 pages with 32 appendices, all her own papers, including research articles, review articles and letters to the editor. Journal searches indicate 90 publications, with 56 as first author. Although they did not overtly acknowledge this with accolades, her male professorial colleagues must have felt very fortunate to have her on the research team.

She was promoted to the title of senior medical research officer but not associate professor, a promotion that should have been awarded given her publication record. In 1992, the clinic closed, and Waal-Manning found herself with neither a job nor an offer of reassignment elsewhere in the university (something her male colleagues allegedly received) despite her substantial contribution to the outputs of this world-renowned research team. She then retrained in general practice and worked as a locum in Port Chalmers, Dunedin, and Alexandra. She retired in 2004 and died in Alexandra in 2022.

JUDITH CHERRY WARDILL (NÉE SMITH)

1957 graduate

Judith Cherry Wardill graduated MB ChB in 1957 and completed her MD in 1964 as part of her training in pathology. The title of her MD thesis was 'Pathology of Human Aortic Valve Homografts'. She was a fellow in pathology at the Mayo Clinic in the United States from 1967 to 1969. On her return to New Zealand, she did part-time clinical work in Russell and Ashburton, and from 1971 to 1974 she worked as a histopathologist at Wellington Hospital. She then moved to the Waikato, where she worked until the end of her career. She had some early publications but focused on a clinical rather than a research career.

PATRICIA MARIE BUCKFIELD

1958 graduate

Patricia Buckfield graduated in 1958 and completed her MD in 1979. Her thesis, 'The Physical Status of New Zealand Infants at Birth and Delineation of Factors Affecting Status', runs to two volumes of 246 and 171 pages, respectively. After house surgeon years and two years as a registrar, she was granted a Department of Health bursary for overseas study. Her time in England from January 1964 to March 1967 included six months of training in neonatal medicine. In April 1967 she returned to Dunedin to a joint clinical/academic role as lecturer with the department of paediatrics and child health at Otago Medical School and as a paediatrician for the Otago Hospital Board.

In 1967 Jim Watt was appointed the first-ever chair of paediatrics and child health in New Zealand at Otago Medical School, and Buckfield became his first staff member. Neonatal intensive care for preterm infants had been established in Dunedin by Donald Malcolm, senior lecturer and later associate professor. When Buckfield arrived in the department, she brought expertise in the use of ventilators for infants with neonatal respiratory disease, and she led the introduction of this technique to New Zealand. She was concerned that while it was one thing to improve neonatal care and decrease perinatal morbidity related to prematurity, it was also important to understand what happened to these infants after discharge.

She studied all the births at Queen Mary Hospital in Dunedin from 1967 to 1973 and recorded the obstetric, perinatal and neonatal histories of more than 10,000 babies and their mothers. This data was documented in her MD thesis and in a paper published in the *New Zealand Medical Journal* in 1978. A successful application to the MRC followed, with a proposal to study 250 four- to five-year-olds born in 1968, half of whom had experienced perinatal problems and half who had not. This study was known as the Queen Mary Multidisciplinary Child Development Study, and Phil Silva was engaged to do the psychological testing.[54] Further publications came from this research. An unexpected finding was that many of the children who did not appear to have risk factors had developed problems early in life. A broader study was therefore planned to investigate a wider range of issues related to children's health and development.

In 1982 Buckfield left her joint clinical academic role and moved to Wellington to take on the role of director of the Puketiro Centre in Porirua, where she worked full-time as a developmental paediatrician. This became her main area of interest, and she did not undertake further substantive research. She died in 1995, just two months short of her 61st birthday, from a haematological malignancy.

Buckfield made her mark on paediatric medicine in New Zealand in two important ways. First, she brought modern neonatal intensive care expertise to New Zealand. Second, she asked pertinent questions about what problems at-risk infants might have as they moved through childhood. This started a chain of multidisciplinary research projects that has now become known as the Dunedin Study, a research programme that has continued since this time and is known about and respected by researchers worldwide.

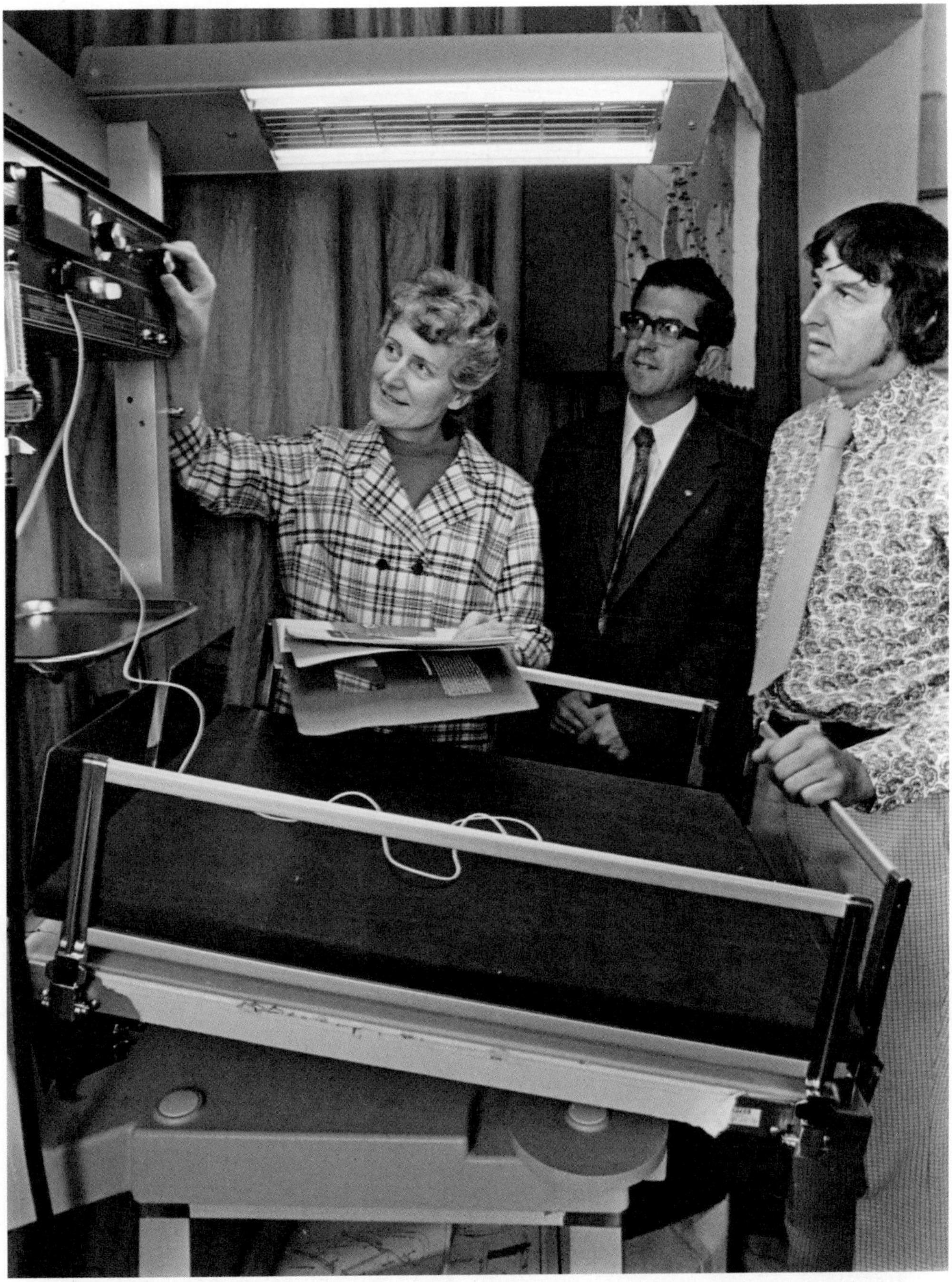

Patricia Buckfield, head of the baby care unit at Queen Mary Hospital, explains the working of a new neonatal unit, donated by the Kiwanis service organisation, to vistors in 1975. *Otago Daily Times*

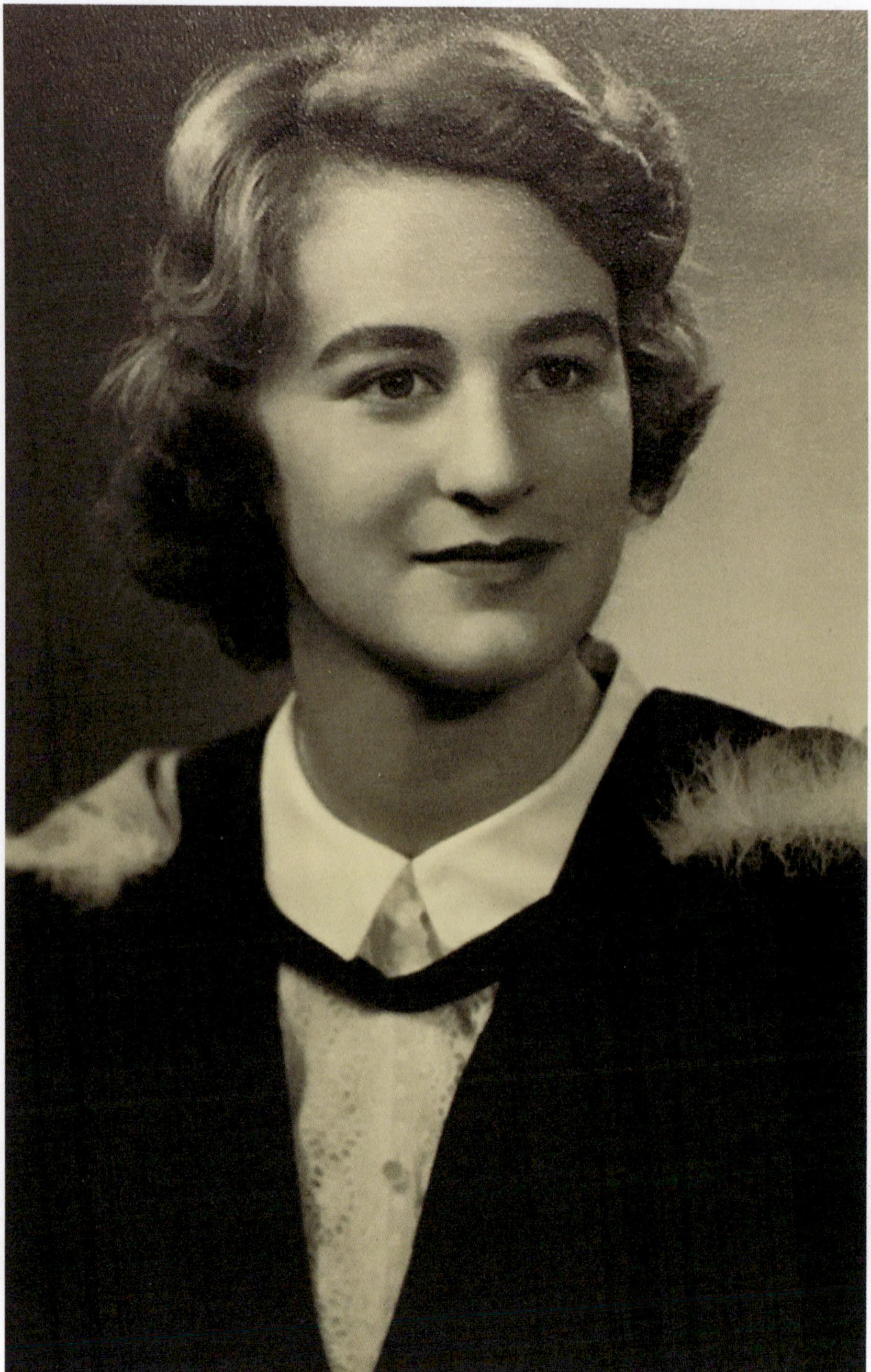

Elizabeth Berry on her graduation from Otago Medical School in 1960. *Courtesy Elizabeth Berry*

ELIZABETH BERRY (NÉE WAUGH-BURNS)

1960 graduate

Elizabeth Berry graduated from Otago Medical School in 1960.[55] She worked in Christchurch in pathology while completing the written examination. She moved to Boston with her husband, who was also a doctor, and trained for two years in haematology at Boston City Hospital. They then moved to Edinburgh, where she worked as a lecturer in haematology at Western General Hospital while she completed the research for a thesis titled 'Cytogenetics of Myeloproliferative Disorders and Other Potentially Leukaemic States'; this was part of her training in her chosen specialty, pathology. After achieving her MD she went to Oxford University, where her research focused on blood coagulation and the management of haemophilia.

When Berry and her husband returned to New Zealand in 1970, it was frustrating to find that her MD qualification was now not required; instead, she was expected to sit and pass two college exams. Luckily, her time overseas prepared her well. She decided not to have children while still training; when children did arrive, haematology was an area where she could have some work flexibility. Berry played a key role in establishing and then directing the first Haemophilia Centre in New Zealand at Auckland City Hospital.[56] She retired in 2002.

NORMA RESTIEAUX

1960 graduate

Norma Restieaux chose to do a BMedSc project during her medical training, as she was interested in research: her thesis was titled 'A Microelectric Study of the Reticular Cells of the Dogfish, *Squalus lebruni*'.[57] She then continued her medical studies and graduated in 1960. After her early postgraduate years, she moved to London to specialise in cardiology. Most of her initial research during this period focused on adults. She passed the Royal College of Physicians exam in 1965 and then moved to Boston, where she took up a position at Boston Children's Hospital.

Here, she expanded her knowledge of cardiology in paediatrics and presented her research at various conferences. Her experience paved the way for other trainee New Zealand doctors to travel to Boston and train at the Children's Hospital.[58]

When she returned to New Zealand in 1970, she took up a position as lecturer at Otago Medical School, teaching mainly students in years four to six. She also worked as a consultant cardiologist, and in 1975 she was appointed head of the cardiology department at Dunedin Hospital. She submitted her MD in 1973 as a monograph titled 'Vectocardiography in Congenital Heart Disease: A Method for Estimating Severity'. She co-authored this with R. Curtis Ellison and, on submission, stated clearly which chapters of the book were her original work.

Restieaux was promoted to associate professor in 1977, one of the first women graduates working both clinically and in research to be promoted to this level. She was an excellent teacher and took the role of mentor seriously, especially for women students and trainees. She notes in her biography that during her final medical school years she appreciated seeing Molly Marples and Barbara Heslop already in teaching roles.

In 1991, Restieaux became the first female president of the New Zealand Medical Association, and in 1992 she was appointed Dame Commander of the Order of the British Empire (DBE) for her contribution to medicine and, in particular, cardiology. In 2000 she was the first New Zealand woman to be elected president of the Royal Australasian College of Physicians, and she held important roles in the college for many years, including as chair of the examining board. She was chair of the medical admission committee of the University of Otago, and she made her mark as one of the first female joint clinical academics at Otago Medical School. She excelled in all the requirements of her role — teaching, research, service and clinical practice — and she set very high standards for those students who aspired to follow in her footsteps.

ROBIN BRIANT

1965 graduate

Robin Briant graduated in 1965 and completed her MD in 1973 while working at Hammersmith Hospital in London.[59] Before going to medical school, she had started

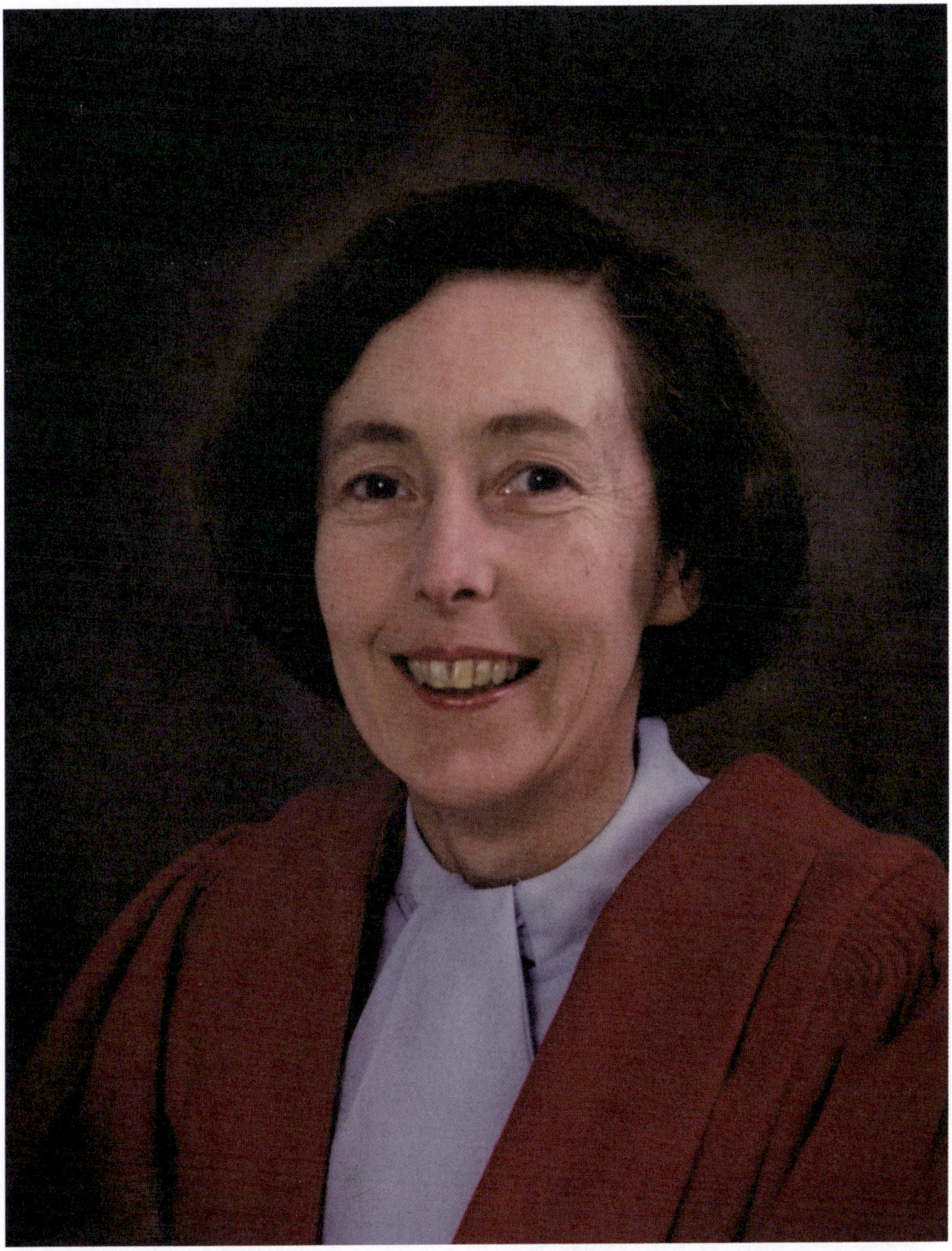

Norma Restieaux in 1981. *Hocken Collections Uare Taoka o Hākena, MS-1537/180*

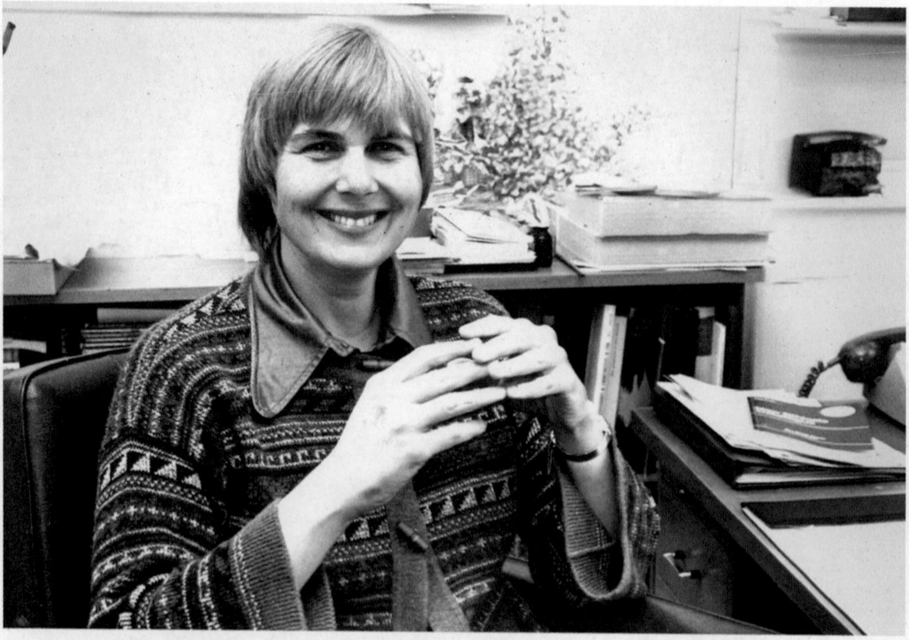

Robin Briant at her medical school desk in 1974. *Courtesy Robin Briant*

training to be a technician in a local laboratory, so she already had some practical science experience. The topic of her MD was 'Metabolism of Isoetherine and Other Bronchodilators in Man and Dog'. The opportunity to do this research arose when she was offered a position at Hammersmith in a well-resourced research team with an experienced leader in Colin Dollery, a clinical pharmacologist who provided good mentorship.

After returning to New Zealand, she took up positions at Auckland Hospital and the University of Auckland, starting as a clinical lecturer in 1974 before being promoted to associate professor in clinical pharmacology. In 1980, she recognised that she preferred lecturing over researching and so decided to drop the research component of her academic career in favour of her many other clinical and teaching interests.[60] Despite this, she published over 40 papers throughout her career.

She later made an important contribution as chair of the New Zealand Medical Council, the first woman in this role, and was awarded a CBE for her services to medicine. By 1999 Briant had given up most of her employment when she was approached by Peter Davis from the School of Population Health at the

University of Auckland to take on the role of clinical director of a public health quality and improvement study throughout New Zealand. The study took two years to complete and remains a landmark study of adverse events in New Zealand hospitals. Although Robin Briant moved on from a research role mid-career, she continued to use those skills throughout the rest of her working life.

There is no doubt the medical women whose stories are told in this book were capable of producing high-quality science, yet many of them did not get the recognition they deserved. Only Barbara Heslop and Beryl Howie were ever promoted to the level of professor during their careers — Howie's promotion was in 1962 in Ludhiana, India, and was more related to her teaching role; and Heslop's was in 1984 in Otago — the only woman graduate to achieve this in New Zealand. Tania Gunn was promoted to honorary professor in semi-retirement. Many failed to get senior academic appointments in the way that we would expect today — and yet they worked with scores of professors over the years, some of whom may have had less distinguished publication and research records.

Even today, with higher numbers of women now in medical school than ever before, they are still underrepresented in some senior positions. For example, despite the fact that there have been women in the role of dean of campus at all three Otago Medical School campuses (Wellington, Christchurch and Dunedin) in the nearly 150 years since the school was founded, there has been only one woman overall dean of Otago Medical School — Linda Holloway held this position between 2005 and 2006, in combination with the pro-vice-chancellor health sciences role. In all its 57 years, there has never been a woman dean at the Faculty of Medicine and Health Sciences at the University of Auckland.

This cohort was among the first wave of women working professionally as clinical doctors, academic teachers and researchers. We salute these women who produced so much excellent work in a medical science environment that was less accommodating than it is today. We thank them for leading the way and making it an easier path to follow for those coming after. Most importantly, we thank them for their substantive research, which led to changes in clinical practice that impacted the lives of their fellow humans in New Zealand and around the world.

Otago Medical School graduates on the steps of St Paul's Cathedral, Dunedin, December 1955. Front row, from left: Unknown, Bronwen Eileen Robinson (née Bloomfield), Gwenyth Marie Allison (née Hookings), unknown, Heather Thomson (née Baillie), unknown, Alison Tarrant, Cathryn Anne McIver, unknown, Constance Marguerita Dennehy, unknown, unknown. *Courtesy Tony Allison*

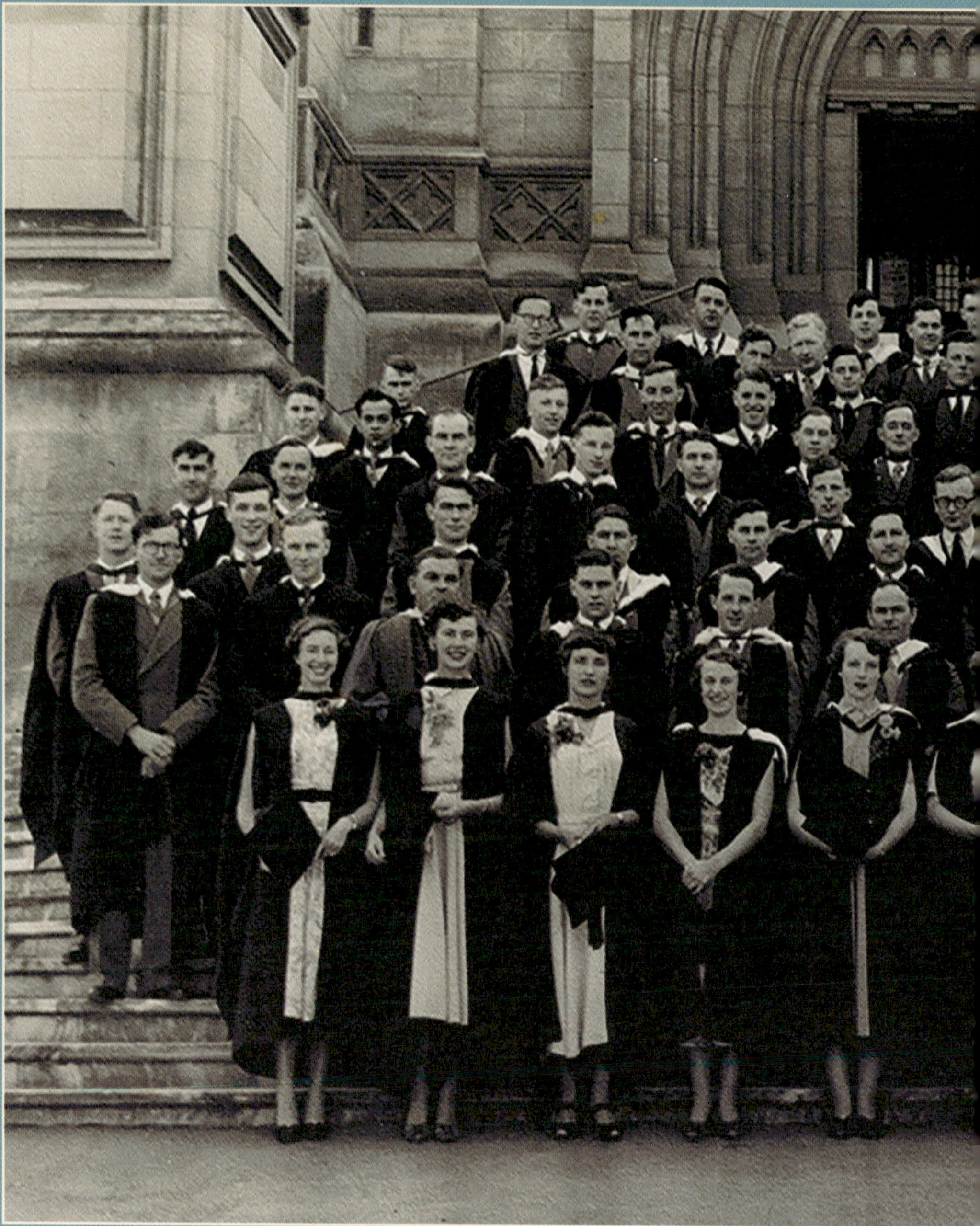

Conclusion

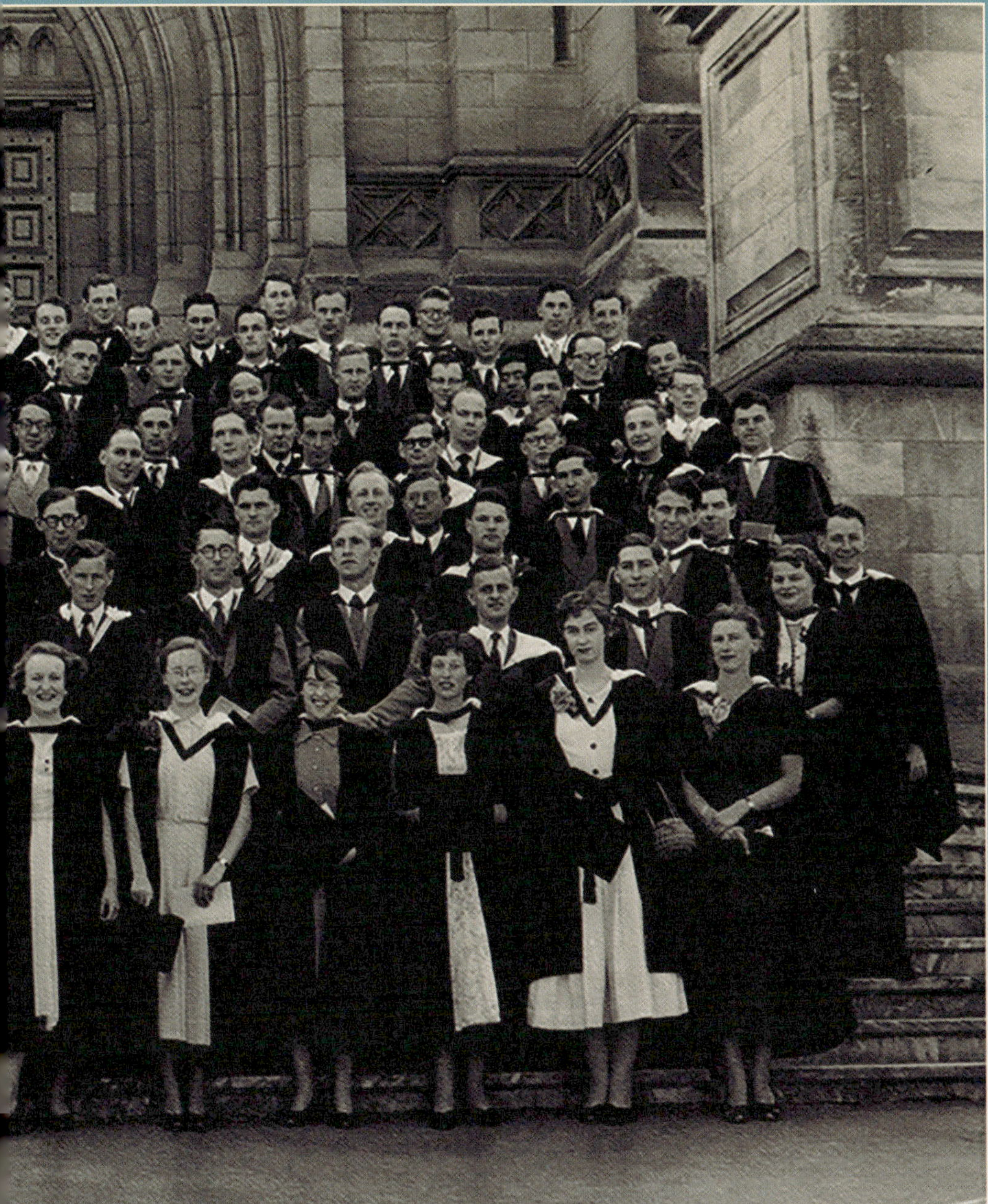

The women who graduated from Otago Medical School between the years of 1896 and 1967 certainly had the odds stacked against them: an average gender ratio of 90 per cent men and 10 per cent women, sexist professors and fellow students, and exclusion from some teaching and clinical placements. And they frequently encountered negative attitudes about their suitability as doctors, and were often told that they had taken the place of men. There was also the common expectation that women medical students who married or had children should give up their studies.

In the light of these challenges it is worth celebrating the achievements of the more than 400 women who graduated MB ChB over these seven decades. The majority subsequently established successful careers and contributed significantly to their fields. Their lives did not get any easier after they graduated. Even as attitudes towards women doctors relaxed and more opportunities arose, they continued to receive negative commentary from colleagues, patients and employers and, in many cases, a level of discrimination that would not be allowed by today's employment laws.

This book illustrates the determination, courage and conviction of early medical women in overcoming these odds. It also highlights the diversity of their experiences and situations across a turbulent century, the communities they built to overcome systemic barriers, and their immense contributions to medical knowledge and practice.

At the beginning of the twentieth century, many New Zealand hospitals refused to employ women doctors because they believed that they were inferior, would give up practice as soon as they married or had children, or would not cope with the long hours. This left few options. In the early years, women doctors were expected to fulfil the roles of both 'ladies' and 'doctors' in their communities — hence the title lady doctor. For some, the only option was working for the School Medical Service, which was regarded as suitable for women doctors because it involved working with children.[1] But working for the SMS was a poor substitute for working as a house officer in a hospital, which was the usual pathway to general practice and specialty training.

A feeling of constantly having to prove themselves to classmates and colleagues in order to be accepted was a common experience for medical women across these seven decades. It was also sometimes a lonely place, as many were the only women on the medical staff.

Although some professors were infamous for their opposition to the very idea of women doctors, others were supportive; they gave advice, encouraged research, employed and promoted women, and made introductions to overseas institutions. When finally, in the 1950s, the teaching staff hosted a welcome event for first-year women medical students, it was a major milestone.

These women came from a range of socioeconomic backgrounds, and some spoke of the divide that created. St Margaret's College offered a place where women could meet, support each other and form lasting friendships, but those who could not afford to stay there often felt they missed out on the opportunity to socialise and bond with others. For many, the friendships established during medical school became lifelong. They held study groups during term time and headed off on tramping trips together in the term breaks. After a few years at St Margaret's, those who developed friendships went flatting together so they could have more freedom and set their own schedules. They were in each other's bridal parties and were members of various community and professional organisations, particularly the Medical Women's Association.

Some women were exposed to racism at medical school and throughout their careers. Kathleen Pih-Chang recalled experiencing racism even though she arrived in New Zealand as a child and grew up here. Lucy Chung (née Chan), who arrived as a refugee from China in 1939 and graduated from medical school in 1964 (one of only two Chinese women to graduate between 1896 and 1967), was required to present

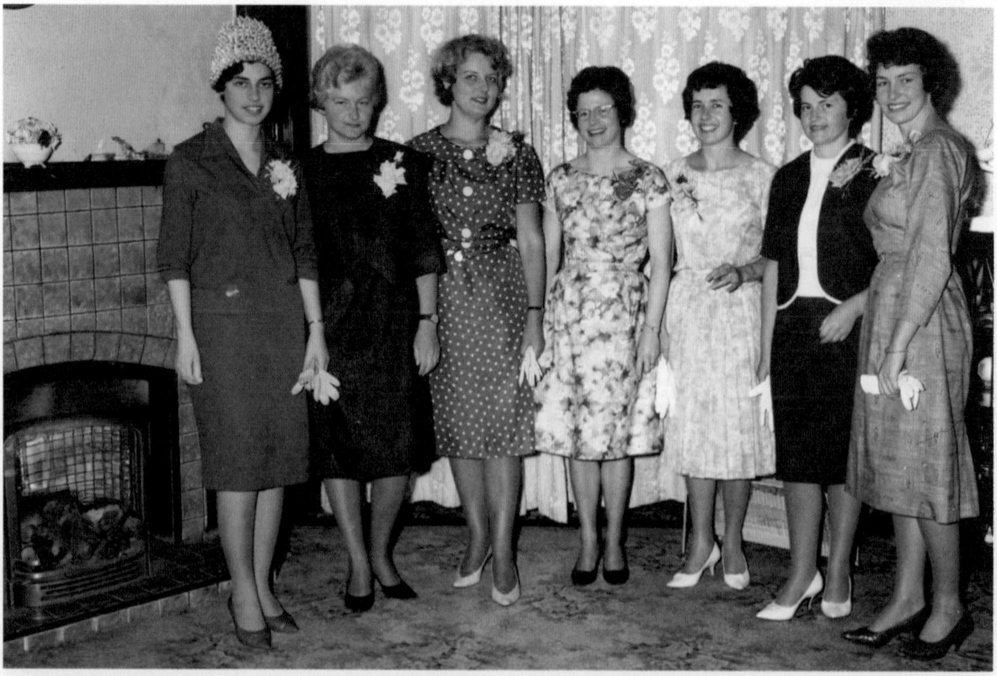

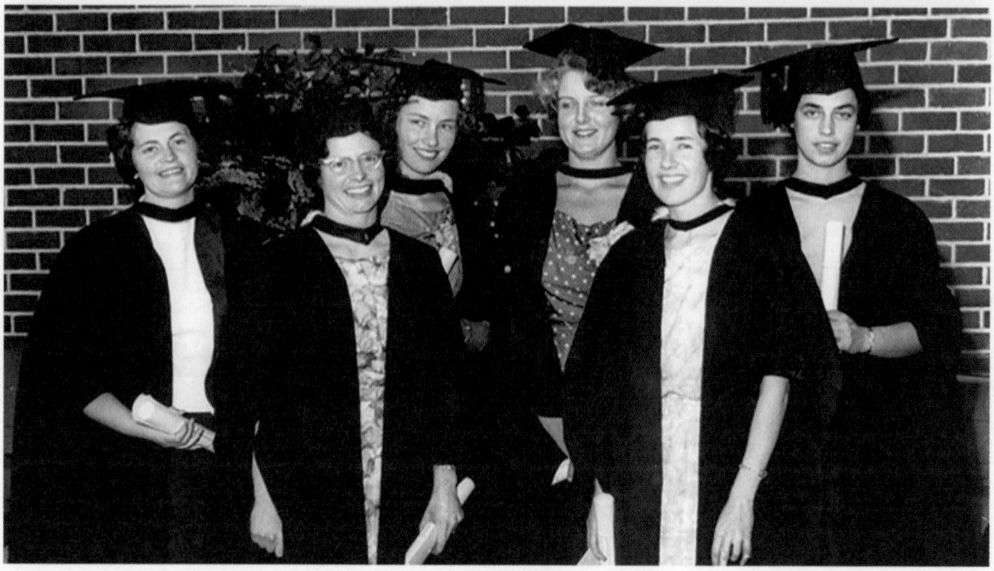

ABOVE: New Zealand Medical Women's Association lunch, 1962. From left: Dorothy Kral, Carol Shand, Haydn Cameron (née Bell), Mary Miller (née Cameron), Maureen Peskett (née Lester), Anne Cowie (née McNulty), Robyn Hewland. *Courtesy Mary Miller*

BELOW: Six of the 10 women who graduated from Otago Medical School in 1962. From left: Anne Cowie (née McNulty), Mary Miller (née Cameron), Robyn Hewland, Haydn Cameron (née Bell), Maureen Peskett (née Lester), Dorothy Kral. *Courtesy Mary Miller*

an Alien Registration Card every time she moved residence. This meant going to the police station each year when she first arrived in Dunedin and then again when she returned to her family in Hamilton for the holidays. For many, the hostility was an unwelcome emotional burden. Selma Ronigar-Hahn, a concentration camp survivor, found that she was retraumatised by 'any form of rejection or criticism [that] revived memories of the fears, punishments and dangers . . . in the camps'. Mirdza Palmer, a refugee from Latvia, spoke of feeling 'distanced from her other classmates . . . partly because of her background and accent'.[2]

The women established vital support networks, both professional and familial, while at medical school and after graduation. The New Zealand Medical Women's Association was established by eight women in 1921 to 'further the interests of Medical Women in New Zealand, and to promote professional association between members by holding meetings at which papers may be given and other matters of interest discussed'.[3] It grew into a strong network, and many women developed helpful collegial relationships through the organisation. Open to all women doctors, by 1993 it had branches in Auckland, Taranaki, Wellington, Christchurch and Dunedin; the national executive was regularly rotated among them. In 1992 there were approximately 280 members. The NZMWA continued for another 10 years, then went into recess in 2003.

Up until the 1950s, most secondary schools were inadequately resourced to teach young women the subjects required to gain entrance to medical school. In the early years, parents often had to organise private tutoring for their daughters in science subjects and in Latin, French or German. By the 1950s, the development of co-educational schools finally offered girls a well-rounded education, including in the sciences, mathematics and languages, that prepared them for medical studies.

The inspiration to study medicine often came from within the family. Daisy Platts-Mills graduated in 1900, and her daughter, Adah Blomfield, was the first daughter of an Otago woman graduate to complete the course in 1930. Blomfield grew up surrounded by medicine: her mother ran her private practice out of their home, and visiting surgeons would come to their home for their own procedures, including the removal of tonsils, adenoids and appendixes. Susanna Williams was the daughter of a medical mother and father and decided to pursue medicine herself. Carol Shand followed her mother Claudia's example and became a doctor.

Lynsie Kerr's (1966) brother entered medical school the year before her and gave her encouragement and advice on what to expect.

Christabel Dickie (née Spence-Sales; 1940) said that her sister Dorothy was the reason she chose to pursue medicine. The sisters were only two years apart during their medical studies, and when they moved to Dunedin their mother Anne came too, and all three lived in a flat together for seven years. Jennifer Wilson (1957) almost did not pursue medicine after watching her sister Meredyth Gunn struggle through the course, eventually taking eight years to complete it. Wilson did not want to repeat that experience, but she enrolled in the medical intermediate nonetheless. In the end she performed so well in the intermediate year that she successfully applied for entry to medical school.

Families also provided financial stability. Most women either received financial support from their parents for board and living costs or, if they were from Otago, continued to live at home. This was the case even after bursaries and scholarships became available. Even later on, the families of women who did not qualify for or could not get a bursary would often provide financial support, even when the funds were limited. Both Shirley Dowding and Susanna Williams were told their families had enough money to support them through each year once; should they fail, there was no money for them to repeat a year. As seen in the stories of Meredyth Gunn, Rina Moore and Margaret Sparrow, families also assisted with childcare so that the students who had children could continue to study or work

Many women doctors from later decades who had families of their own told us that they would not have been able to achieve as much as they did without paid home help. But in earlier decades women were expected to end their studies — and their careers — when they married, or when they had children. However, not all women who left practice were forced out, and not all regretted their choice to leave.

The relationships established during training were important for those who travelled overseas — as many did. Until the 1940s, the lack of postgraduate training opportunities in New Zealand meant newly qualified doctors had to apply to programmes in Edinburgh, London, Vienna or in the United States. Those who had gone before opened the doors for later women. Kathleen Todd, Augusta Klippel and Sylvia Chapman all reunited in Vienna where they were doing their postgraduate studies; Diana Mason studied at Great Ormond

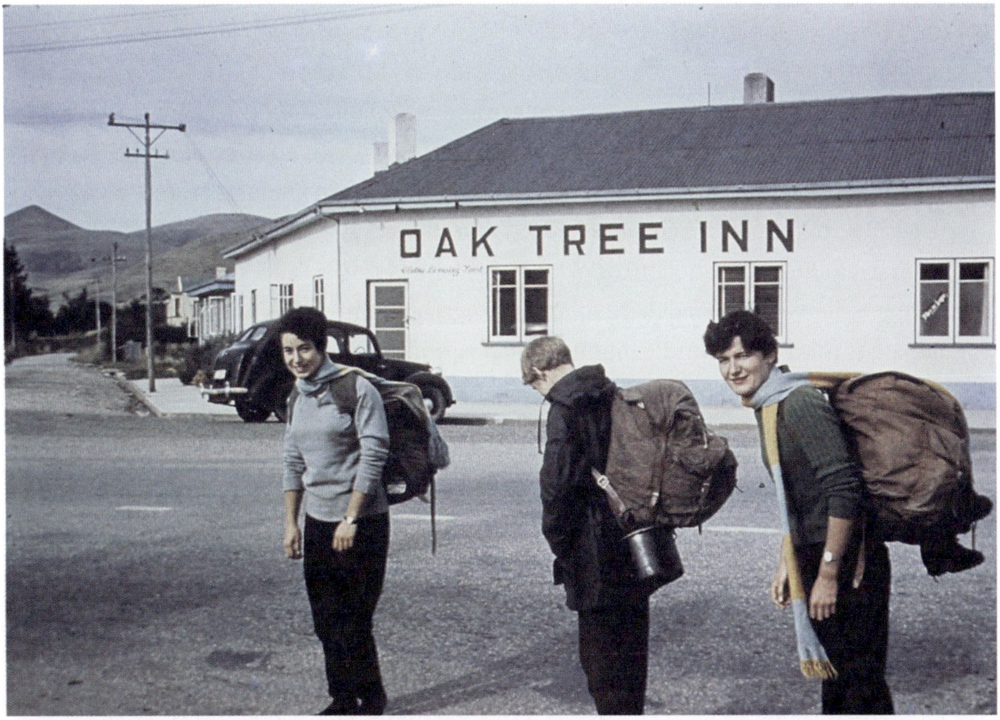

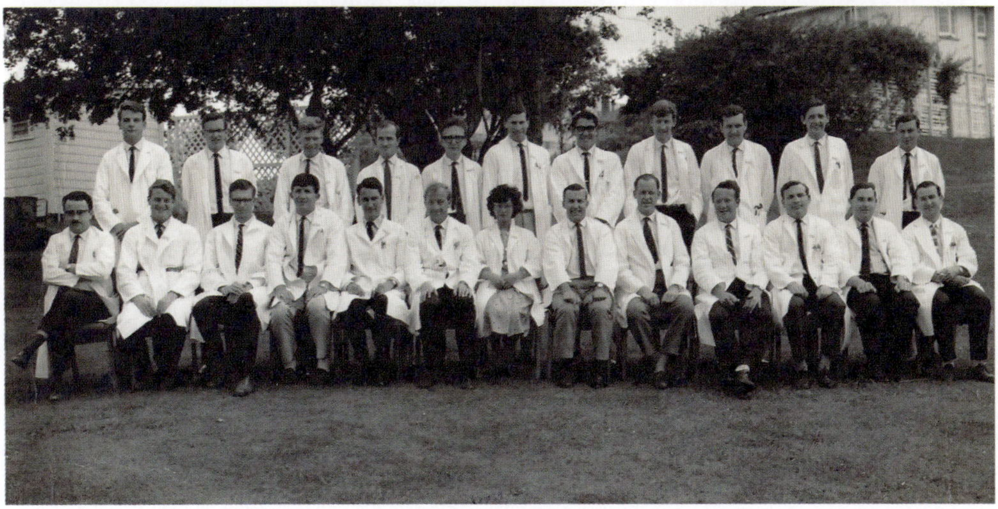

ABOVE: Miriam Frank, Rachel Senn and Patricia Houghton on a tramping holiday in Australia in 1959, between their fifth and sixth years at Otago Medical School. *Courtesy Miriam Frank*

BELOW: Resident doctors at Waikato Hospital in 1965–66. Lucy Chung is seated in the middle. *Family collection*

Street Hospital alongside three other Otago women graduates. Norma Restieaux enabled later women graduates to train in cardiology at Boston Children's Hospital.

Before air travel became commonplace and affordable it took several weeks to get to Europe, Asia or the United States from New Zealand, but New Zealand was not completely cut off from global connections, and women graduates made strong use of these to progress their careers.

The graduates tended to look out for one another and provide support where possible. Emily Siedeberg employed Agatha Monfries as a locum after she graduated, until she found a permanent position. When Margaret Guthrie first moved to Dunedin for her medical studies, she boarded with 1921 graduate Moana Gow until she could organise a more permanent solution. Glenys Smart (née Arthur; 1960) offered Judy Barfoot (née Radcliffe; 1960) a room in the flat she was renting in London.[4]

Kathleen Todd, who spent most of her career in and around the London area, stayed with two other Otago graduates — Beatrix Bakewell (1920) and Edith Mayo (1923) — on her first trip there while she was working as a house surgeon. When Todd returned to London after a short stint back in New Zealand, she established a permanent home in Hampstead that always had an open door to New Zealand doctors who were travelling through London.[5] Later, Todd funded Ruth Schell's (née Stevenson; 1964) studies, which finally made medicine a possibility for her.[6] Miriam Frank changed her specialty from general practice to anaesthetics when fellow Otago graduate Patricia Wood (née Houghton; 1960) advised her that London hospitals were starting to offer part-time positions in anaesthesia for women doctors.[7]

Early New Zealand medical women played a leading role in improvements in healthcare and reproductive rights, and developing scientific and medical knowledge. Ada Paterson pushed for improved child healthcare, and Alice Bush and Margaret Sparrow worked to educate the public about the realities of sex. Carol Shand and Robyn Hewland fought for better support for sexual abuse survivors; Viopapa Annandale-Atherton and Beryl Howie worked to improve healthcare and teaching overseas, and both provided advice to the World Health Organization. Patricia Hill was part of the team that sought to make healthcare more affordable through the development of the inner-city low-cost Te Aro Health Centre.

These early graduates were also involved in research and science. Muriel Bell's nutrition research played a key role in raising awareness about the country's dietary needs, from children to mountain climbers. Helen Deem reformed the Plunket system, making it more evidence-based. Barbara Heslop headed the transplantation research group in Dunedin from 1964 and was well respected in Australia and New Zealand for her postgraduate training programmes. Senga Whittingham investigated autoimmune diseases, while Patricia Buckfield brought modern neonatal intensive care to New Zealand.

Some of this work was commemorated in the form of awards, medals, damehoods, honorary doctorates or public structures. A statue of Margaret Cruickshank was erected in Waimate in 1922, and a street in Dunedin is named for Emily Siedeberg. In Ludhiana, an O&G block is dedicated to Beryl Howie. The legacies of some of this work is cemented in institutions today, in the form of, for example, the Dr Emily Hancock Siedeberg Scholarship, the Alice Bush Memorial Prize, the Barbara Heslop Memorial Scholarship, the Mercia Barnes Trust for research in O&G, and the Margaret Neave Trust for charity work with children in need.

But barriers still existed that restricted women's involvement in research and leadership. In 1987, Barbara Heslop analysed the realistic situation for women who wished to pursue a career in medicine. Despite the changes to women's health and their access to better family planning, women were still bound to abide by a system that was designed for men. She noted that, even at the time of writing, the intensive training courses for specialisation did not adequately cater to women who already had families or who intended to have them. The demands of training were high, even if a woman was permitted to study part-time. This meant that unless a woman decided to have children before specialising, she tended either not to have children at all or to have them much later.

Moreover, the demands of motherhood, even if a woman took only a short maternity leave, placed women behind on the work–time scale. Heslop argued: 'It is a medical commonplace (although rather hard to verify) that professionally one moves either forwards or backwards; one does not stand still. It is generally assumed that a no-work period represents backwards movement.'[8]

It is possibly for this reason, coupled with continued sexism in the workplace, that there are still very few women in positions of medical leadership nearly 40 years after Heslop's report.[9] A study of medical women in Australia and New Zealand published in 2020 found that gender disparity remained a 'pervasive

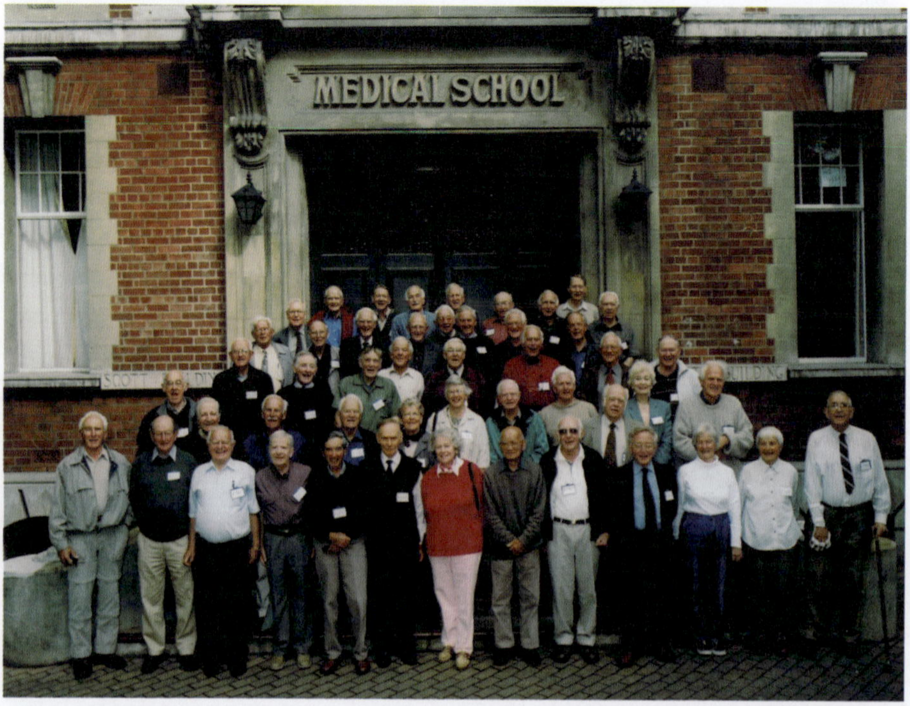

The fiftieth reunion of the Otago Medical School class of 1955 in November 2005. From front left: Margaret Maxwell, Constance Dennehy, Charlotte Robertson. Second row: Gwenyth Allison, Heather Thomson, Bronwen Robinson. *Courtesy Gwenyth Allison*

---

issue' in the field of medicine in both academia and specialty colleges. Of the 13 specialties analysed, women are still underrepresented in all specialist fields, with the exception of medical oncology and geriatric medicine (women make up 47 per cent of specialists in both fields) and endocrinology (46 per cent).[10]

The lowest representation is in cardiology, where women comprise only 15 per cent of the total body of specialists; in the subspecialty of interventional cardiology it is below 5 per cent. The 13 specialties analysed were specifically not those in which women have traditionally been prominent, such as obstetrics and gynaecology.[11] In comparison, an analysis of the New Zealand specialist workforce argued that the 'feminisation' of specialties has occurred at a greater rate in those that had an early uptake of woman doctors — including psychiatry, where women make up 52 per cent of the workforce, general practice (60 per cent), pathology (61 per cent), paediatrics (73 per cent) and obstetrics and gynaecology (the highest at

84 per cent).[12] Women in medicine have made major strides in the last half-century, but these figures show that there is still a long way to go.

There has been little in this book about Māori medical graduates. Over the seven decades, only two Māori women graduated, Rina Moore (née Rōpiha) in 1949 and Judith Hall (née Karaitiana) in 1956. We don't know if there were more who enrolled. The number of Māori men graduates was not much better, although some very notable Māori leaders graduated in the very early years. In 1951, a 'preferential' entry system was introduced, offering priority entry to two Māori students. Fortunately, since then many changes have been made and now each year approximate 15 per cent of Otago medical graduates identify as Māori.

Although the experiences documented in this book were shaped by societal and world events, they were also defined by the women themselves, who were prepared to push boundaries and challenge the norms of the day. The over 400 women who graduated from the Otago Medical School between 1896 and 1967 did not have one singular experience. For some, discrimination fuelled a fight for equality in their careers. But some claimed to have experienced no discrimination during their studies; rather, they found acceptance, support and love among their male colleagues. Some went on to become world-renowned researchers and doctors who pushed medical practices into the future, while others focused their attention on their families and communities.

The journey of the women graduates of Otago Medical School from 1896 to 1967 is a story of resilience, progress and enduring impact. Despite encountering many obstacles they paved the way for future generations through their courage and determination. Their stories highlight not only the barriers they encountered but also their remarkable achievements. These pioneering women did more than just break into a male-dominated profession; they redefined it. Their legacy is one of perseverance, hard work and the pursuit of equality, and it continues to inspire and guide women in medicine today.

The history of medicine in Aotearoa New Zealand is richer and more inclusive because of the invaluable contributions these women have made, reminding us that progress is built on the foundations laid by those who dared to challenge the established order, against all odds.

Graduates and their qualifications
Notes
Bibliography
Acknowledgements
About the authors
Index

Graduates and their qualifications

Names in bold indicate that a biography for this graduate has been written and published on the Early Medical Women of New Zealand website: www.earlymedwomen.auckland.ac.nz

1891–1913

Emily Hancock Siedeberg-McKinnon (née Siedeberg), MB ChB 1896; LRCP 1896; BSc 1901; CBE 1949
Margaret Barnett Cruickshank, MB ChB 1897; MD 1903
Constance Helen Frost, BA 1892; MB ChB 1900
Daisy Elizabeth Platts-Mills (née Platts), MB ChB 1900; OStJ 1929
Alice Horsley (née Woodward), MB ChB 1900; OBE 1939
Jane Kinder, MB ChB 1900
Jessie Clarkson Maddison, MB ChB 1902; LRCP 1902
Eleanor Southey Baker McLaglan (née Baker), MB ChB 1903; LM
Agatha Helen Jane Monfries (née Adams), MB ChB 1904
Winifrede Ismay Bathgate, BSc 1896; MB ChB 1904
Emily Helen Violetta Nées (née Ridley), MB ChB 1904
Ada Gertrude Paterson, MB ChB 1906; LM 1908
Ina Burnman Moody (née Dugleby), MB ChB 1910
Catherine Louisa Brookfield (née Will), MB ChB 1911

1914–1919

Doris Clifton Gordon (née Jolly), MB ChB 1915; DPH, FRCSE 1925; OBE 1935; FRCOG 1936
Mary Francesca Compere Dowling, MB ChB 1915
Glady Margaret Wilkes Shaw, MB ChB 1916
Irene Woodhouse, MB ChB 1916
Mabel Aileen Christie (née Hanron), MB ChB 1917
Grace Stevenson, MB ChB 1918; DPH 1924
Marion King Bennie Cameron (née Whyte), MB ChB 1918; DA RCP & RCS 1939; FFARACS 1954
Mary Phoebe Wilson, MB ChB 1918
Emma Gertrude Atmore (née Applegate), MB ChB 1919

1920–1938

Beatrix 'Tui' Helen Bakewell, MB ChB 1920; DPH 1937; D Obst RCOG 1938
Elspeth Mary Fitzgerald (née Cameron), MB ChB 1920
Moana Maru Gow (née Anderson), MB ChB 1921; BEM 1974
Sylvia Gytha de Lancey Chapman, MB ChB 1921; DGO 1924; LM 1924; MD 1934; Hon FRCGP 1967
Rosina Dorothy Richards (née Crawley), MB ChB 1921
Eva Esther Hill (née Day), MB ChB 1921
Rita Ethel Osborne Gardner (née Gillies), MB ChB 1921
Muriel Emma Bell, MB ChB 1922; MD 1926; FNZIC 1941; FRSNZ 1952; FRACP 1959; CBE 1959; Hon DSc 1968

Eily Elaine Gurr, MB ChB 1922; LM (Dublin), Hon FRNZCGP 1983; OStJ 1954
Grace Helena Proude (née Kime), MB ChB 1922
Frances Isabella Preston (née McAllister), MB ChB 1922
Augusta Klippel (née Manoy), MB ChB 1922
Zealanda Aitken (née Marshall), MB ChB 1922
Phyllis Mather, MB ChB 1922
Hessie McDermid (née Morton), MB ChB 1922
Hazel Rebecca Bryan Allison (née Patterson), MB ChB 1922; DA 1926
Marion Aroha Radcliffe-Taylor (née Taylor), MB ChB 1922; FRCSEd 1930
Susannah Catherine Campbell Sinclair (née McKnight), MA 1902; MSc 1907; MB ChB 1922
Phyllis Haddow, MB ChB 1923; DTM 1928
Ruth Marjorie Cruickshank Barclay, MB ChB 1923; DMRE 1927
Mollie Christie (née Fisher), MB ChB 1923; DMRE 1926; MBE 1971
Isabella Wise (née Gault), MB ChB 1923
Elizabeth Kate Hughes (née Jary), MB ChB 1923; OBE 1974
Elizabeth Pretoria Hall (née Lumsden), MB ChB 1923
Edith Annie Mayo, MB ChB 1923
Marjorie Smith-Wilson, MB ChB 1923; DPH (England) 1936
Caroline Morrow Stenhouse, MB ChB 1923; DOMS
Kathleen Mary Gertrude Todd, MB ChB 1923; DPM 1929
Mary Anderson Champtaloup, MB ChB 1924
Winifred Ethel Morton (née Cox), MB ChB 1924
Muriel Helen Deem (née Easterfield), MB ChB 1924; MD 1928; D Obst RCOG 1935; DPH (London) 1935; OBE 1952
Gladys Murison Bremner (née MacAlister), MB ChB 1924
Margaret Joan Williams (née Mayfield), MB ChB 1924
Alice Campbell Tallerman (née Rose), MB ChB 1924; MRCP 1927; DA 1942
Dorothy McKeefry (née Sweeney), MB ChB 1924
Jeanie Gardner Fougere (née Wood), MB ChB 1924
Catherine Ellen Weppener Anderson, MB ChB 1925
Cecily Mary Aroha Wise Pickerill (née Clarkson), MB ChB 1925; OBE 1958; DBE 1977
Mary Douglas, MB ChB 1925
Theodora Clemens Hall (née Easterfield), MB ChB 1925; MRCP 1932; FRACP 1974
Nina Catherine Muir (née Howard), MB ChB 1925; DGO 1950
Ella Connolly (née Langley), MB ChB 1925
Effie Muriel Morgan, MB ChB 1925
Uriti May Strack-Torrie (née Strack), BHSc 1911; MB ChB 1925
Eleanor Kathleen Abbott, MB ChB 1926; DMR 1937
Margaret Marion Vida Lemon (née Grater), MB ChB 1926; DA, RCS 1944; FFARCS 1960
Janette Muir King (née Grave), MB ChB 1926
Phyllis Maude Babington (née Moir), MB ChB 1926
Sarah Margaret Felicia Walmsley, MB ChB 1926; DPH 1931
Helen Edith Lochhead (née Dougall), MB ChB 1927
Jessie Burnett (née Alexander), MB ChB 1927; FFARACS 1966
Barbara Hay Roche (née Henry), MB ChB 1927
Beryl Jessie Lawrence, MB ChB 1927; DCH 1938; DPH 1942; DCP 1945
Alexandra Carson Mathieson, MB ChB 1927
Mary Jane Hulse Russell, MB ChB 1927

Pauline Catherine Simcock (formerly Witherow, née Aitken), MB ChB 1927; D Bact 1931
Nellie Isabel Houghton, MB ChB 1928
Bettina Matraves Hamilton (née Collier), MB ChB 1929
Nola Mary Ivory, MB ChB 1929
Rosalind Brackenbury Latter, MB ChB 1929; MRCP 1935
Kathleen Anuei Chang (Bi Zhen-Wah) (née Pih), MB ChB 1929; DOMS 1937
Dorothy Barnard Kelly (née Smith), MB ChB 1930
Ellen Gough Boddy (née Heycock), MB ChB 1930; DPH 1934
Elfie Néedham (formerly Connall, née McCaskill), MB ChB 1930
Adah Hamilton Evelyn Blomfield (née Platts-Mills), MB ChB 1930; D Obst 1934
Anne Margaret Thomson, MB ChB 1930
Anna Lydia Nannestad (née Hansen), MB ChB 1931
Katherine Milner Hastie, MB ChB 1931
Florence Aileen Craig, MB ChB 1932
Teresa Imelda Thompson (née Craig), MB ChB 1932
Martha Kirkland Gregory (née Grigor), MB ChB 1932
Meredith Conley Moore, MB ChB 1932; FRCS 1937
Margaret Ruth Sneddon, MB ChB 1932
Marie Payne Buchler (née Stringer), MB ChB 1932
Beryl Eveline G. Douglas (née Bowden), MB ChB 1933
Zoe Cuff Mason (née Rutherford), MB ChB 1933; DMRE 1939; MCRA 1949; FCRA 1950
Dorothy Marian Stewart, MB ChB 1933; D Obst RCOG 1937; MRCOG 1938; MRCP 1939; FRCOG 1957
Ruth Margaret Hill (née Boyd-Wilson), MB ChB 1934
Evelyn Joyce Lester (née Burley), MB ChB 1934
Elizabeth Vivien Whitta (née Newlands), MB ChB 1934
Marion Kerr Steven, MB ChB 1934; MA 1942
Mary Watson, MB ChB 1934; DA RCP & RCS 1947; FFARCS 1954
Gertrude Aphra Morley (née Willis), MB ChB 1934
Margaret Annie Begg (née Birks), MB ChB 1935
Mavel Collis Laing (née Wood), MB ChB 1935
Margaret Elizabeth Wilson MacDonald (née Christie), MB ChB 1936
Gertrude Louisa Brosnahan (née Galliers), MB ChB 1936
Margaret Stuart Smith (née Riddell), MB ChB 1936; DA RCP & RCS 1939; FFARACS 1952; OBE 1990
Alice Grace Armour (née Stanley), MB ChB 1936
Dora Mary Young (née Stevenson-Wright), MB ChB 1936; DA RCP & RCS 1946; FFARACS 1956
Myrtle Inez Hill (née Thew), BA; MB ChB 1936
Claudia Lillian Shand (née Weston), MB ChB 1936
Annie Hayes Berry, MB ChB 1937; OBE 1962
Margaret Robina Chieffi (née Jackson), MB ChB 1937
Beatrice Esther Schuchard (née Nelson), MB ChB 1937
Alice Mary Bush (née Stanton), MB ChB 1937; MRACP 1946; MRCP 1949; DCH, RCP & RCS 1949; FRACP 1956; FRCP 1970
Margaret Fraser Gatman (née Hunter), MB ChB 1938
Dorothy Spence-Sales, MB ChB 1938; FFARCS 1953
Molly Smith (née Wagstaff), MB ChB 1938

1939–1948

Alison Jean Marshall, MB ChB 1939
Norma May Witters (née Morey), MB ChB 1939
Jean Mary Sandel, MB ChB 1939; FRCS 1947; FRACS 1957
Norma Beatrice Benson, MSc; MB ChB 1940
Eunice Janet Loan (née McLean), MB ChB 1940
Anne Helen Morgan-Coakle (née Morgan), MB ChB 1940
Christabel Mary Dickie (formerly Wallace, née Spence-Sales), MB ChB 1940; D Obst RCOG 1949
Irene Glenwynne Rhodes (née Burford), MB ChB 1941
Elsie Craig Gibbons, MB ChB 1941; DCH, RCP & RCS 1947; MRCP (London) 1947; MRCP (Edinburgh) 1948
Cecilia Ellen Hands, MB ChB 1941
Mavis Laline MacDougall (née McClymont), MB ChB 1941; D Ven 1971
Catherine Newman (née Weisz), MD (Vienna) 1933; Special Exam 1941; MB ChB (Ad Eundem) 1947
Olga Wilhelmina Lina Semon, MD 1929; Special Exam 1941; MB ChB 1947
Mary Lorraine Talbot, MB ChB 1941
Margaret McBeth Buxton (née Beedie), MB ChB 1942
Elizabeth Rae McFarlane Brown, MB ChB 1942
Roma Holbrook Roberts (née Chatfield), MB ChB 1942
Marjorie Elizabeth Macready (née Cuttle), MB ChB 1942; MCCM 1980
Margaret Isabel Giles (née Elliott), MB ChB 1942
Hilda Berdach Fleischl (née Barber), MD 1939; Special Exam 1942; MB ChB (Ad Eundem) 1947
Iris Mabel Emily Hamlin, MB ChB 1942; MC Path 1964
Nancy Jocelyn Gruar (née Hunter), MB ChB 1942
Marjorie Dorothea Rohan, MB ChB 1942
Margaret Isabel Wishart (née Moore), MB ChB 1942
Molly Joan Woodroffe (née Boyes), MB ChB 1943
Patricia Rae McDonald (née Ford), MB ChB 1943; DA RCP & RCS 1952; FFARCS 1954; FFARACS 1956
Alison Hunter, MB ChB 1943; DCH, RCP & RCS 1949; MRCP 1954; MRACP 1973; FRCP 1977
Jean Dudley Margaret Savage (née Jerram), MB ChB 1943
Joan Katherine Griggs (née McDougall), MB ChB 1943; DPH, RCP & RCS 1949
Aileen Nada Maxwell, MB ChB 1943
Margaret Isobel Erskine Neave, MB ChB 1943; MRCP 1951; DCH, RCP & RCS 1951; FRACP 1965
Monica Annie Neville (née Ongley), MB ChB 1943
Ada Maisie Gilling, MB ChB 1944; D Obst 1962
Joyce May Emery Merriman (née Gones), MB ChB 1944
Mary Joyce Marples, MB ChB 1944; MD 1951; DTM&H, RCP & RCS 1956
Daphne Phyllis Adams (née Morrison), MB ChB 1944
June Esther Kriechbaum (née Reid), MB ChB 1944
Flora Smith, MB ChB 1944; MC Path 1963
Maureen Bell (formerly Dingwall, née Bridgman), MB ChB 1945
Shirley Juliette Dowding (née Appleton), MB ChB 1945; QSM 1993
Shirley Lyford Tonkin (née Curtis), MB ChB 1945; DCH, RCP & RCS 1953; MCCM 1980
Jean Winsome McLean (née Isdale), MB ChB 1945
Helen Maxwell Jeans, DHSc; MB ChB 1945
Joan Eleanor Walton (née Robertson), MB ChB 1945; DCH, RCP & RCS 1953; QSM 1993
Diana Manby Mason (née Shaw), MB ChB 1945; DCH, RCP & RCS 1950; MRCGP 1957; FRCGP 1970
Norma Claire Campbell Kent (née Shepherd), MB ChB 1945; PhD 1955; MANZCP 1963

Phyllis Mary Armstrong (née Stockdill), MB ChB 1945; D Obst 1960
Patricia Hunter Cook (née Will), MB ChB 1945; DCH, RCP & RCS 1950
Juliet Carleton Harrison (née Williams), MB ChB 1945
Mollie Marmion Pryor (née Wood), MB ChB 1945
Nancy Serena Geddis Butt-Kwan (née Butt), MB ChB 1946; FFARCS 1954
Margaret Mary Clayton (née Isdale), MB ChB 1946
Sheila Frances Hurrell (née Wilding), MB ChB 1946
Ngaire Alexander Woods, MB ChB 1946
Stephanie Joy Ellis (née Wylie), MB ChB 1946
Judy Ann David Wilson (née Collins), MB ChB 1947
Winifred Mary Staple (née Croke), MB ChB 1947; DPM 1971; MRC Psych 1973
Judith (Judy) Moyra de Vernot McCann (née Faris), MB ChB 1947; QSO 2004
Prudence Anne Abrahams (née Fitzgerald), MB ChB 1947
Barbara McLeod Allen (née Graham), MB ChB 1947
Edith Jean Patricia Lyness, MB ChB 1947
Jean Boyd (née MacDonald), MB ChB 1947
Diana Marcia Smith (née Morton), MB ChB 1947
Nancy Margaret Saunders (née Salmond), MB ChB 1947
Maire Jean Smith (née Tait), MB ChB 1947
Mary Alice Theodore Tolley, MB ChB 1947; MRCOG 1958; FRCS 1958; FRCOG 1974
Helen Rarity McCreanor (née Young), MB ChB 1947; MD 1972; MRACP 1973; FRACP 1977
Fay Young (née Booth), MB ChB 1948
Helen Kathleen Borg, MB ChB 1948; D Obst RCOG 1951; DCH, RCP & RCS 1953; MRCOG 1971
Barbara Farnsworth Heslop (née Cupit), MB ChB 1948; MD 1954; FRCP Path 1964; FRC Path 1971; FRACS 1976; FRSNZ 1990; CBE 1991
Marianne Fillenz, MB ChB 1948; DPhil 1955; DSc 2000
Maxine Winslow Wanty (née Gray), MB ChB 1948
Mary Coldham (née Hanafin), MB ChB 1948
Elaine Valerie Osmond (née Hulse), MB ChB 1948
Rachel Monk/Munk, MD 1932; MB ChB 1948
Diana Edwards (née Montgomery), MB ChB 1948; MRCOG 1958; FRCOG 1975; FRNZCOG 1986
Rina Winifred Moore (née Rōpiha), MB ChB 1948; MANZCP 1968
Shirley Blyth Robertson, MB ChB 1948; MRCOG 1961; FRCOG 1978
Olga Dorothea Batt (née Skousgaard), MB ChB 1948
Zoë Petronella During (née Smuts-Kennedy), MB ChB 1948; MCCM 1980
Linnie Bryant Calvert (née Tombleson), MB ChB 1948; DTM&H 1954
Dorothy Field Potter (née Usher), MB ChB 1948; DO, RCP & RCS 1952; CBE 1993
Patricia MacKay (née Wilson), MB ChB 1948; DA 1952; DA, RCS 1953; FFARCS 1954; FFARACS 1955

1949–1967

Ruth Evelyn Mitchell (née Adams), BMedSc 1946; MB ChB 1949; DCH, RCP & RCS 1953; MD 1968
Margaret Shirley Tennent (née Andrews), MB ChB 1949; MRCGP 1960; MRNZCGP 1974
June Barclay, MB ChB 1949; DCH, RCP & RCS 1954; MRCP 1969
Thelma Constance Becroft, MB ChB 1949
Beverley Jean Luke (née Brown), MB ChB 1949
Noeline Burn (née Clemens), MB ChB 1949; DCH, RCP & RCS 1953
Rosemary Agatha Faull (née Clendon), MB ChB 1949
Stella Lindsay Johnstone (née Horwell), MB ChB 1949

Beryl Overton Howie, MB ChB 1949; MRCOG 1955; FRCOG 1966; FRACS 1970; RNZCOG 1984; RANZCOG 1984
Jane Munro (née Aylward), MB ChB 1950
Kathleen Elsie Wake (née Brown), MB ChB 1950
Mary Litster O'Halloran (née Burnet), BA; MB ChB 1950
Keitha Farmer (née Corlett), MB ChB 1950; DCH, RCP & RCS 1955; MRCP 1958; MRACP 1960; PhD 1963; FRACP, FRCP 1972
Shirley Elizabeth Entrican, MB ChB 1950
Susi Ruth Levene (née Levinsohn), MB ChB 1950
Margaret Elizabeth Coop (née Rudd), MB ChB 1950; DO, RCS & P 1955; MACO 1972
Helen Florence Wood (née Salkeld), MB ChB 1950; D Obst RCOG 1966
Deirdre Morag Airey, MB ChB 1951; QSM 1979
Patricia Elizabeth Gardner, MB ChB 1951
Anne Priscilla McKinnon (formerly Jarvis, née Pearson), MB ChB 1951
Marjorie Joyce Seymour (née King), MB ChB 1951
Shona Hodgson (née McLeod), MB ChB 1951; D Phys Med 1960
Jane Harrison (née Munro), MB ChB 1951
Teresa Patricia Riordan, MB ChB 1951; FFARCS 1964
Marie Margaret Simpson, MB ChB 1951; FFARCS 1960; FFARACS 1968
Margaret Winn Guthrie (formerly Wray, née Hoodless), BSc 1945; MB ChB 1951; CNZM 1997
Marjorie Rose Young, MB ChB 1951
Meredyth Colston Gunn (née Wilson), MB ChB 1952
Edith Ruth Black (née Blumenthal), BA; MB ChB 1952; CBE 1980
Joan Dorothy Anne Casserley, MB ChB 1952; FFARCS 1959
Muriel Blanche Elizabeth Berney Mason (née Falcon), BSc; MB ChB 1952
Mary Lillian David Skinner, BA; MB ChB 1952
Margaret Phear (née Woods), MB ChB 1952
Phyllis Muriel Brass, BHSc 1934; MB ChB 1953
Colleen Anne Hall (née Conyngham), MB ChB 1953; MRACP 1958; DPM, RCP & RCS 1963; MANZCP 1968; FRACP 1972; FRANZCP 1975
Margot Ronson Gardner (née Craw), MB ChB 1953; FFARCS 1957
Adrienne Lorraine Gibson (née Croucher), BSc; MB ChB 1953
Joan Jessep Presland (formerly Fitchett, née Kay), MB ChB 1953
Eva Ruth Seelye (née Hersch), BA; MB ChB 1953; FFARCS 1961; FFARACS 1968
Helen Margaret Irwin Liley (née Hunt), BSc 1948; MB ChB 1953; MRCOG 1955; FROCOG 1966
Clara Elizabeth (Betty) Rawley (née Jackson), BSc 1949; MB ChB 1953; QSM 1987
Mary Max Patrick, MB ChB 1953
Selma Ronigar-Hahn, MB ChB 1953
Kathleen Rose Standage, MB ChB 1953
Senga Florence Whittingham, MB ChB 1953; DCP 1963; RCPA, RACP 1966;PhD 1970
Irene Therese Valentine (née Abrahamsohn), MB ChB 1954
Elizabeth Naylor (née Beauchamp), MB ChB 1954
Patricia Ann Weston (née Coates), MB ChB 1954; DA RCP & RCS 1958
Margaret Miriam Belton (formerly Fanselow, née Hart), MB ChB 1954
Kathleen Audrey Bradford (née Johnstone), MB ChB 1954; DPM 1965; MRANZCP 1966; FRANZCP 1976; MCCM 1980; MBE 1989; FAFPHM (RACP) 1994
Evelyn Belle Lind, MA; MB ChB 1954; DPM, RCP & RCS 1959; MANZCP 1966; FRANZCP 1975
Natalia Venetz (née Pachomov), MB ChB 1954

Margaret Clare Gibberd (née Sidey), MB ChB 1954; MRCP 1959
Katharine Helen Campbell Bowden (née Thomson), MB ChB 1954; MNZOM 2001
Heather Thomson (née Baillie), MB ChB 1955; D Obst 1973l; MNZM 2007
Mercia Annette Barnes, MB ChB 1955; MRCOG 1962
Patricia Bassett, MB ChB 1955
Bronwen Eileen Robinson (née Broomfield), BMedSc 1952; MB ChB 1955; MRCP 1962
Charlotte Lilian Robertson (née Christie), MB ChB 1955; DA RCP & RCS 1959; FFARCS 1963; CRCP(C) 1967; FRACP(C) 1973
Constance Marguerita Dennehy, MB ChB 1955; MRCP 1960
Gwenyth Marie Allison (née Hookings), MB ChB 1955; DPM 1977
Margaret Iris Meffan (née King), MB ChB 1955
Cathryn Anne Christie (née McIver), MB ChB 1955
Patricia Claire Cairney (née Meikle), MB ChB 1955
Clarice Lora Main (née Moore), MB ChB 1955
Margaret Dawn Maxwell (née Parsonage), MB ChB 1955
Alison Myra Gaitonde (née Tarrant), MB ChB 1955
Tatiana (Tania) Roberta Gunn (née Tarulevicz), MB ChB 1955; MD 1989
Elizabeth Anne Bowie, MB ChB 1956; MRCP 1964; MRACP 1975; FRACP 1978
Elizabeth Mary Irvine (née Corbett), BSc; MB ChB 1956; DA RCP & RCS 1960
Pamela Mary McGruer (née Dawe), MB ChB 1956
Judith Hall (née Karaitiana), MB ChB 1956
Annie Moy (née Low), MB ChB 1956
Ngaire Margaret Walsh (née McKerrow), MB ChB 1956; MD 1963
Jocelyn Valerie Hay (née Bell), MB ChB 1957
Joan Shirley Chapple, MB ChB 1957; FRACS 1963; CNZM 2001
Patricia Mary Clarkson, MB ChB 1957; MRACP 1969; Dip Amer Board Pediatrics 1965; Ped Cardiol 1966; FRACP 1974
Simme Alterman (née Coggin), MB ChB 1957; D Obst 1961
Lesley Kathleen Doak (née Harries), MB ChB 1957
Susanna Renate Williams (née Lemchen), MB ChB 1957
Elizabeth Margaret Rich, MB ChB 1957; DPM, RCP & RCS; MRC Psych 1973
Judith Cherry Wardill (née Smith), MB ChB 1957; MD 1967; FRCPA 1974
Hendrika (Enny) Jacoba Waal-Manning, MB ChB 1957; BMedSc 1956; MD 1982
Jennifer Colston Wilson, MB ChB 1957; D Obst 1960; MRCOG 1963; FRCOG 1979
Helen Beaumont Angus, MB ChB 1958; FRCPA 1967
Pamela Jones (née Brown), MB ChB 1958; MRCP 1967; MRACP 1970; FRACP 1974; FRCP 1991
Patricia Marie Buckfield, MB ChB 1958; DCH 1953; MRCPE 1964; MRCP 1965; MRACP 1975; FRACP 1978; MD 1979; FRCPE 1983; FRCP 1985
Annetta Elsie Alexandra Gillies, MB ChB 1958; D Phys Med, RCP & RCS 1963
Helen Maud Bichan (née Simpson), MB ChB 1958; DPM 1975; MRANZCP 1979; DHA 1982; FRANZCP 1981; MCCM 1986; ONZM 2002
Elizabeth Ramage (née Aitken), MB ChB 1959
Kathleen Mary Lawther (née Christian), MB ChB 1959
Rosalie Davida-Horvath, MD 1945 (Budapest); MB ChB 1959
Jean Bryant (née Fyfe), MB ChB 1959
Viola Cornelia Palmer (née Heine), MB ChB 1959; DA RCP & RCS 1963
Braida Merle Hopper, MB ChB 1959
Janice Marion McKay, MB ChB 1959

Rosalie Helen Sneyd (née McPherson), MB ChB 1959
Glenys Patricia Smart (née Arthur), MB ChB 1960; MRACP 1974; FRACP 1978; FAFRM 1983; CNZM 2002
Elizabeth Berry (née Waugh-Burns), MB ChB 1960; MD 1972; FRCPA 1972; FRACP 1978; QSM 1988
Miriam Frank, MB ChB 1960; FRCS 1975
Elizabeth Ann Hewitt (née Hodge), MB ChB 1960; DMRD 1969; FFR 1971
Patricia Wood (née Houghton), MB ChB 1960; DA RCP & RCS 1966
Alison Jean Sommerville (née Knox), MB ChB 1960; MCRA 1966
Isla Ellen Frew (née Lonie), MB ChB 1960; DPM (ANZCP) 1967; MANZCP 1967
Heather Leslie (née Macallan), MB ChB 1960
Kantha Soni (née Madhavji), MB ChB 1960
Judith Anne Barfoot (née Radcliffe), MB ChB 1960; FFARCS 1967
Norma Restieaux, BMedSc 1957; MB ChB 1960; MRACP 1964; MRCP 1965; FRACP 1971; FRCP 1982; MD 1973; DBE 1992
Rachel Emily Maule (née Senn), MB ChB 1960; DPM RCP & RCS 1964; MRC Psych 1974; MNZM 2003
Ailsa Mary Morrison-Galt (née Smith), MB ChB 1960; DMRD, RCP & RCS 1968; MRACR 1977; FRANZCR 1985
Elaine Mary O'Brien (née Tutchen), MB ChB 1960
Noeline Lillian Beatrice Carrington (née Walker), MB ChB 1960; DPM, RCP & RCS 1971
Roma Agnes Wilson, MB ChB 1960
Pauline Anne Blue (née Ellis), MB ChB 1961; DMRD, RCP & RCS 1968; MRACR 1977
Tatyana (Tania) Hillerby (née Godyaew), MB ChB 1961
Mirdza Palmer (née Robins), MB ChB 1961
Janis Lorin Oliver (née Sutherland), MB ChB 1961; D Obst RCOG 1967
Phyllis Margaret Charlton (née Taylor), MB ChB 1961; MRCP 1969; D Phys Med 1970; D Com Health 1982
Dorothy Haydn Cameron (née Bell), MB ChB 1962
Helen Robyn Hewland, MB ChB 1962; DPM, RCP & RCS 1972; MRC Psych 1972; MRANZCP 1975
Dorothy Jean Kral, MB ChB 1962; MANZCP 1970; MRC Psych 1973; FRANZCP 1980
Maureen Joan Peskett (née Lester), MB ChB 1962; FFRACS 1968; FFARACS 1977
Cecily Anne Cowie (née McNulty), MB ChB 1962; D Obst 1968
Mary Victoria Miller (née Cameron), MB ChB 1962; D Obst 1980; FRCPA 1985
Meon Carolyn (Carol) Shand, MB ChB 1962; RACP (AChSHM) 1985; FNZCGP, CNZM 2008
Lorraine Elsa Smith, MB ChB 1962
Helen Brading MacNeill (née Foreman), MB ChB 1963
Florence Anne Fraser, MB ChB 1963; MRCOG 1969
Hester Nina Squire (née Grudnoff), MB ChB 1963
Mary Robertson Heyhoe, MB ChB 1963
Janet Rickord McCall Smith (née Irwin), MB ChB 1963; AM 1991
Jocelyn Mabel MacKnight, BMedSc 1960; MB ChB 1963
Maureen Anne Bassili (née O'Brien), MB ChB 1963; DA 1967; FFARACS 1979
Lesley Anne Smith (née Palmer), MB ChB 1963
Billie Rosemary Jane Campbell (née Porter), MB ChB 1963
Katherine Jean Lennane (née Scott), MB ChB 1963; MRACP 1969; DPM, RCP & RCS 1973; FRACP 1974
Margaret June Sparrow (née Muir), BSc 1955; MB ChB 1963; D Ven 1976; MBE 1987; DCNZM 2002; DBE 2009
Ngaire Jean Jeffreys (née Twose), MB ChB 1963
Viopapa 'Vio' Annandale-Atherton, MB ChB 1964; DTM&H 1976; LLD (Hon)

Marion Ruth Fromm (née Bucens), MB ChB 1964; FRCPA 1981
Lucy Fong King Chung (née Chan), MB ChB 1964
Judith Anne Driscoll (née Daniels), MB ChB 1964
Marion Joy Carey-Smith (née Dewar), MB ChB 1964; D Obst 1968; MRCOG 1970; FRNZCOG 1982; FRCOG 1983
Winifred Anne Kennedy (née Fisher), MB ChB 1964
Karen Thelma Palmer (née France), BSc 1960; MB ChB 1964; MRACP 1970; FRACP 1978; G Dip Sc 2006
Anthea Helen Wheeler (née Hatfield), MB ChB 1964; DA RCP & RCS 1970; FFRACS 1974; FFARACS 1980
Helen Ann James, MB ChB 1964; FRCS 1973; Am Board Plastic Surgery 1986
Marion Joan Boock (née Kral), MB ChB 1964
Marion McInnes (née Hamilton), MB ChB 1964
Margaret Alison Rainer (née McLaglan), MB ChB 1964
Evelyn Jean Mander (née Martindale), MB ChB 1964; D Obst 1967
Ruth Harriet Schell (née Stevenson), MB ChB 1964
Karen Deborah Williams (née Zelas), MB ChB 1964; MRC Psych 1973; MANZCP 1975
Robin Helen Briant, MB ChB 1965; RACP, MRCP 1968; MD 1973; CBE 1995
Gael Brook (née McLean), BMedSc 1962; MB ChB 1965; D Obst 1968; FRCR 1976
Margaret Christine Croxson (née Cunningham), MB ChB 1965
Dorothy Edith Stevens (née Dowd), MB ChB 1965
Beth Janice Leslie Synek (née MacGregor), MB ChB 1965
Ann Elizabeth Minnie Steele, MB ChB 1965; D Obst 1969
Gabrielle Brett Doyle (née Collison), MB ChB 1966; DPH 1972; DIH 1977, MCCM 1980
Joan Lorraine Wilson (née Faoagali), MB ChB 1966; DCP 1972; FRCPA 1974
Suzanne Helen East (née Hatch), MB ChB 1966
Anna Astrid Orgill (née Holst), MB ChB 1966
Jill Juanita Calveley (née Kelly), MB ChB 1966; QSM 2008
Lynsie Ruth Kerr (née Kitchen), MB ChB 1966
Barbara Jean Hooker (née Rusbatch), MB ChB 1966; DA 1973
Marise Anne Thacker, MB ChB 1966; DA, RCS 1967; FFARCS 1978
Karen Margaret Leslie Ward, MB ChB 1966
Mary Anthea Wright (née Ellis), BA; MB ChB 1966
Ailsa Clyne Heath Barker, MB ChB 1967; D Obst 1970; MRCP 1973; DTM&H, RCP & RCS 1973
Doreen Constance Bolton, MB ChB 1967
Noeline Margaret Butcher, MB ChB 1967
Patricia Dorothy Hill (née Cruickshank), MB ChB 1967; DTM&H 1971; D Obst RCOG 1972
Ynys Tamazin Douglas, MB ChB 1967
Ann Lang (née Philipp), MB ChB 1967
Beryl 'Monica' Lewis (née Moody), MB ChB 1967
Janet Antonoff Dunlop (née Lewis), BSc; MB ChB 1967
Elizabeth Celia Purves, BMedSc 1964; MB ChB 1967
Jocelyn Mary Williams, MB ChB 1967; D Obst 1971; FRACS 1977
Wendy Hadden (née Fitzwilliam), MB ChB 1968; RACR 1984

KEY

AChSHM: Australasian Chapter of Sexual Health Medicine
AM: Member of the Order of Australia

BA: Bachelor of Arts
BEM: British Empire Medal
BHSc: Bachelor of Home Science
BMedSc: Bachelor of Medical Science
BSc: Bachelor of Science
CBE: Commander of the Order of the British Empire
CNZM: Companion of the New Zealand Order of Merit
CRA: College of Radiologists of Australia
CRCP(C): Certificate of Royal College of Physicians Canada
D Bact: Diploma in Bacteriology
D Comm Health: Diploma in Community Health
D Obst: Diploma in Obstetrics
D Phys Med: Diploma in Physical Medicine
D Ven: Diploma in Venereology
DA: Diploma in Anaesthetics
DBE: Dame Commander of Order of the British Empire
DCH: Diploma in Child Health
DCP: Diploma in Clinical Pathology
DGO: Diploma in Gynaecology and Obstetrics
DHA: Diploma in Health Administration
DHSc: Diploma in Health Sciences
DIH: Diploma in Industrial Health
DMR: Diploma in Medical Radiology
DMRD: Diploma in Medical Radio-diagnosis
DMRE: Diploma in Medical Radiology and Electrology
DO: Diploma in Ophthalmology
DOMS: Diploma in Ophthalmic Medicine and Surgery
DPH: Diploma in Public Health
DPM: Diploma in Psychological Medicine
DSc: Doctor of Science
DTM&H: Diploma in Tropical Medicine and Hygiene
FAFPHM: Fellow of the Australasian Faculty of Public Health Medicine
FAFRM: Fellow of the Australasian Faculty of Rehabilitation Medicine
FCRA: Fellow of the College of Radiologists of Australia
FFARACS: Fellow of the Faculty of Anaesthetists of the Royal Australasian College of Surgeons
FFARCS: Fellow of the Faculty of Anaesthetists of the Royal College of Surgeons
FFR: Fellow of the Faculty of Radiology
FNZIC: Fellow of the New Zealand Institute of Chemistry
FRACP: Fellow of the Royal Australasian College of Physicians
FRACS: Fellow of the Royal Australasian College of Surgeons
FRANZCP: Fellow of the Royal Australian and New Zealand College of Psychiatrists
FRANZCR: Fellow of the Royal Australian and New Zealand College of Radiologists
FRCA: Fellow of the Royal College of Anaesthetists
FRCGP: Fellow of the Royal College of General Practitioners
FRCOG: Fellow of the Royal College of Obstetricians and Gynaecologists
FRCP: Fellow of the Royal College of Physicians
FRCP(C): Fellow of the Royal College of Physicians Canada
FRCPA: Fellow of the Royal College of Pathologists of Australasia

FRCPE: Fellow of the Royal College of Physicians of England
FRCR: Fellow of the Royal College of Radiologists
FRCS: Fellow of the Royal College of Surgeons
FRCSE: Fellow of the Royal College of Surgeons of England
FRCSEd: Fellow of the Royal College of Surgeons of Edinburgh
FRNZCGP: Fellow of the Royal New Zealand College of General Practitioners
FRNZCOG: Fellow of the Royal New Zealand College of Obstetricians and Gynaecologists
FRSNZ: Fellow of the Royal Society of New Zealand
G Dip Sc: Graduate Diploma in Science
LLD (Hons): Honorary Doctor of Laws
LM: Licentiate in Midwifery
LRCP: Licentiate of the Royal College of Physicians
MA: Master of Arts
MACO: Member of the Australian College of Opthalmologists
MANZCP: Member of the Australian and New Zealand College of Psychiatrists
MB ChB: Bachelor of Medicine, Bachelor of Surgery
MBE: Member of the Order of the British Empire
MC Path: Member of the Royal College of Pathologists
MCCM: Member of the New Zealand College of Community Medicine
MCRA: Member of the College of Radiologists of Australia
MD: Doctor of Medicine
MNZOM: Member of the New Zealand Order of Merit
MRACP: Member of the Royal Australasian College of Physicians
MRACR: Member of the Royal Australasian College of Radiologists
MRANZCP: Member of the Royal Australian and New Zealand College of Psychiatrists
MRC Psych: Member of the Royal College of Psychiatrists
MRCGP: Member of the Royal College of General Practitioners
MRCOG: Member of the Royal College of Obstetricians and Gynaecologists
MRCP: Member of the Royal College of Physicians
MRCPE: Member of the Royal College of Physicians Edinburgh
MSc: Master of Science
OBE: Officer of the Order of the British Empire
OStJ: Officer of the Order of St John
QSM: Queen's Service Medal
RACP: Royal Australasian College of Physicians
RACR: Royal Australian College of Radiologists
RANZCOG: Royal Australian and New Zealand College of Obstetrics and Gynaecology
RCA: Royal College of Anaesthetists
RCGP: Royal College of General Practitioners
RCO: Royal College of Ophthalmologists
RCOG: Royal College of Obstetricians and Gynaecologists
RCP: Royal College of Physicians
RCPA: Royal College of Pathologists of Australasia
RCS: Royal College of Surgeons
RCS & P: Royal College of Surgeons and Physicians
RNZCOG: Royal New Zealand College of Obstetricians and Gynaecologists

Notes

ABBREVIATIONS

EMWoNZ Early Medical Women of New Zealand

INTRODUCTION

1 Lucy Goodman, interview with Marion Joy Carey-Smith (née Dewar), 2019, EMWoNZ.

2 Diana Brown, *The Unconventional Career of Dr Muriel Bell* (Dunedin: Otago University Press, 2018).

3 Moira Lynch, interview with Robyn Hewland, 2019, EMWoNZ; Claire Gooder, interview with Jennifer Colston Wilson, 2016, EMWoNZ.

4 Rennae Taylor, interview with Beryl 'Monica' Lewis (née Moody), 2022, EMWoNZ.

5 Michaela Selway, 'Miriam Frank', *Early Medical Women of New Zealand* (blog), 4 November 2021, www.earlymedwomen.auckland.ac.nz/2021/11/04/miriam-frank; Miriam Frank, *My Innocent Absence: Tales from a Nomadic Life* (London: Arcadia Books, 2010), 140.

6 Julia Margaret Anne Hanna, interview by Zana Bell, 2 February 2002, Interviews about Alice Horsley, Auckland's First Woman Doctor, Alexander Turnbull Library, OHInt-0862-01; Ross Galbreath and Todd Corporation, *Enterprise and Energy: The Todd Family of New Zealand* (Wellington: Todd Corporation, 2010), 145.

7 Cynthia Farquhar and Michaela Selway, interview with Sam Bufton, 2021, EMWoNZ.

8 Lucy Goodman, interview with Susan Cambridge, 2019, EMWoNZ.

9 Examples include Margaret Guthrie, Marion Carey-Smith, Alice Horsley, Muriel Bell, Robyn Hewland, Elizabeth Berry, Carol Shand, Judith Driscoll, Marion McInnes, Katharine Bowden, Jennifer Wilson, Miriam Frank, Viola Palmer and Karen Palmer.

10 Frances I. Preston, *Lady Doctor, Vintage Model* (Wellington: A. H. & A. W. Reed, 1974); Cynthia Farquhar and Lucy Goodman, interview with Ann Gluckman, 2020, EMWoNZ; Nora Lynch, interview with Robyn Hewland, 2019, EMWoNZ.

11 Dorothy Page, 'Dissecting a Community: Women Medical Students at the University of Otago, 1891–1924', in *Communities of Women: Historical Perspectives*, eds Barbara Brookes and Dorothy Page (Dunedin: Otago University Press, 2002), 126; Kathleen Anderson, 'Beyond the Pioneer Woman Doctor: A Study of Women Doctors in Auckland 1900–1960' (MA thesis, University of Auckland, 1992), 47.

12 Notably, the first two women medical graduates and the first woman law graduate in New Zealand came from Otago Girls' High School when Alexander Wilson was the rector. Dorothy Page, 'The First Lady Graduates: Women with Degrees from Otago University, 1885–1900', in *Women in History 2: Essays on Women in New Zealand*, eds Barbara Brookes, Charlotte Macdonald and Margaret Tennant (Wellington: Bridget Williams Books, 1992), 105.

13 Ruth Fry, *It's Different for Daughters: A History of the Curriculum for Girls in New Zealand Schools, 1900–1975*, Educational Research Series, no. 65 (Wellington: New Zealand Council for Educational Research, 1985), 45.

14 Beryl Hughes and Sheila Ahern, *Redbrick and Bluestockings: Women at Victoria, 1899–1993* (Wellington: Victoria University Press, 1993), 15.

15 'Differentiation of the Curricula between the Sexes in Secondary Education', Report of the Consultative Committee to the Board of Education (the Hadow Report) (London: HMSO, 1923), 1–2; Fry, *It's Different for Daughters*, 21.

16 Fry, *It's Different for Daughters*, 13; Mrs Steadman Aldis, 'The Present Development of Women's Education in New Zealand', in *Women and Empire 1750–1939*, Vol. II: New Zealand, ed. Caroline Daley (London: Routledge, 2009), 276.

17 Fry, *It's Different for Daughters*, 11.

18 Ibid., 18.

19 Ibid., 47.

20 Ibid., 47.

21 Ibid., 50.

22 Ibid., 58.

23 Dudley William Carmalt Jones, *Annals of the University of Otago Medical School, 1875–1939* (Wellington: A. H. & A. W. Reed, 1945), 43–44.

24 The University of New Zealand was first established in Christchurch in 1870 and, after it absorbed the University of Otago in 1874, it became the only degree-granting university in New Zealand until 1961. The university followed the collegiate system and had various colleges around New Zealand: Otago, Christchurch, Auckland, Wellington, Lincoln and Palmerston North. Otago negotiated a degree of separation from the other colleges and so maintained its title as a university, even though students were awarded degrees by the wider association — the University of New Zealand. As the University of New Zealand expanded to other colleges, these colleges also adopted the policy of accepting women students. Page, 'Dissecting a Community', 111; Hughes and Ahern, *Redbrick and Bluestockings*, 9.

25 Gordon Parry, *Otago Medical School 1875–1975: An Historical Sketch* (Dunedin: University of Otago Medical School, 1975), 10; Arthur Porritt, 'The History of Medicine in New Zealand', *Medical History* 11, no. 4 (October 1967): 340, https://doi.org/10.1017/S0025727300012485

26 Page, 'The First Lady Graduates', 98; Hughes and Ahern, *Redbrick and Bluestockings*, 11.

27 The full list of women who graduated from Otago University between 1885 and 1900 can be found in the appendix of Page, 'The First Lady Graduates'.

28 'University Council', *Otago Daily Times*, 10 May 1882, p.3.

29 Jones, *Annals*, 103.

30 Dorothy Page, *Anatomy of a Medical School: A History of Medicine at the University of Otago, 1875–2000* (Dunedin: Otago University Press, 2008), 48.

31 Jones, *Annals*, 109; R. G. Robinson, 'The Otago Medical School, 1875–1975', *British Medical Journal* 1, no. 5954 (1975): 379.

32 Jones, *Annals*, 107.

33 Ibid., 45.

34 Jennifer Curtin, 'New Zealand: A Country of Firsts in Women's Political Rights', in *The Palgrave Handbook of Women's Political Rights*, eds Susan Franceschet, Mona Lena Krook and Netina Tan (London: Palgrave Macmillan, 2019), 132, https://doi.org/10.1057/978-1-137-59074-9_9; Irma Sulkunen, 'An International Comparison of Women's Suffrage: The Cases of Finland and New Zealand in the Late Nineteenth and Early Twentieth Century', *Journal of Women's History* 27, no. 4 (December 2015): 97, https://doi.org/10.1353/jowh.2015.0040

35 Curtin, 'New Zealand', 134.

36 Raewyn Dalziel, 'The Colonial Helpmeet: Women's Role and the Vote in Nineteenth-Century New Zealand', *New Zealand Journal of History* 11, no. 2 (1977): 113; Anderson, 'Beyond the Pioneer Woman Doctor', 3.

37 *Daybreak*, 6 July 1895, p.2; Patricia Ann Sargison, '"Essentially a Woman's Work": A History of General Nursing in New Zealand, 1830–1930' (PhD thesis, University of Otago, Dunedin, 2001), 60.

38 Sulkunen, 'An International Comparison of Women's Suffrage', 106.

39 Dalziel, 'The Colonial Helpmeet'.

40 Michael Belgrave, 'A Subtle Containment: Women in New Zealand Medicine, 1893–1941', *New Zealand Journal of History* 22, no. 1 (1988): 45.

41 Page, 'Dissecting a Community', 117; Anderson, 'Beyond the Pioneer Woman Doctor', 27–28.

42 Sargison, '"Essentially a Woman's Work"', 49, 58.

43 Ibid., 55.

44 In the first year of the Auckland School of Medicine, 20 per cent of the class were women. While this was noted as low, one of the lecturers from the school, Graham White, mentioned that the school had not received a high number of female applicants. By 1974, women made up 42 per cent of the class. See 'Students', Faculty of Medical and Health Sciences History, https://fmhs-history.blogs.auckland.ac.nz/admissions

45 Charles Hercus and Gordon Bell, *The Otago Medical School Under the First Three Deans* (Edinburgh and London: E. & S. Livingstone, 1964), 159.

46 Jones, *Annals*, 104.

47 Belgrave, 'A Subtle Containment'; Anderson, 'Beyond the Pioneer Woman Doctor'; John Armstrong, 'The "Common-Health" and Beyond: New Zealand Medical Specialists and the International Medical Network, 1945–85', *Health and History* 14, no. 1 (2012); Page, 'The First Lady Graduates'; Page, 'Dissecting a Community'.

48 Margaret D. Maxwell, *Women Doctors in New Zealand: An Historical Perspective, 1921–1986* (Auckland: IMS NZ, 1990).

49 Jill McIlraith, *The Goods' Train Doctors: Stories of Women Doctors in New Zealand 1920–1993* (Dunedin: New Zealand Medical Women's Association, 1994).

50 The interviews are with Diana Mason, Dorothy Potter, Margaret Sparrow, Susi Williams, Diana Edwards, Tamsin Hayter and Maire Smith.

51 For example, refugee organisations and church groups.

52 https://paperspast.natlib.govt.nz/newspapers/all#year

53 Alistair Thomson and Robert Perks, *Oral History*, eds Paul Atkinson et al. (London: Sage, 2020), 1.

54 Ann Beaglehole, *A Small Price to Pay: Refugees from Hitler in New Zealand 1936–46* (Wellington: Bridget Williams Books, 2015), 6–7.

1. THE PIONEERS 1891 – 1913

1 Letter, 10 March 1891, from Emily Siedeberg, York Place, to the Chancellor of the University of Otago [first & second page], from 'Scrapbook of autograph letters and photographs of Otago University Medical School staff', MS-1689/001, University of Otago Medical Library Historical Collection.

2 John H. Scott, *Without Parade or Fuss: A Biographical Memoir of John Halliday Scott, M.D.* (Christchurch: Admin Services, 1996), 51; Dudley William Carmalt Jones, *Annals of the University of Otago Medical School, 1875–1939* (Wellington: A. H. & A. W. Reed, 1945), 86.

3 Barbara Brookes, 'A Corresponding Community: Dr Agnes Bennett and Her Friends from the Edinburgh Medical College for Women of the 1890s', *Medical History* 52, no. 2 (April 2008): 240, https://doi.org/10.1017/S0025727300002374

4 Barbara Brookes, 'Emily Siedeberg, New Zealand's First Woman Doctor', *Corpus* (blog), 3 April 2017, https://corpus.nz/emily-siedeberg-new-zealands-first-woman-doctor

5 Emily Olga Host, 'Emily H. Siedeberg-McKinnon', in *Women Doctors in New Zealand: An Historical Perspective, 1921–1986* (Auckland: IMS NZ, 1990), 140.

6 More information about this abuse can be found in her biography. Michaela Selway, 'Emily Hancock Siedeberg-McKinnon', *Early Medical Women of New Zealand* (blog), 9 March 2021, www.earlymedwomen.auckland.ac.nz/2021/03/09/emily-hancock-siedeberg-mckinnon

7 Charlotte Macdonald, Merimeri Penfold and Bridget R. Williams (eds), *The Book of New Zealand Women — Ko Kui Ma Te Kaupapa* (Wellington: Bridget Williams Books, 1991).

8 There was only one graduate in 1896 and 1897, no graduates until 1900 when there were four, then only one in 1902 and in 1903. There were none until one woman in 1906, and a larger gap until one woman in 1910 and in 1911.

9 Otago Girls' High School graduates: Emily

Siedeberg, Margaret Cruickshank, Daisy Platts-Mills, Jane Kinder, Eleanor McLaglan, Agatha Monfries, Winifrede Bathgate, Emily Nees and Ada Paterson; Braemar House graduate: Catharine Will.

10 'Dr Jessie Maddison', *Press*, 29 November 1975.

11 Patricia Whitford, *Woodward Questions* (self-published, n.d.), 39; Horsley Family, 'Life in 1900: Dr. Alice Horsley, Auckland's First Woman Doctor', *Journal of the Auckland Historical Society* 32 (n.d.): 29.

12 'Civil Service Examinations', *New Zealand Herald*, 21 January 1905.

13 Dorothy Page, 'Dissecting a Community: Women Medical Students at the University of Otago, 1891–1924', in *Communities of Women: Historical Perspectives*, eds Barbara Brookes and Dorothy Page (Dunedin: Otago University Press, 2002), 112.

14 Kathleen Anderson, 'Constance Frost in New Zealand and Australia: A Trans-Tasman Look at Colonial Medicine', in *New Countries and Old Medicine: Proceedings of an International Conference on the History of Medicine and Health, Auckland, New Zealand, 1994*, eds Linda Bryder and Derek Dow (Auckland: Pyramid Press, 1994), 219; V. Sherwood, 'Dr Constance Helen Frost: General Practitioner, Bacteriologist, Pathologist', *Prospect* 14 (2015): 32.

15 Page, 'Dissecting a Community', 114.

16 Jones, *Annals*, 130.

17 Julia Margaret Anne Hanna, interview by Zana Bell, 2 February 2002, Interviews about Alice Horsley, Auckland's First Woman Doctor, Alexander Turnbull Library, OHInt-0862-01; Whitford, *Woodward Questions*, 42.

18 Eleanor Southey Baker McLaglan, *Stethoscope and Saddlebags: An Autobiography* (Auckland: Collins, 1965).

19 Ibid.

20 Dorothy Page, *Anatomy of a Medical School: A History of Medicine at the University of Otago, 1875–2000* (Dunedin: Otago University Press, 2008), 50.

21 Kathleen Anderson, 'Beyond the Pioneer Woman Doctor: A Study of Women Doctors in Auckland 1900–1960' (MA thesis, University of Auckland, 1992), 31.

22 Page, 'Dissecting a Community', 119.

23 Dunedin: Winifrede Bathgate, Emily Nees, Ina Moody and Catharine Will; Auckland: Constance Frost and Alice Horsley; Christchurch: Jessie Maddison.

24 Women who opened their own practice: Emily Siedeberg, Constance Frost, Daisy Platts-Mills, Alice Horsley, Eleanor McLaglan and Winifrede Bathgate. Agatha Monfries bought a practice.

25 Anderson, 'Beyond the Pioneer Woman Doctor', 41.

26 'Danger of Goitre: School Doctor's Warning', *Ashburton Guardian*, 23 July 1927; Charles Hercus and Eleanor Southey Baker, 'Statistical Study of the Incidence of Goitre Amongst the School-children of Canterbury and the West Coast', *New Zealand Medical Journal* (1921): 116–21.

27 Michael Belgrave, 'A Subtle Containment: Women in New Zealand Medicine, 1893–1941', *New Zealand Journal of History* 22, no. 1 (1988): 48–49.

28 Anderson, 'Beyond the Pioneer Woman Doctor', 64–65.

29 Page, 'Dissecting a Community', 119.

30 Belgrave, 'A Subtle Containment', 48.

31 Ibid.

32 Charles Hercus and Gordon Bell, *The Otago Medical School Under the First Three Deans* (Edinburgh and London: E. & S. Livingstone, 1964), 165; Dorothy Page, 'The First Lady Graduates: Women with Degrees from Otago University, 1885–1900', in *Women in History 2: Essays on Women in New Zealand*, eds Barbara Brookes, Charlotte Macdonald and Margaret Tennant (Wellington: Bridget Williams Books, 1992), 110.

33 This trend was also witnessed in Britain by Mary Ann Elston, who explained that the second and third generation of women medical graduates found it harder to combine a career with marriage. Brookes, 'A Corresponding Community', 250.

34 Host, 'Emily H. Siedeberg-McKinnon', 139.

35 National Council of Women of New Zealand, *A New Earth: Pioneer Women of New Zealand* (Wellington: National Council of Women of New Zealand, 1975), 62; Host, 'Emily H. Siedeberg-McKinnon', 139.

36 Mary R. S. Creese and Thomas M. Creese, *Ladies in the Laboratory III: South African, Australian, New Zealand, and Canadian Women in Science: Nineteenth and Early Twentieth Centuries: A Survey of their Contributions* (Lanham, MD: Scarecrow Press, 2010), 146; David Murray, 'Emily Siedeberg's House', *Built in Dunedin* (blog), 25 July 2016, https://builtindunedin.com/2016/07/25/emily-siedebergs-house

37 Host, 'Emily H. Siedeberg-McKinnon'.

38 Mrs Steadman Aldis, 'The Present Development of Women's Education in New Zealand', in *Women and Empire 1750–1939*, Vol. II: New Zealand, ed. Caroline Daley (London: Routledge, 2009), 275

39 Ibid.

40 Patricia Ann Sargison, *Notable Women in New Zealand Health, Te Hauora Ki Aotearoa: Ōna Wāhine Rongonui* (Auckland: Longman Paul, 1993), 13; Host, 'Emily H. Siedeberg-McKinnon', 139.

41 See the Introduction for information on the reaction to Mary Tracey, the first woman to request entrance to the Otago Medical School.

42 National Council of Women of New Zealand, *A New Earth*, 62.

43 Patricia A. Sargison, 'Emily Hancock Siedeberg', *Te Ara — the Encyclopedia of New Zealand*, 1996, https://teara.govt.nz/en/biographies/3s16/siedeberg-emily-hancock; Page, *Anatomy of a Medical School*, 48.

44 National Council of Women of New Zealand, *A New Earth*, 63.

45 Host, 'Emily H. Siedeberg-McKinnon', 140.

46 Brookes, 'Emily Siedeberg, New Zealand's First Woman Doctor'.

47 Jill Leichter, 'Emily Siedeberg', *Jewish Online Museum* (blog), www.jewishonlinemuseum.net/emily-siedeberg; Host, 'Emily H. Siedeberg-McKinnon', 139.

48 National Council of Women of New Zealand, *A New Earth*, 63; Page, *Anatomy of a Medical School*, 48.

49 Creese and Creese, *Ladies in the Laboratory III*; Leichter, 'Emily Siedeberg'.

50 Creese and Creese, *Ladies in the Laboratory III*, 146; 'Emily Siedeberg', *Royal Society, Te Aparangi* (blog), www.royalsociety.org.nz/150th-anniversary/150-women-in-150-words/1867-1917/emily-siedeberg

51 Sargison, *Notable Women in New Zealand Health*, 14.

52 Murray, 'Emily Siedeberg's House'; Sargison, *Notable Women in New Zealand Health*, 14.

53 Brookes, 'Emily Siedeberg, New Zealand's First Woman Doctor'; Monica Cronin, 'The Great Women of Anaesthesia: Emily Hancock Siedeberg McKinnon', Geoffrey Kaye Museum of the Australian and New Zealand College of Anaesthetists, 8 June 2017, www.geoffreykayemuseum.org.au/the-great-women-of-anaesthesia-emily-hancock-siedeberg-mckinnon

54 Sargison, *Notable Women in New Zealand Health*, 14.

55 Ibid.

56 National Council of Women of New Zealand, *A New Earth*, 62; Sargison, *Notable Women in New Zealand Health*, 15.

57 Sargison, *Notable Women in New Zealand Health*, 15.

58 Host, 'Emily H. Siedeberg-McKinnon', 144.

59 Brookes, 'Emily Siedeberg, New Zealand's First Woman Doctor'; Cronin, 'The Great Women of Anaesthesia,' 9.

60 Host, 'Emily H. Siedeberg-McKinnon', 145.

61 Charlotte Macdonald, 'Emily's Dream: A Women's Memorial Building and a History Without Walls: Citizenship and the Politics of Public Remembrance in 1930s–40s New Zealand', in *Women's Rights and Human Rights: International Historical Perspectives*, eds Patricia Grimshaw, Katie Holmes and Marilyn Lake (New York: Palgrave Macmillan, 2001), 169.

62 Michael Belgrave, 'A Subtle Containment: Women in New Zealand Medicine, 1893–1941', *Journal of New Zealand History* 22, no. 1 (1988).

63 Ibid.; David R. Lockyer, *Beyond the Splendours of the Sunset — To the One Satisfying Goal: A Biography of Margaret Barnett Cruickshank, M.B., Ch. B., University of N.Z., 1897*, ed. Daphne Mackenzie (Christchurch: David R. Lockyer, 2014).

64 Mike Houlahan, 'Heroic Woman Doctor Succumbed to Flu', *Otago Daily Times*, 23 November 2018.

65 'Dr Margaret Barnett Cruickshank', Timaru District Council Te Kaunihera ā-Rohe o Te Tihi o Maru, 16 September 2021, www.timaru.govt.nz/community/our-district/hall-of-fame/category-three/dr-margaret-cruickshank; Lockyer, *Beyond the Splendours of the Sunset*; Nancy Cooke, 'A Remarkable Woman: Margaret Barnet Cruickshank', *New Zealand Genealogist* 51, no. 382 (2020): 60–63.

66 Elizabeth Jamieson Morrison, *Dr Margaret Barnett Cruickshank, M.D. : First Woman Doctor in New Zealand* (Christchurch: Whitcombe & Tombs, 1923).

67 Macdonald, Penfold and Williams, *The Book of New Zealand Women*; Lockyer, *Beyond the Splendours of the Sunset*; 'Margaret Cruickshank'.

68 Lockyer, *Beyond the Splendours of the Sunset.*

69 Houlahan, 'Heroic Woman Doctor Succumbed to Flu'.

70 Lockyer, *Beyond the Splendours of the Sunset.*

71 Ibid.; Morrison, *Dr Margaret Barnett Cruickshank.*

72 Christchurch City Council Libraries, 'Dr Margaret Cruickshank'; Hughes, 'Margaret Barnet Cruickshank'.

73 Morrison, *Dr Margaret Barnett Cruickshank*; Lockyer, *Beyond the Splendours of the Sunset.*

74 Timaru District Council, 'Dr Margaret Barnett Cruickshank'; Christchurch City Council Libraries, 'Dr Margaret Cruickshank'.

75 Morrison, *Dr Margaret Barnett Cruickshank.*

76 This biography is based on multiple interviews with Alice's family members. The interviews with Anne Hanna (née Morris), Graham Mandeno, John Hughlings Jackson, Alice Walker and Mary Daphne (Bobbie) Woodward were conducted by Zana Bell for the Alice Horsley Project in 2002 and accessed in 2021 by the EMWoNZ project at the National Library. Cindy Farquhar and Michaela Selway conducted another interview with Anne Hanna in February 2021 for the EMWoNZ Project.

77 Julia Margaret Anne Hanna, interview by Zana Bell, 2 February 2002, Interviews about Alice Horsley, Auckland's First Woman Doctor, Alexander Turnbull Library, OHInt-0862-01.

78 John Hughlings Jackson, interview by Zana Bell, 28 April 2002, Interviews about Alice Horsley, Auckland's First Woman Doctor, Alexander Turnbull Library, OHC-015935; *Mangere Bridge School Centennial Record 1889–1989* (Auckland: Mangere Bridge School Centennial Committee, 1989), 9.

79 Bobbie Woodward, interview by Zana Bell, 1 February 2002, Interviews about Alice Horsley, Auckland's First Woman Doctor, Alexander Turnbull Library, OHC-015939; Jackson, interview by Zana Bell, 28 April 2002.

80 Cindy Farquhar and Michaela Selway, interview with Anne Hanna, 13 January 2021, EMWoNZ; Whitford, *Woodward Questions*, 37.

81 Jackson, interview by Zana Bell, 28 April 2002.

82 Whitford, *Woodward Questions.*

83 Hanna, interview by Zana Bell, 2 February 2002; Whitford, *Woodward Questions*, 41.

84 Ibid.

85 Farquhar and Selway, interview with Anne Hanna, 13 January 2021; Whitford, *Woodward Questions*, 42.

86 Whitford, *Woodward Questions*, 42.

87 Anderson, 'Alice Woodward Horsley'; Royal Society, 'Alice Woodward Horsley', 150 Women in 150 Words, Royal Society Te Aparangi, www.royalsociety.org.nz/150th-anniversary/150-women-in-150-words/1867-1917/alice-woodward-horsley

88 Walker, interview by Zana Bell, 1 April 2002.
89 Whitford, *Woodward Questions*, 42.
90 Jackson, interview by Zana Bell, 28 April 2002.
91 Farquhar and Selway, interview with Anne Hanna, 13 January 2021.
92 Sherwood, 'Dr Constance Helen Frost', 32.
93 Anderson, 'Constance Frost in New Zealand and Australia'; Sherwood, 'Dr Constance Helen Frost', 32;.
94 Sherwood, 'Dr Constance Helen Frost', 33.
95 Anderson, 'Constance Frost in New Zealand and Australia', 220.
96 Ibid., 219; Anderson, 'Beyond the Pioneer Woman Doctor', 85.
97 Anderson, 'Constance Helen Frost'.
98 Sherwood, 'Dr Constance Helen Frost', 33.
99 Ibid., 35.
100 Anderson, 'Constance Frost in New Zealand and Australia', 220.
101 Anderson, 'Beyond the Pioneer Woman Doctor', 87–88.
102 Ibid., 93.
103 Ibid., 103.
104 Sherwood, 'Dr Constance Helen Frost', 34–35.
105 Anderson, 'Beyond the Pioneer Woman Doctor', 7.
106 Anderson, 'Constance Frost in New Zealand and Australia', 221.
107 'N.Z. University Scholarships', *Evening Star*, 27 January 1897.
108 'Advertisements Column 4', *Evening Star*, 5 October 1904, p.1.
109 'Obituary Dr Agatha Adams-Monfries', *The Outlook*, 7 March 1911.
110 Margaret Tennant, 'Ada Gertrude Paterson', *Te Ara — the Encyclopedia of New Zealand*, 1996, https://teara.govt.nz/en/biographies/3p13/paterson-ada-gertrude
111 Tennant, 'Ada Gertrude Paterson'.
112 Amanda Kennedy, 'Ada Paterson (1880–1937)', The Northern Cemetery, 2022, www.northerncemetery.org.nz/biography/?id=43
113 'Dr Ada Paterson, Obituary'; Hester Maclean, *Nursing in New Zealand: History and Reminiscences* (Wellington: Tolan Printing, 1932), 96.
114 Kennedy, 'Ada Paterson (1880–1937)'.
115 'Breaking Up. Napier District School', *Daily Telegraph*, 19 December 1899, p.3; 'Town Edition,' *Daily Telegraph*, March 9, 1900, p.8.
116 'Town Edition.'
117 'Napier School Committee. Special Meeting,' *Hawke's Bay Herald*, 20 April 1901, p.4; 'Breaking-Up. Napier Main School', *Daily Telegraph*, 18 December 1900.
118 Aldis, 'The Present Development of Women's Education in New Zealand'.
119 'Advertisements', *Poverty Bay Herald*, 28 January 1910, p.3.
120 'Personal', *Clutha Leader*, 23 March 1910.
121 'Accidents and Fatalities', *Otago Daily Times*, 11 May 1910, p.3.
122 'Personal', *Hawke's Bay Tribune*, 21 October 1912, p.5.
123 'Personal', *Manawatu Standard*, 2 April 1913, p.5.
124 'Obituary. Dr I. B. Moody' *Auckland Star*, 17 February 1930, p.3.
125 Catharine Brookfield's great-grandson, John McMillan, and her granddaughters, Judith McMillan and Linden Hart, provided an early family history written by Brookfield's son, Melville. The spelling of her first name varied in her birth, marriage and death registrations and her medical degree diploma; the family have asked for Catharine to be used.
126 'Shipwreck Relief', *Otago Daily Times*, 10 February 1911.

2. THE WAR YEARS 1914–1919

1 Sarah Luxford, 'Passengers for the War? The Involvement of New Zealand Women in Employment during the Great War 1914–1918' (MA thesis, Massey University, 2005).
2 Melanie Nolan, '"Keep New Zealand Home Fires Burning": Gender, Welfare and the First World War', in *New Zealand's Great War*, eds John Crawford and Ian McGibbon (Auckland: Exisle, 2007), 494.
3 Ibid., 12, 496.
4 Ibid., 499.
5 Kate Hunter, 'Women's Mobilization for

War (New Zealand)', *1914–1918-Online. International Encyclopedia of the First World War*, 2015, 6, https://doi.org/10.15463/IE1418.10768

6 Nolan, 'Keep New Zealand Home Fires Burning', 497.

7 Hunter, 'Women's Mobilization for War'.

8 Margaret Tennant, *Across the Street, Across the World: A History of the Red Cross in New Zealand 1915–2015* (Wellington: New Zealand Red Cross, 2015), 30.

9 Hunter, 'Women's Mobilization for War', 16; Nolan, 'Keep New Zealand Home Fires Burning', 498.

10 Beryl Hughes, 'Margaret Barnet Cruickshank', *Te Ara — the Encyclopedia of New Zealand*, 1996, https://teara.govt.nz/en/biographies/3c41/cruickshank-margaret-barnet

11 Hunter, 'Women's Mobilization for War', 30.

12 Doris Gordon, *Backblocks Baby-Doctor: An Autobiography* (Wellington: Whitcombe & Tombs, 1955).

13 Ross Galbreath and Todd Corporation, *Enterprise and Energy: The Todd Family of New Zealand* (Wellington, New Zealand: Todd Corporation, 2010), 143.

14 Susannah Grant, *Vision for the Future: A Centennial History of St Margaret's College, Dunedin 1911–2011* (Dunedin: St Margaret's College, 2010).

15 Gordon Parry, *Otago Medical School 1875 1975: An Historical Sketch* (Dunedin: University of Otago Medical School, 1975), 12.

16 Dudley William Carmalt Jones, *Annals of the University of Otago Medical School, 1875–1939* (Wellington: A. H. & A. W. Reed, 1945), 129, 140, 141–42.

17 Augusta Klippel, interview by Shirley Ross, 1989, Auckland Jewish Oral History Project, Auckland Libraries Heritage Collection, OH_1434.

18 Linda Bryder, '"Lessons" of the 1918 Influenza Epidemic in Auckland', *New Zealand Journal of History* 16, no. 2 (1982): 99.

19 Geoffrey Rice and Linda Bryder, *Black November: The 1918 Influenza Pandemic in New Zealand*, revised and enlarged second edition (Christchurch: Canterbury University Press, 2016); Geoffrey Rice, 'Christchurch in the 1918 Influenza Epidemic: A Preliminary Study', *New Zealand Journal of History* 13, no. 2 (1979): 109–37.

20 David R. Lockyer, *Beyond the Splendours of the Sunset — To the One Satisfying Goal: A Biography of Margaret Barnett Cruickshank, M.B., Ch. B., University of N.Z., 1897*, ed. Daphne Mackenzie (Christchurch: David R. Lockyer, 2014).

21 Tennant, *Across the Street*, 32; Hunter, 'Women's Mobilization for War', 33.

22 Lauris Edmond and Carolyn Milward (eds), *Women in Wartime: New Zealand Women Tell Their Story* (Wellington: Government Printers, 1986), 100.

23 W. A. Anderson, *Doctor in the Mountains* (Wellington: A. H. & A. W. Reed, 1965), 49.

24 The family never confirmed where this military hospital was located, only that it was within walking distance from Alice Horsley's home in Auckland CBD. It was potentially the Ranfurly Hospital, which had been established in 1903, but it was most likely a temporary hospital set up for the war years. Bobbie Woodward, interview by Zana Bell, 1 February 2002, Interviews about Alice Horsley, Auckland's First Woman Doctor, Alexander Turnbull Library, OHC-015939; Horsley Family, 'Life in 1900: Dr. Alice Horsley, Auckland's First Woman Doctor', *Journal of the Auckland Historical Society* 32 (n.d.): 30.

25 Alice Walker, interview by Zana Bell, 1 April 2002, Interviews about Alice Horsley, Auckland's First Woman Doctor, Alexander Turnbull Library, OHC-015938.

26 Frances I. Preston, *Lady Doctor, Vintage Model* (Wellington: A. H. & A. W. Reed, 1974).

27 Galbreath and Todd Corporation, *Enterprise and Energy*, 144.

28 Michaela Selway, 'Moana Maru Gow (née Anderson)', *Early Medical Women of New Zealand* (blog), 3 June 2021,

www.earlymedwomen.auckland.ac.nz/2021/06/03/moana-maru-gow-nee-anderson-biography/#_ftn6

29 John Barrett, *Cancer and Cure: A Doctor's Story* (London: Bachman & Turner, 1976).

30 Gordon, *Backblocks Baby-Doctor*.

31 Galbreath and Todd Corporation, *Enterprise and Energy*, 12.

32 Kathleen Anderson, 'Constance Frost in New Zealand and Australia: A Trans-Tasman Look at Colonial Medicine', in *New Countries and Old Medicine: Proceedings of an International Conference on the History of Medicine and Health, Auckland, New Zealand, 1994*, eds Linda Bryder and Derek Dow (Auckland: Pyramid Press, 1994), 221.

33 Gordon, *Backblocks Baby-Doctor*.

34 Preston, *Lady Doctor*.

35 This biography has drawn heavily on the information from Doris Gordon's two autobiographies, *Backblocks Baby-Doctor* and *Doctor Down Under*. Her grandson Tony Gordon supplied valuable information on the early history of the Jolly family; also he and her granddaughter Nicky Gordon supplied several photos. We are grateful for the assistance of Ronald W. Jones, current chairman of the Doris Gordon Memorial Trust, who kindly lent us the first two volumes of the minutes of the Obstetrical Society (BMA NZ Branch).

36 Gordon, *Backblocks Baby-Doctor*.

37 Ibid.

38 Ibid.

39 Ibid.

40 'Personal', *Taranaki Herald*, 13 June 1919.

41 Gordon, *Backblocks Baby-Doctor*.

42 Linda Bryder, 'Gordon, Doris Clifton', *Te Ara — the Encyclopedia of New Zealand*, 1998, https://teara.govt.nz/en/biographies/4g14/gordon-doris-clifton

43 Gordon, *Backblocks Baby-Doctor*.

44 Ibid.

45 Bryder, 'Gordon'.

46 'Double Medical Pass', *Auckland Star*, 14 May 1925.

47 Gordon, *Backblocks Baby-Doctor*.

48 Ibid.

49 The NZOS was renamed the New Zealand Obstetrical and Gynaecological Society (NZOGS) in 1935.

50 'Dr Doris Gordon', *Manawatu Standard*, 22 February 1933; 'Invested with O.B.E', *Stratford Evening Post*, 23 March 1936.

51 *History of National Women's Hospital* (Auckland: Auckland District Health Board, 2010).

52 Linda Bryder, *The Rise and Fall of National Women's Hospital: A History* (Auckland: Auckland University Press, 2014).

53 *History of National Women's Hospital*.

54 Doris C. Gordon, *Doctor Down Under* (London and Christchurch: Faber & Faber and Whitcombe & Tombs, 1957).

55 Gordon, *Doctor Down Under*.

56 R. W. Jones, 'Doris Gordon: Foundation of a Legacy', *New Zealand Medical Journal* 129, no. 1437 (2016): 71–76.

57 'Local Craftsmanship. High School Honours Board', *Taranaki Herald*, 17 December 1908; 'Successful Students. Taranaki Matriculation Passes', *Hawera & Normanby Star*, 20 January 1909.

58 Gordon, *Backblocks Baby-Doctor*.

59 'Medical Examination. The Successful Candidates', *Evening Post*, 13 September 1915.

60 'The Social Round', *Sun*, 13 October 1915.

61 Gordon, *Backblocks Baby-Doctor*.

62 'St Patrick's Day Sports', *Taihape Daily Times*, 15 March 1917.

63 Beryl Hughes, 'Margaret Barnet Cruickshank', *Te Ara — the Encyclopedia of New Zealand*, 1996, https://teara.govt.nz/en/biographies/3c41/cruickshank-margaretbarnet

64 N. Hanron, 'The Hanrons: Background to the Hanron Family in Ireland, India and New Zealand' (unpublished family monograph, 1994), 43.

65 Ibid.

66 Ibid., 54.

67 P. Thomas, 'The Samoan Women's Health Committees: A Study of Community Vulnerability and Resilience' (NZ Development Network Conference, Otago

University, 2014), http://devnet.org.nz/sites/default/files/Thomas%20Paper%20for%20Devnet%20Conf%202014%20for%20NZDEVNET%20website.pdf

68 Hanron, 'The Hanrons'.

69 Nora Lynch, 'Mabel Aileen Christie (née Hanron)', *Early Medical Women of New Zealand* (blog), 22 May 2020, www.earlymedwomen.auckland.ac.nz/2020/05/22/mabel-aileen-christie-nee-hanron

70 'Late Rev. A. Whyte Memorial Service at Columba College', *Evening Star*, 11 November 1919; R. D. J. Brown, 'Funeral of Dr Marion (Whyte) Cameron', in *First Church of Otago, and How It Got There*, ed. Arthur Louis Salmond (Dunedin: Otago Heritage, 1983), 3.

71 'Scholarship Results', *Evening Star*, 22 January 1908.

72 Jim Clayton, *The History of Anaesthesia in Dunedin Hospital* (Dunedin: Dunedin Hospital and Otago Medical School, 2006).

73 Grant, *Vision for the Future.*

74 This biography is largely based on family reminiscences written by Gertrude Atmore's son-in-law, Richard Bush. Lois and Richard's two sons, Tony and Chris Bush, also supplied a collection of articles and Bush family photos.

75 B. McLellan, 'Doctor Gertrude Atmore: Beloved Physician', *Otaki Historical Journal* 10 (1987): 40–41.

76 Ibid.

77 McLellan, 'Doctor Gertrude Atmore: Beloved Physician'; 'Hospital: 19 Buffalo Beach Rd, Mercury Bay, Whitianga', Heritage New Zealand Pouhere Taonga, 11 March 2018, www.heritage.org.nz/list-details/4631/Listing

78 Palmerston North City Library, 'Otaki Sanatorium', Manawatu Heritage, 2021, https://manawatuheritage.pncc.govt.nz/item/e5ecc592-c713-4fb5-955f-f7f330b44feb#tab-item-description

79 R. T. Roach, 'The Brave and Modest Charles Atmore', *Otaki Historical Journal* 34 (2012): 18–20.

80 McLellan, 'Doctor Gertrude Atmore: Beloved Physician'.

81 'Obituary: Emma Gertrude Atmore', *New Zealand Medical Journal* 58 (1959): 398–99.

82 Richard Bush, email to EMWoNZ, 'Personal correspondence regarding Emma Gertrude Atmore', 2021.

83 B. McLellan, 'Woman Doctor Remembered', *Evening Post*, 9 June 1987.

3. THE INTERWAR YEARS 1920–1938

1 James Belich, *Paradise Reforged: A History of the New Zealanders from the 1880s to the Year 2000* (Auckland: Allen Lane, 2001).

2 Barbara Brookes, *A History of New Zealand Women* (Wellington: Bridget Williams Books, 2016).

3 Diane B. Paul, John Stenhouse and Hamish G. Spencer (eds), *Eugenics at the Edges of Empire: New Zealand, Australia, Canada and South Africa* (Cham: Palgrave Macmillan, 2018.

4 Katie Pickles, 'Empire Settlement and Single British Women as New Zealand Domestic Servants During the 1920s', *New Zealand Journal of History* 31, no. 1 (2001): 22–44.

5 Brookes, *A History of New Zealand Women,* 217. See also Carolyn Daley and Deborah Montgomerie (eds), *The Gendered Kiwi* (Auckland: Auckland University Press, 1999).

6 Brookes, *A History of New Zealand Women,* 421

7 Ibid.

8 Michael Belgrave, 'A Subtle Containment: Women in New Zealand Medicine, 1893–1941', *New Zealand Journal of History* 22, no. 1 (1988): 48

9 Margaret Tennant, 'Missionaries of Health: The School Medical Service during the Inter-war Period', in *A Healthy Country: Essays on the Social History of Medicine in New Zealand,* ed. Linda Bryder (Wellington: Bridget Williams Books, 1991).

10 George Weisz, *Divide and Conquer: A Comparative History of Medical Specialization* (Oxford: Oxford University Press, 2005).

11 Mareeta Dolling, interview with Alwyn Dolling, 2021, EMWoNZ.

12 Dorothy Page, *Anatomy of a Medical School: A History of Medicine at the University of Otago, 1875–2000* (Dunedin: Otago University Press, 2008),

13 Brookes, *A History of New Zealand Women*, 215.

14 Fay Hercock, *Alice: The Making of a Woman Doctor, 1914–1974* (Auckland: Auckland University Press, 1999).

15 Ibid.; Tim Frank, 'Bread Queues and Breadwinners: Gender in the 1930s', in *The Gendered Kiwi*, eds Carolyn Daley and Deborah Montgomerie (Auckland: Auckland University Press, 1999).

16 Ruth Newton, interview with Molly Smith (née Wagstaff), 2019, EMWoNZ.

17 Rennae Taylor, 'Alice Mary Bush (née Stanton)', *Early Medical Women of New Zealand* (blog), 13 October 2021, www.earlymedwomen.auckland.ac.nz/2021/10/13/alice-mary-bush-nee-stanton

18 Rennae Taylor, 'Margaret Stuart Smith (née Riddell)', *Early Medical Women of New Zealand* (blog), 15 August 2021, www.earlymedwomen.auckland.ac.nz/2021/08/15/margaret-stuart-smith-nee-riddell

19 According to New Zealand Jewish law, Judaism follows matrilineal descent. This means that anyone with a Jewish mother automatically obtains Jewish status even if they themselves are not practising. Emily Siedeberg's father was Jewish, but her mother was not Jewish and Siedeberg was not practising, so she is not considered the first Jewish woman graduate.

20 This biography is based on an interview with and material produced by Augusta Klippel's daughter, Ann Gluckman. This material includes an interview with Augusta Klippel in 1988.

21 Cynthia Farquhar and Lucy Goodman, interview with Ann Gluckman, 2020, EMWoNZ.

22 Augusta Klippel, interview by Shirley Ross, 1989, Auckland Jewish Oral History Project, Auckland Libraries Heritage Collection, OH_1434.

23 Ann Gluckman, *Identity and Involvement, Volume III: Auckland Jewry, Past and Present* (Palmerston North: Dunmore Press, 1990).

24 Farquhar and Goodman, interview with Ann Gluckman.

25 Ibid.

26 Ibid.

27 Ibid.

28 Ross Galbreath and Todd Corporation, *Enterprise and Energy: The Todd Family of New Zealand* (Wellington: Todd Corporation, 2010).

29 Ibid., 144.

30 Ibid.

31 Ibid.

32 Bronwyn Labrum, 'Kathleen Mary Gertrude Todd', *Te Ara — the Encyclopedia of New Zealand*, 2000. https://teara.govt.nz/en/biographies/5t15/todd-kathleen-mary-gertrude

33 Labrum, 'Kathleen Mary Gertrude Todd'.

34 This biography is based on secondary literature written about Kathleen Pih-Chang by close friends. The majority of the information comes from the chapter on Pih-Chang in Manying Ip, *Home Away from Home: Life Stories of Chinese Women in New Zealand* (Auckland: New Women's Press, 1990), which is primarily a transcript of Manying's interview with Pih-Chang.

35 Eva Wong, 'Kathleen Anuei Pih-Chang' [obituary], *New Zealand Medical Journal* (March 1991); Margaret D. Maxwell, *Women Doctors in New Zealand: An Historical Perspective, 1921–1986* (Auckland: IMS NZ, 1990).

36 Maxwell, *Women Doctors in New Zealand*; Manying Ip, 'The Story of Kathleen Pih-Chang', in *Home Away from Home*, 28–49.

37 Wong, 'Kathleen Anuei Pih-Chang'.

38 Ip, 'The Story of Kathleen Pih-Chang', 35–36.

39 Ibid., 37.

40 Maxwell, *Women Doctors in New Zealand*; Ip, 'The Story of Kathleen Pih-Chang'.

41 Ip, 'The Story of Kathleen Pih-Chang', 37.
42 Wong, 'Kathleen Anuei Pih-Chang'; 'Social Items From London', *Evening Star*, 23 May 1936; 'Mission Enterprise', *New Zealand Herald*, 11 July 1936; Maxwell, *Women Doctors in New Zealand.*
43 Ip, 'The Story of Kathleen Pih-Chang', 46.
44 Ibid., 49.
45 Rennae Taylor, 'Florence and Teresa Craig', *Early Medical Women of New Zealand* (blog), 27 July 2021, www.earlymedwomen.auckland.ac.nz/2024/07/27/florence-and-teresa-craig
46 C. H. Leng, 'Health Status and the Development of Health Services in a Colonial State: The Case of British Malaya', *International Journal of Health Services* 12, no. 3 (1982): 397–417.
47 'Story of Heroism, New Zealand Sisters at Singapore', *Otago Daily Times*, 6 June 1942, p.7.
48 'Lives of the Fellows: Margaret Stuart Smith (Riddell)', Geoffrey Kaye Museum of Anaesthetic History, 2007, www.geoffreykayemuseum.org.au/fellows/home/margaret-stuart-smith
49 Rennae Taylor, 'Margaret Stuart Smith (née Riddell)', *Early Medical Women of New Zealand* (blog), 15 August 2021, www.earlymedwomen.auckland.ac.nz/2021/08/15/margaret-stuart-smith-nee-riddell
50 'Lives of the Fellows: George "Eric" Frederick Vernon Anson', Geoffrey Kaye Museum of Anaesthetic History, 1969, www.geoffreykayemuseum.org.au/fellows/home/george-eric-anson
51 'The Professional Career of Dr Margaret Stuart Smith, OBE, QJM', *Curriculum Vitae*, ed. Shelia Weston (2004).
52 'Obituary: Dr Mary Dowling', *Hawera & Normanby Star*, 22 November 1918.
53 Ibid.
54 Hercock, *Alice.*
55 Fay Hercock, 'No Talents Wasted . . . No Time Misspent: An Account of the Early Life and Career of Alice Mary Bush' (MA thesis, University of Auckland, 1988).
56 Hercock, *Alice.*
57 A. Hunter and B. Quin, 'Dr Alice Mary Bush' [obituary], *New Zealand Medical Journal* (1974).
58 H. Smyth, *Rocking the Cradle: Contraception, Sex, and Politics in New Zealand* (Wellington: Steele Roberts, 2000).
59 Hunter and Quin, 'Dr Alice Mary Bush'.
60 Hercock, *Alice.*
61 Lucy Goodman, interview with Ruth Newton, 2019, EMWoNZ. The entirety of this biography is based on this interview.

4. THE 'PRIVILEGE OF BEING STUDENTS' 1939–1948

1 Dorothy Page, 'Dissecting a Community: Women Medical Students at the University of Otago, 1891–1924', in *Communities of Women: Historical Perspectives*, eds Barbara Brookes and Dorothy Page (Dunedin: Otago University Press, 2002); Barbara Brookes, *A History of New Zealand Women* (Wellington: Bridget Williams Books, 2016).
2 Jill McIlraith (ed.), *The Goods' Train Doctors: Stories of Women Doctors in New Zealand, 1920–1993* (Dunedin: New Zealand Medical Women's Association, 1993). 10.
3 Ibid.
4 Cynthia Farquhar and Michaela Selway, interview with Nigel Wilson, 2021, EMWoNZ.
5 Michael Kelly, *Carry On: A Biography of John Wilson* (Wellington: Wilson Family, 2012).
6 Dorothy Page, *Anatomy of a Medical School: A History of Medicine at the University of Otago, 1875–2000* (Dunedin: Otago University Press, 2008), 117.
7 Deborah Montgomerie, 'Man-powering Women: Industrial Conscription During the Second World War', in *Women in History 2: Essays on New Zealand Women*, eds Barbara Brookes, Charlotte Macdonald and Margaret Tennant (Wellington: Bridget Williams Books, 1992).
8 Montgomerie, 'Man-powering Women'; Carolyn Daley and Deborah Montgomerie (eds), *The Gendered Kiwi* (Auckland: Auckland University Press, 1999).

9 Deborah Montgomerie, *The Women's War: New Zealand Women, 1939–45* (Auckland: Auckland University Press, 2001), 99.
10 Caroline Daley, 'Colonial Helpmeets, Carnival Queens and Beauty Contestants: Multiple Femininities in Twentieth-Century New Zealand', *New Zealand Journal of History* 51, no. 1 (2017): 164–83.
11 Brookes, *A History of New Zealand Women.*
12 McIlraith, *The Goods' Train Doctors.*
13 Michaela Selway, 'Meon Carolyn (Carol) Shand', *Early Medical Women of New Zealand* (blog), 24 April 2023, www.earlymedwomen.auckland.ac.nz/2023/04/24/meon-carolyn-carol-shand-biography
14 Rennae Taylor, 'Joan Eleanor Walton (née Robertson)', *Early Medical Women of New Zealand* (blog), 28 September 2021, www.earlymedwomen.auckland.ac.nz/2021/09/28/joan-eleanor-walton-nee-robertson
15 Selway, 'Diana Manby Mason (née Shaw)', *Early Medical Women of New Zealand* (blog), 27 July 2024, www.earlymedwomen.auckland.ac.nz/2024/07/27/diana-manby-mason-nee-shaw
16 Lucy Goodman, 'Maire Jean Smith (née Tait)', *Early Medical Women of New Zealand* (blog), 23 May 2020, www.earlymedwomen.auckland.ac.nz/2020/05/23/maire-jean-smith-nee-tait
17 Farquhar and Selway, interview with Nigel Wilson.
18 Farquhar and Selway, interview with Alexandra Moira Recordon and Katherine Mary Didsbury, 2021, EMWoNZ.
19 Bruce Hadden, *Eye Surgeons and Surgery in New Zealand* (Auckland: Wairau Press, 2012).
20 Brookes, *A History of New Zealand Women*, 273.
21 Ibid., 331.
22 Selway, 'Diana Manby Mason (née Shaw)'.
23 Farquhar and Selway, interview with Nigel Wilson; Selway and Taylor, interview with Catherine Wishart and John Wishart, 2021, EMWoNZ.
24 McIlraith, *The Goods' Train Doctors.*
25 Norma Harris, 'Norma Beatrice Benson', *Early Medical Women of New Zealand* (blog), 29 September 2020, www.earlymedwomen.auckland.ac.nz/2020/09/29/norma-beatrice-benson
26 Farquhar and Selway, interview with Alexandra Moira Recordon and Katherine Mary Didsbury.
27 Hadden, *Eye Surgeons and Surgery*, 139.
28 This biography is largely based on an oral interview with Isabel Wishart's daughter Catherine (Kitty) Wishart and son John Wishart in May 2021 for the EMWoNZ project.
29 'Captain P. W. Wishart, N.Z.M.C.', Auckland War Memorial Museum, 2017, www.aucklandmuseum.com/war-memorial/online-cenotaph/record/142744
30 Selway and Taylor, interview with Catherine Wishart and John Wishart.
31 Ibid.
32 This biography is primarily drawn from a biography Daphne Adams' children wrote for the EMWoNZ project in 2020. Margie Adams, John Adams and Jenny Schurer, 'Daphne Phyllis Adams (née Morrison)', *Early Medical Women of New Zealand* (blog), 23 May 2020, www.earlymedwomen.auckland.ac.nz/2020/05/23/daphne-phyllis-adams-nee-morrison
33 This biography is primarily based on an interview with Diana Mason conducted in 1998 for the Stories of Diversity and Success Oral History Project, conducted by Tree Cocks on behalf of the NZMWA. Reference number: OHInt-0780-01.
34 Sarah Burgess, 'Mason, Diana Manby — Biography', *Dictionary of New Zealand Biography*, 2020, *Te Ara — the Encyclopedia of New Zealand*, https://teara.govt.nz/en/biographies/6m8/mason-diana-manby; 'Diana Manby Mason', *New Zealand Medical Journal* 120, no. 1257 (2007).
35 Cocks, interview with Diana Mason.
36 Margaret Clark, *Beyond Expectations: Fourteen New Zealand Women Write About their Lives* (Wellington: Bridget Williams Books, 2017), 21–36.

37 Cocks, interview with Diana Mason.

38 Ibid.

39 Burgess, 'Mason, Diana Manby'.

40 Clark, *Beyond Expectations*; Cocks, interview with Diana Mason.

41 Clark, *Beyond Expectations.*

42 Cocks, interview with Diana Mason.

43 Selway, 'Diana Manby Mason (née Shaw)'.

44 Clark, *Beyond Expectations.*

45 This biography is based on an interview with Judy Wilson's son Nigel Wilson in May 2021 for the EMWoNZ project. Further information and photographs were sourced from Michael Kelly, *Carry On: A Biography of John Wilson* (Wellington: Wilson Family, 2012).

46 Two others from her year graduated from medicine in the same year as Judy, and they met up at medical reunions from then on. Farquhar and Selway, interview with Nigel Wilson.

47 Farquhar and Selway, interview with Nigel Wilson.

48 Kelly, *Carry On*, 165.

49 Ibid., 123.

50 Ibid., 175.

51 Ibid., 128, 174; B. J. Taylor, E. A. Mitchell and R. P. K. Ford, 'Preventing Cot Death in New Zealand', *Therapeutic Notes*, no. 210, Department of Health (1991).

52 Ibid., 175.

53 'Qualifies as Doctor: First Maori Woman', *Gisborne Herald*, 15 April 1948, p.6.

54 K. Beatson, 'Rina Moore', in *The Book of New Zealand Women — Ko Kui Ma Te Paupapa*, eds Carolyn Macdonald, Merimeri Penfold and Bridget R. Williams (Wellington: Bridget Williams Books, 1991), 772.

55 Selway, 'Rina Winifred Moore (née Rōpiha)', *Early Medical Women of New Zealand* (blog), 16 May 2024. www.earlymedwomen.auckland.ac.nz/2024/05/16/rina-winifred-moore-nee-ropiha

56 Ibid.

57 Beatson, 'Rina Moore'.

58 Selway, 'Rina Winifred Moore (née Rōpiha)'.

5. REFUGEES OF WAR 1941–1967

1 Armin Nolzen, 'The Nazi Party and Its Violence Against the Jews, 1933–1939: Violence as a Historiographical Concept', *Yad Vashem Studies* 31 (2003): 245–86.

2 Ann Beaglehole, *A Small Price to Pay: Refugees from Hitler in New Zealand 1936–46* (Wellington: Bridget Williams Books, 2015), 13.

3 Dorothy Page, *Anatomy of a Medical School: A History of Medicine at the University of Otago, 1875–2000* (Dunedin: Otago University Press, 2008), 119; James N. Bade and James Braund (eds), *Out of the Shadow of War: The German Connection with New Zealand in the Twentieth Century* (Melbourne: Oxford University Press, 1998), 33.

4 Bade and Braund, *Out of the Shadow of War*, 25.

5 'Refugees Displaced by World War II', National Archives of Australia, www.naa.gov.au/explore-collection/immigration-and-citizenship/migrant-stories/refugees/refugees-displaced-world-war-ii

6 Michaela Selway and Cindy Farquhar, interview with Marion Boock (née Kral), 2024, EMWoNZ.

7 'Woman Killed: Fall From Cliff at Sumner', *Press*, 16 November 1956.

8 Anthony Grenville and Swen Steinberg (eds), 'Restricted Refuge: Medical Refugees in New Zealand 1933–1945', in *Refugees from Nazi-Occupied Europe in British Overseas Territories* (Leiden: Brill Rodopi, 2020), 103–04; Beaglehole, *A Small Price to Pay*, 13.

9 Susanna Williams, 'Jewish Doctors in New Zealand 1933–1945', Holocaust Centre of New Zealand, September 2008, www.holocaustcentre.org.nz/uploads/1/2/2/4/122437058/jewish_doctors_in_new_zealand_1933_-1945_2.pdf; 'Eva Ruth Seelye', *New Zealand Medical Journal* 124, no. 1328 (2011): 138–39.

10 *Lives Remembered: 'Exile in New Zealand'*, vol. 7 (Vienna: Nationalfonds der Republik Österreich für Opfer des Nationalismus, 2022).

11 At the time, the BMA was the only medical association in New Zealand. Its purpose was to represent doctors and medical students in New Zealand. It was originally founded in 1886 at Dunedin Hospital and was only challenged in the 1960s by medical refugee Erich Geiringer, who accused the association of being extremely problematic, largely due to racism and conservatism. Geiringer, in response, founded a new medical association called the New Zealand Medical Association (NZMA) since the name was technically available.

12 Ibid., 116, 119.

13 Page, *Anatomy of a Medical School*, 116.

14 'Doctors from Abroad. Medical School. Thirteen To Be Admitted', *Evening Post*, 22 March 1939.

15 Beaglehole, *A Small Price to Pay*, 15.

16 Bade and Braund, *Out of the Shadow of War*, 25.

17 Beaglehole, *A Small Price to Pay*, 9–11, 18–19.

18 Ann Gluckman (ed.), *Identity and Involvement, Vol. 1: Auckland Jewry, Past and Present* (Palmerston North: Dunmore Press, 1990), 136.

19 'Free Access: Africa, Asia and Europe, Passenger Lists of Displaced Persons, 1946–1971', Passenger Lists of Displaced Persons, 1949.

20 Cynthia Farquhar and Michaela Selway, interview with Hendrika (Enny) Waal-Manning, 2021, EMWoNZ.

21 Cynthia Farquhar, interview with Mirdza Palmer (née Robins), 2022, EMWoNZ.

22 'Fremantle, Western Australia, Passenger Lists, 1897–1963', 23 October 1948.

23 Bade and Braund, *Out of the Shadow of War*, 201.

24 Susanna Renate Williams, interview by Tree Cocks, 11–16 May 1998, Stories of Diversity and Success Oral History Project, Alexander Turnbull Library, OHInt-0780-04.

25 Ibid.; Bade and Braund, *Out of the Shadow of War*, 26.

26 Grenville and Steinberg, 'Restricted Refuge', 100; Bade and Braund, *Out of the Shadow of War*, 201.

27 Selway and Farquhar, interview with Marion Boock.

28 Michaela Selway, 'Miriam Frank', *Early Medical Women of New Zealand* (blog), 4 November 2021, www.earlymedwomen.auckland.ac.nz/2021/11/04/miriam-frank

29 Bade and Braund, *Out of the Shadow of War*, 26.

30 Beaglehole, *A Small Price to Pay*, 92; Miriam Frank, *My Innocent Absence: Tales from a Nomadic Life* (London: Arcadía Books, 2010).

31 Farquhar and Selway, interview with Enny Waal-Manning.

32 Grenville and Steinberg, 'Restricted Refuge', 108.

33 Rennae Taylor, 'Hilda Berdach Fleischl (née Barber)', *Early Medical Women of New Zealand* (blog), 16 May 2024, www.earlymedwomen.auckland.ac.nz/2024/05/16/hilda-berdach-fleischl-nee-barber

34 Grenville and Steinberg, 'Restricted Refuge', 108.

35 Georg Lemchen, for example, failed his final exam in the one-year course purely on account of his poor control of the English language. He was given a 'special' the following year which he passed. Instances like these were one of the arguments for a three-year course as it assumed the refugees would have more time to catch up.

36 Jillian Rothwell, *Against All Odds: The Dramatic Story of Escape from the Horrors of Nazi-Occupied Vienna to a Life in New Zealand* (Auckland: David Ling Publishing, 2020), 120.

37 Taylor, 'Hilda Berdach Fleischl'.

38 Ann Gluckman, Deb Levy Friedler and Lindy Davis (eds), *Identity and Involvement, Vol. III: Auckland Jewry into the 21st Century* (Nelson: Renaissance Publishing, 2020), 137–38.

39 Selway and Farquhar, interview with Marion Boock.

40 Farquhar and Selway, interview with Enny Waal-Manning.

41 'Eva Ruth Seelye'.

42 'Degrees Conferred at University Ceremony', *Otago Daily Times*, 12 May 1948; 'Degree

Examinations', *Otago Daily Times*, 8 November 1947; 'Examinations in Medicine', *Press*, 20 November 1953.

43 John Stein, 'Obituary: Marianne Fillenz (1924–2013)', *Physiology News* (January 2013): 53, https://doi.org/10.36866/pn.93.53
44 Farquhar and Selway, interview with Enny Waal-Manning.
45 Farquhar, interview with Mirdza Palmer.
46 Farquhar and Selway, interview with Viola Cornelia Palmer.
47 'Eva Ruth Seelye'.
48 R. O'Regan, 'Obituary: Hilda Fleischl', *New Zealand Medical Journal* (1962): 2.
49 It should be noted that this was not a universal experience. Margaret Gibberd (1954), for example, was let go from her practice in London when she announced that she was pregnant.
50 Jill McIlraith (ed.), *The Goods' Train Doctors: Stories of Women Doctors in New Zealand, 1920–1993* (Dunedin: New Zealand Medical Women's Association, 1993), 6.
51 'Dr Catherine Newman,' *Press*, 16 July 1960.
52 'Frank Monk', Holocaust Centre of New Zealand, www.holocaustcentre.org.nz/uploads/1/2/2/4/122437058/frank_monk_1.pdf
53 Grenville and Steinberg, 'Restricted Refuge', 115.
54 'Auguste Friedburg 1879', Stolpersteine Hamburg, 2023, www.stolpersteine-hamburg.de/en.php?MAIN_ID=7&BIO_ID=1157
55 Frank, *My Innocent Absence*, 158.
56 Selway, 'Miriam Frank'.
57 Mike Crean, 'Margaret Stuart Smith' [obituary], *New Zealand Medical Journal* 20, no. 1261 (2007): 85–86.
58 Selway and Farquhar, interview with Marion Boock.
59 'Fresh Start', *Press*, 11 December 1959.
60 O'Regan, 'Obituary: Hilda Fleischl'.
61 *Lives Remembered: 'Exile in New Zealand'*.
62 Ruth Black, 'A Reputable Member of the Profession', in McIlraith, *The Goods' Train Doctors*, 44–45.
63 A. Newland, 'Short Biographies: Ruth Black CBE', in Gluckman, Friedler and Davis, *Identity and Involvement Vol. III*, 163–65.
64 Black, 'A Reputable Member of the Profession'.
65 Ibid.
66 This biography is based on an interview with Hendrika Waal-Manning in 2021 for the EMWoNZ project.
67 Cynthia Farquhar and Michaela Selway, interview with Hendrika (Enny) Waal-Manning, 2021, EMWoNZ.
68 This biography is based on an interview with Viola Palmer in 2021 for the EMWoNZ project.
69 During the Second World War, people the government considered 'enemy aliens' and a potential security risk were imprisoned in the former quarantine barracks on Matiu Somes Island in Wellington Harbour; most of them were German.
70 Frank, *My Innocent Absence*, 83.
71 Ibid., 140.
72 Selway, 'Miriam Frank'.
73 Frank, *My Innocent Absence*, 262.
74 Selway, 'Miriam Frank'.
75 Ibid.
76 This biography is largely based on an oral interview with Mirdza Palmer and David Palmer conducted in March 2022 for the EMWoNZ project.

6. AGENTS OF CHANGE 1948–1967

1 Barbara Brookes, Claire Gooder and Nancy De Castro, '"Feminine as Her Handbag, Modern as Her Hairstyle": The Uptake of the Contraceptive Pill in New Zealand', *New Zealand Journal of History* 47, no. 2 (2013): 223.
2 Michaela Selway, interview with Margaret Gibberd, 2022, EMWoNZ.
3 Ailsa Morrison-Galt and Michaela Selway, 'Ailsa Mary Morrison-Galt (née Smith)', *Early Medical Women of New Zealand* (blog), www.earlymedwomen.auckland.ac.nz/2021/08/20/ailsa-mary-morrison-galt-nee-smith
4 Tree Cocks, interview with Diana Mason, 1998, Stories of Diversity and Success Oral

History Project, Alexander Turnbull Library, OHInt-0780-01.

5 Rennae Taylor, 'Joan Eleanor Walton (née Robertson)', *Early Medical Women of New Zealand* (blog), 28 September 2021, www.earlymedwomen.auckland.ac.nz/2021/09/28/joan-eleanor-walton-nee-robertson

6 Claire Gooder, interview with Helen Maud Bichan (née Simpson), 2016, EMWoNZ.

7 Cynthia Farquhar, interview with Katharine Helen Campbell Bowden (née Thomson), 2018, EMWoNZ.

8 Fay Hercock, *Alice: The Making of a Woman Doctor 1914–1974* (Auckland: Auckland University Press, 1999).

9 Tree Cocks, interview with Margaret June Sparrow, 1998, Stories of Diversity and Success Oral History Project, Alexander Turnbull Library, OHInt-0780-03.

10 Cynthia Farquhar, interview with Meon Carolyn (Carol) Shand, 2020, EMWoNZ.

11 Margaret Sparrow, *Abortion Then and Now: New Zealand Abortion Stories from 1940 to 1980* (Wellington: Victoria University Press, 2010), 203.

12 For more information read: R v. Davidson (Supreme Court of Victoria 26 May 1969); 'R. v. Davidson', Legal Information Institute, www.law.cornell.edu/women-and-justice/resource/r_v_davidson; Barbara Baird, 'Abortion and the Limits of the Personal Becoming Political', *Australian Feminist Studies* 33, no. 95 (January 2018): 137–38, https://doi.org/10.1080/08164649.2018.1498735; Kate Gleeson, 'The Other Abortion Myth: The Failure of the Common Law', *Journal of Bioethical Inquiry* 6 (2009): 73, https://doi.org/10.1007/s11673-008-9131-4; 'R v Wald 28 October 1971', *Legal Helpdesk Lawyers* (blog), 27 October 2014, https://legalhelpdesklawyers.com.au/2014/10/28/r-v-wald-28-october-1971

13 Cocks, interview with Margaret June Sparrow.

14 Ibid.

15 Ibid.

16 'Ewart Hospital Nurses' Home (Former)', Wellington City Council Me Heke ki Poneke, 20 April 2017, https://wellingtoncityheritage.org.nz/buildings/1-150/59-ewart-hospital-nurses-home-former

17 Margaret J. Sparrow, 'The Contraceptive Practice of One Thousand Abortion Patients', *New Zealand Medical Journal* 95, no. 722 (December 1982): 885–87.

18 Cindy Farquhar and Lucy Goodman, interview with Winifred Anne Kennedy (née Fisher), 2019, EMWoNZ.

19 Farquhar, interview with Meon Carolyn (Carol) Shand, 2020.

20 Nora Lynch, interview with Robyn Hewland, 2019, EMWoNZ.

21 Margaret W. Guthrie, *Different Stars for Different Times: Memoirs of a Woman Doctor* (Auckland: Margaret Guthrie, 2014), 67.

22 Beryl Harris, *A Dame We Knew: A Tribute to Dame Cecily Pickerill* (Wellington: Beryl Harris, 2014).

23 Address at Mercia Barnes Funeral, 18 April 1994, personal communication.

24 Cynthia Farquhar, interview with Lady Helen Margaret Irwin Liley (née Hunt), 2020, EMWoNZ.

25 *Staphylococcus aureus* is a bacteria present on the skin that, if transferred, can cause serious harm to babies because of their undeveloped immune systems.

26 Sylvia Yang Yuan, '"Kiwis" in the Middle Kingdom: A Sociological Interpretation of the History of New Zealand Missionaries in China from 1877 to 1953 and Beyond' (PhD thesis, Massey University, Auckland, 2013), 224, https://mro.massey.ac.nz/server/api/core/bitstreams/71dd07e5-7ad7-4c5b-911d-eff15af87d31/content

27 Ailsa Barker, 'Teologi, Studi Biblika, Dan Misi', *Indonesian Journal of Theology* 5, no. 1 (July 2017): 99–131, https://doi.org/10.46567/ijt.v5i1.36

28 Michael Gill, *Himalayan Hospitals: Sir Edmund Hillary's Everest Legacy* (Nelson: Potton and Burton, 2011).

29 Cynthia Farquhar and Rennae Taylor, interview with Viopapa Annandale-

Atherton, 2023, EMWoNZ; Adel Fruean, 'Papalii Dr Viopapa Atherton', *Samoa Observer*, 2024, www.samoaobserver.ws/category/article/41849

30 'A Woman of the Pacific', University of Otago Ōtākou Whakaihu Waka, www.otago.ac.nz/otagomagazine/issue50/profiles/a-woman-of-the-pacific

31 This biography is primarily based on information from Harris, *A Dame We Knew*; and Harvey Brown, *Pickerill: Pioneer in Plastic Surgery, Dental Education, and Dental Research* (Dunedin: Otago University Press, 2007). Approval for this biography was given by Cecily's niece, Fay Hope. We are grateful to Beryl, Harvey and Fay for their support of this project.

32 This biography is based on oral interviews with Patricia Mackay's two daughters, Colyn and Indi Mackay, conducted in Melbourne for the EMWoNZ project, and secondary material in the public domain, including two interviews for professional bodies.

33 V. Paterson, 'Top Anaesthetist Visits Home Town', *Otago Daily Times*, 1 February 1991; 'Business Announcements: Professional', *Otago Daily Times*, 30 December 1948, p.1.

34 K. Dulhunty, 'Trail-blazing Leader in Anaesthetics Was a Pioneer for Patient Safety — and a Great Cook', *Sydney Morning Herald*, 23 October 2015, www.smh.com.au/national/trailblazing-leader-in-anaesthetics-was-a-pioneer-for-patient-safety–and-a-great-cook-20151023-gkhc2j.html; C. Ball, interview with Dr Patricia Mackay, OAM, 2013, ANZCA, www.anzca.edu.au/about-us/our-history-and-heritage/oral-histories

35 Rennae Taylor, 'Patricia Mackay (née Wilson)', *Early Medical Women of New Zealand* (blog), 14 July 1948, www.earlymedwomen.auckland.ac.nz/2024/07/14/patricia-mackay-nee-wilson

36 Taylor, 'Patricia Mackay (née Wilson)'.

37 Ball, interview with Dr Patricia Mackay, 2013.

38 'Mackay, Patricia (1926–)', *Melbourne: Encyclopedia of Australian Science and Innovation*, www.eoas.info/biogs/P004343b.htm

39 W. B. Runciman, 'Lessons from the Australian Patient Safety Foundation: Setting Up a National Patient Safety Surveillance System — Is This the Right Model?', *Quality & Safety in Health* 11, no. 3 (2002).

40 Ball, interview with Patricia Mackay, 2013.

41 Paterson, 'Top Anaesthetist Visits Home Town'.

42 This biography is based on information from the biography by Bartha Finna Hill, *Teaching Hundreds to Heal Millions: The Story of Dr Beryl Howie, Medical Missionary in India* (Auckland: Daystar Books, 2013). Howie's nephew and niece have provided further information on their Ngāi Tahu lineage and access to family photos.

43 Susannah Grant, *Vision for the Future: A Centennial History of St Margaret's College, Dunedin 1911–2011* (Dunedin: St Margaret's College, 2010).

44 D. Troughton, R. Troughton and M. Laigesen, 'Obituary: Beryl Overton Howie', *New Zealand Medical Journal* 126, no. 1370 (2013).

45 'Beloved Professor Remembered', *Ludhiana CMC US Review*, 2013.

46 This biography is primarily based on the two autobiographies written by Margaret Guthrie: *Different Stars for Different Times*; and *An Enduring Savour* (Porirua: MWG Publishing, n.d.).

47 Guthrie, *An Enduring Savour*, 144.

48 Ibid., 194.

49 This biography is based on an interview with Helen (Margaret) Liley in 2020 for the EMWoNZ project. Farquhar, interview with Margaret Liley.

50 This biography is based on an interview with Margaret Maxwell in 2019 for the EMWoNZ project.

51 This biography is based on an interview with Helen Angus in 2019 for the EMWoNZ project. Nora Lynch, interview with Helen Beaumont Angus, 2019, EMWoNZ.

52 This biography is based on an interview with Carol Shand conducted in 2020 for the EMWoNZ project and biographical material included in the family history: Farquhar, interview with Carol Shand; Ann Green, *Virtue Leads, Fortune Follows: A Short History of the Shand Family from Scotland to New Zealand* (Rotorua: Ann Green, 2013); Carol Shand, *Things I Remember or Was Told: A Memoir* (Wellington: Writes Hill Press, 2022).

53 This biography is largely based on an interview between Dame Margaret Sparrow and Dr Tree Cocks from 12 May 1998. The interview was recorded as part of the New Zealand Medical Women's Association Oral History Project, Stories of Diversity and Success, and is held at the National Library of New Zealand in Wellington. Permission to use this interview was granted by Dame Margaret Sparrow and the National Library. Tree Cocks, interview with Margaret June Sparrow, 1998, Stories of Diversity and Success Oral History Project, Alexander Turnbull Library, OHInt-0780-03.

54 This biography is largely based on an interview with Papali'i Viopapa Annandale-Atherton and her son James on 27 April 2023. Farquhar and Taylor, interview with Viopapa Annandale-Atherton.

55 'Rising to the Challenge — First Pacific Graduate Paves the Way', *Otago Bulletin Board Uni News*, 2019, www.otago.ac.nz/otagobulletin/news/otago709868.html; A. Richardson, 'Profiles: A Woman of the Pacific', *University of Otago Magazine*, 2019.

56 Lafi Sanerivi, 'Samoa', in Mark Bray and Lucy Steward, *Examination Systems in Small States: Comparative Perspectives on Policies, Models and Operations*, Educational Development in the Small States of the Commonwealth (Commonwealth Secretariat, 1998), 306; J. M. Barrington, 'The United Nations and Educational Development in Western Samoa during the Trusteeship Period 1946–1961', *International Review of Education / Internationale Zeitschrift Für Erziehungswissenschaft / Revue Internationale de l'Education* 19, no. 2 (1973): 255–61.

57 'Rising to the Challenge'.

58 D. Lythgoe, 'A Study of Annandale Families — Dr John Atherton', 2021, https://annandale.one-name.net/getperson.php?personID=I2156&tree=annandale

59 Richardson, 'Profiles'.

60 Farquhar and Taylor, interview with Viopapa Annandale-Atherton.

61 This biography is based on an interview between Cindy Farquhar and Wendy Hadden in 2018 for the EMWoNZ project. Cynthia Farquhar, interview with Wendy Hadden (née Fitzwilliam), 2018, EMWoNZ.

62 Farquhar, interview with Wendy Hadden.

63 Ibid.

7. MAKING THEIR MARK IN RESEARCH 1896–1967

1 Emphasis is our own. Gordon Parry, *Otago Medical School 1875–1975: An Historical Sketch* (Dunedin: University of Otago Medical School, 1975).

2 Dorothy Page, *Anatomy of a Medical School: A History of Medicine at the University of Otago, 1875–2000* (Dunedin: Otago University Press, 2008), 126.

3 C. Elizabeth Le Couteur, 'Dentist, Doctor, Dean: Professor Sir Charles Hercus and His Record of Fostering Research at the Otago Medical School, 1921–1958' (PhD thesis, University of Canterbury, 2013), 78.

4 Page, *Anatomy of a Medical School*, 127.

5 Ibid., 126.

6 Le Couteur, 'Dentist, Doctor, Dean', 118–19.

7 Ibid., 121.

8 Claire Gooder, interview with Helen Maud Bichan (née Simpson), 2016, EMWoNZ.

9 Cynthia Farquhar and Michaela Selway, interview with Hendrika (Enny) Waal-Manning, 2021, EMWoNZ.

10 Page, *Anatomy of a Medical School*, 133.

11 Ibid.

12 Esther Irving, 'Sylvia Gytha de Lancey Chapman', *Te Ara — the Encyclopedia of New Zealand*, 1998, https://teara.govt.nz/en/biographies/4c17/chapman-sylvia-gytha-de-lancey

13 Diana Brown, *The Unconventional Career of*

Dr Muriel Bell (Dunedin: Otago University Press, 2018).
14 Ibid.
15 Ibid.
16 Ibid.
17 Ibid.
18 Elizabeth Gregory et al., *Good Nutrition: Principles and Menus* (Wellington: Government Printer, 1956).
19 'Scholarships and Prizes', University of Otago Ōtākou Whakaihu Waka, www.otago.ac.nz/humannutrition/study/scholarships-prizes
20 D. K. Mackay, *An Appetite for Wonder: Cawthron Institute 1921–2011, 90th Anniversary* (Nelson: Cawthron Institute, 2011).
21 Linda Bryder, *A Voice for Mothers: The Plunket Society and Infant Welfare, 1907–2000* (Auckland: Auckland University Press, 2003).
22 Ibid.
23 Marie Stringer Buchler, 'An Analysis of 20,319 Obstetrical Case Records of the New Zealand Obstetrical and Gynaecological Society' (MD thesis, University of Otago, Dunedin, 1938).
24 'Nursing Service', *Otago Daily Times*, 13 June 1936.
25 Christine Daniell, *A Doctor at War: A Life in Letters, 1914–43* (Masterton: Fraser Books, 2001), 170, 180, 188.
26 Marie Buchler, 'Pulmonary Tuberculosis in Wellington: A Radiological Investigation Among Office and Factory Workers and Secondary School Children', *New Zealand Medical Journal* 43 (1944): 73–81.
27 'Advertisements', *Evening Post*, 27 April 1943.
28 'The Inside Story', Microbiology Memoirs: The History of the Microbiology Department, 28 April 2017, https://otagomicrobes.com/category/The-inside-story/?order=asc
29 '"Influenzial" Career', University of Otago Ōtākou Whakaihu Waka, www.otago.ac.nz/otagomagazine/issue44/features/influenzial-career
30 'Helen Rarity McCreanor', Te Whatu Ora Health New Zealand, 31 October 2016, www.ccdhb.org.nz/about-us/history/wellington-hospital-smo-archive/appointments-made/1961-1980/medical-admin-clinical-support-services/pathology/mccreanor-helen-r
31 'John Donal McCreanor', Royal College of Physicians, https://history.rcplondon.ac.uk/inspiring-physicians/john-donal-mccreanor
32 'Obituary: Helen McCreanor (née Young)', *New Zealand Medical Journal* 89 (1979): 402–03.
33 This biography is largely based on Barbara Heslop's own written reflections of her life as well as an interview with her two daughters, Helen and Hilary Heslop, on 27 March 2023 for the EMWoNZ project.
34 Helen Heslop and Hilary Heslop, 'Obituary of John Herbert Heslop', Royal Australasian College of Surgeon, 2014, www.surgeons.org/about-racs/about-the-college-of-surgeons/in-memoriam/obituaries/john-herbert-heslop
35 Edwin Nye, *Medical Research in Otago, 1922–1997: As Portrayed by 75 Years of the Proceedings of the University of Otago Medical School* (Dunedin: Otago Medical School Research Society, 1998), 145.
36 Ibid., 145.
37 'Barbara and John Heslop Medal', Royal Australasian College of Surgeons, www.surgeons.org/about-racs/about-the-college-of-surgeons/awards-lectures-prizes/awards/distinguished-awards/barbara-and-john-heslop-medal
38 'Graduation', *Evening Star*, 14 May 1946.
39 'Advertisements', *Press*, 6 January 1949.
40 'Marianne Fillenz', Department of Physiology, Anatomy and Genetics, www.dpag.ox.ac.uk/women-in-physiology-anatomy-genetics/marianne-fillenz
41 'Marianne Fillenz Memorial Lecture Series', Department of Physiology, Anatomy and Genetics, www.dpag.ox.ac.uk/named-lectures/marianne-fillenz-lecture
42 Eric Clarke, Karen Clarke and Sue Clarke, 'John Clarke Obituary', *Guardian*, 8

July 2010, www.theguardian.com/education/2010/jul/08/john-clarke-obituary

43 Peter Calder, 'Sir Edmund Hillary's Life', *New Zealand Herald*, 10 January 2008, www.nzherald.co.nz/nz/sir-edmund-hillarys-life/CS3E7VXPDQNZBZ43XWAMCMV6PA

44 The biography is based on an oral interview with Senga Whittingham conducted in 2023 for the EMWoNZ project.

45 This biography is largely based on an oral interview with Tania Gunn's son, Professor Alistair Gunn, and her daughter-in-law, Dr Diana Rabone, conducted in October 2022 for the EMWoNZ project.

46 Cynthia Farquhar, interview with Alistair Gunn and Diana Rabone, 2022, EMWoNZ.

47 Ibid.

48 Ibid.

49 'Obituary: Ngaire Margaret Walsh (nee McKerrow)', *New Zealand Medical Journal* 95 (January 1982): 52.

50 B. F. Heslop et al., 'Women in Medicine in New Zealand', *New Zealand Medical Journal* 77, no. 491 (1973): 219–29.

51 Page, *Anatomy of a Medical School*, 130.

52 Parry, *Otago Medical School 1875–1975*, 20.

53 Many of Hendrika's articles that she published through this clinic can be found in Nye, *Medical Research in Otago, 1922–1997*; Farquhar and Selway, interview with Hendrika (Enny) Waal-Manning, 2021.

54 'The Dunedin Study', Dunedin Multidisciplinary Health and Development Research Unit, https://dunedinstudy.otago.ac.nz/studies/assessment-phases

55 This biography is based on an interview with Elizabeth Berry in 2016 for the EMWoNZ project.

56 Ibid.

57 This biography is based on an interview with Norma Restieaux in 2017 for the EMWoNZ project.

58 This concurs with John Armstrong, who argued that the networks were self-perpetuating, and those that were given a foot in the door would often pass this on to other New Zealanders. Laurence Monnais-Rousselot and David Wright (eds), 'A System of Exclusion: New Zealand Women Medical Specialists in International Medical Networks, 1945–1975', in *Doctors Beyond Borders: The Transnational Migration of Physicians in the Twentieth Century* (Toronto: University of Toronto Press, 2018), 121.

59 This biography is based on an interview with Robin Briant in 2017 for the EMWoNZ project.

60 Nora Lynch, interview with Robin Helen Briant, 2017, EMWoNZ.

CONCLUSION

1 Michael Belgrave, 'A Subtle Containment: Women in New Zealand Medicine, 1893–1941', *New Zealand Journal of History* 22, no. 1 (1988): 44–55; Margaret Tennant, 'Missionaries of Health: The School Medical Service during the Inter-War Period', in *A Healthy Country: Essays on the Social History of Medicine in New Zealand*, edited by Linda Bryder (Wellington: Bridget Williams Books, 1991).

2 Cynthia Farquhar, interview with Mirdza Palmer (née Robins), 2022, EMWoNZ.

3 Kathleen Anderson, 'New Zealand Medical Women's Association, 1921–2003', New Zealand History — Nga Korero a Ipurangi o Aotearoa, 1993, https://nzhistory.govt.nz/women-together/new-zealand-medical-womens-association

4 Claire Gooder, interview with Judith Anne Barfoot (née Radcliffe), 2016, EMWoNZ.

5 John Armstrong, 'The "Common-Health" and Beyond: New Zealand Medical Specialists and the International Medical Network, 1945–85', *Health and History* 14, no. 1 (2012): 176, https://doi.org/10.5401/healthhist.14.1.0165; Ross Galbreath and Todd Corporation, *Enterprise and Energy: The Todd Family of New Zealand* (Wellington: Todd Corporation, 2010).

6 Cynthia Farquhar and Lucy Goodman, interview with Ruth Harriet Schell (née Stevenson), 2019, EMWoNZ.

7 Michaela Selway, 'Miriam Frank', *Early Medical Women of New Zealand* (blog),

4 November 2021, www.earlymedwomen.auckland.ac.nz/2021/11/04/miriam-frank

8 Barbara Heslop, 'For Better or for Worse? Women Doctors at the End of the Decade', *New Zealand Medical Journal*, 25 March 1987: 178.

9 Ibid., 176–77.

10 These 13 specialties analysed were: general physicians, endocrinology, geriatric medicine, medical oncology, rheumatology, infectious disease, nephrology, respiratory medicine, neurology, gastroenterology, cardiology, general surgery, orthopaedics.

11 Sonya Burgess et al., 'Gender Equity within Medical Specialties of Australia and New Zealand: Cardiology's Outlier Status', *Internal Medicine Journal* 50, no. 4 (April 2020): 415–16, https://doi.org/10.1111/imj.14406

12 ASMS Toi Mata Hauora, 'Demographic and Attitudinal Change in the New Zealand Specialist Workforce', ASMS Research Brief, 2016.

Bibliography

Primary sources

INTERVIEWS

Angus, Helen Beaumont. Interview with Nora Lynch Angus, 2019. EMWoNZ.

Annandale-Atherton, Papali'i Viopapa. Interview with Cynthia Farquhar and Rennae Taylor, 2023. EMWoNZ.

Barfoot (née Radcliffe), Judith Anne. Interview with Claire Gooder, 2016. EMWoNZ.

Berry (née Waugh-Burns), Elizabeth. Interview with Lucy Goodman, 2016. EMWoNZ.

Bichan (née Simpson), Helen Maud. Interview with Claire Gooder, 2016. EMWoNZ.

Boock (née Kral), Marion. Interview with Cynthia Farquhar and Michaela Selway, 2024. EMWoNZ.

Briant, Robin Helen. Interview with Helen Beaumont Angus, 2017. EMWoNZ.

Bufton, Sam. Interview with Cynthia Farquhar and Michaela Selway, 2021. EMWoNZ.

Cambridge, Susan. Interview with Lucy Goodman, 2019. EMWoNZ.

Campbell Bowden (née Thomson), Katharine Helen. Interview with Cynthia Farquhar, 2018. EMWoNZ.

Carey-Smith (née Dewar), Marion Joy. Interview with Lucy Goodman, 2019. EMWoNZ.

Dickie, John. Interview with Cynthia Farquhar and Michaela Selway, 2021. EMWoNZ.

Doak, Phil. Interview with Michaela Selway, 2021. EMWoNZ.

Driscoll (née Daniels), Judith Anne. Interview with Cynthia Farquhar, 2020. EMWoNZ.

Gluckman, Ann. Interview with Cynthia Farquhar and Lucy Goodman, 2020. EMWoNZ.

Hadden (née Fitzwilliam), Wendy. Interview with Cynthia Farquhar, 2018. EMWoNZ.

Hanna, Anne. Interview with Cynthia Farquhar and Michaela Selway, 2021. EMWoNZ.

Hanna, Julia Margaret Anne. Interview with Zana Bell, 2002. Interviews about Alice Horsley, Auckland's First Woman Doctor, Alexander Turnbull Library, OHInt-0862-01.

Hewland, Robyn. Interview with Helen Beaumont Angus, 2019. EMWoNZ.

Jackson, John Hughlings. Interview with Zana Bell, 2002. Interviews about Alice Horsley, Auckland's First Woman Doctor, Alexander Turnbull Library, OHC-015935.

Kennedy (née Fisher), Winifred Anne. Interview with Cynthia Farquhar and Lucy Goodman 2019, EMWoNZ.

Klippel, Augusta. Interview with Shirley Ross, 1989, Auckland Jewish Oral History Project, Auckland Libraries Heritage Collection, OH_1434.

Lewis (née Moody), Beryl 'Monica'. Interview with Rennae Taylor, 2022. EMWoNZ.

Liley (née Hunt), Lady Helen Margaret Irwin. Interview with Cynthia Farquhar, 2020. EMWoNZ.

Mackay, Patricia. Interview with C. Ball, 2013. ANZCA. www.anzca.edu.au/about-us/our-history-and-heritage/oral-histories

Mason, Diana. Interview with Tree Cocks, 1998. Stories of Diversity and Success Oral History Project, Alexander Turnbull Library, OHInt-0780-01.

McInnes (née Hamilton), Marion. Interview with Cynthia Farquhar and Michaela Selway, 2021. EMWoNZ.

Newton, Ruth. Interview with Lucy Goodman, 2019. EMWoNZ.

Palmer (née France), Karen Thelma. Interview with Claire Gooder, 2017. EMWoNZ.

Palmer (née Robins), Mirdza. Interview with Cynthia Farquhar, 2022. EMWoNZ.

Palmer (née Heine), Viola Cornelia. Interview with Cynthia Farquhar and Michaela Selway, 2021. EMWoNZ.

Rabone, Diana, and Alistair Gunn. Interview with Cynthia Farquhar, 2022. EMWoNZ.

Recordon, Alexandra Moira, and Katherine Mary Didsbury. Interview with Cynthia Farquhar and Michaela Selway, 2021. EMWoNZ.

Schell (née Stevenson), Ruth Harriet. Interview with Cynthia Farquhar and Lucy Goodman, 2019. EMWoNZ.

Shand, Meon Carolyn. Interview with Cynthia Farquhar, 2020. EMWoNZ.

Sparrow, Margaret June. Interview with Tree Cocks, 1998. Stories of Diversity and Success Oral History Project, Alexander Turnbull Library, OHInt-0780-03.

Waal-Manning, Hendrika (Enny). Interview with Cynthia Farquhar and Michaela Selway, 2021. EMWoNZ.

Walker, Alice. Interview with Zana Bell, 2002. Interviews about Alice Horsley, Auckland's First Woman Doctor, Alexander Turnbull Library, OHC-015938.

Whittingham, Senga. Interview with Cynthia Farquhar, 2023. EMWoNZ.

Williams, Susanna Renate. Interview with Tree Cocks, 1998. Stories of Diversity and Success Oral History Project, Alexander Turnbull Library, OHInt-0780-04.

Wilson, Jennifer Colston. Interview with Claire Gooder, 2016. EMWoNZ.

Wishart, Catherine, and John Wishart. Interview with Cynthia Farquhar and Michaela Selway, 2021. EMWoNZ.

Woodward, Bobbie. Interview with Zana Bell, 2002. Interviews about Alice Horsley, Auckland's First Woman Doctor, Alexander Turnbull Library, OHC-015939.

ARCHIVAL SOURCES AND ORAL HISTORIES

Ancestry. 'Electoral Rolls, Auckland, Waitakere', 1949.

——. 'England and Wales Civil Registration Marriage Index, 1916–2005', 1939.

——. 'Free Access: Africa, Asia and Europe, Passenger Lists of Displaced Persons, 1946–1971', Passenger Lists of Displaced Persons, 1949.

——. 'Fremantle, Western Australia, Passenger Lists, 1897–1963', 1939.

——. 'Fremantle, Western Australia, Passenger Lists, 1897–1963', 23 October 1948.

——. 'Irene Therese Abrahamsohn Valentine Family Tree', www.ancestry.com.au/family-tree/person/tree/9513351/person/25803772691/facts?_phsrc=vZE186&_phstart=successSource

——. 'New Zealand, Naturalisations, 1843–1981', 15 August 1947.

——. 'New Zealand, Naturalisations, 1843–1981', 5 April 1956.

——. 'Tatyana Godyaew', Brisbane State High School, 16 May 1950. Brisbane State High School Admission Register.

——. 'Tatyana Godyaew', New Zealand Naturalisations, 1843–1981, 21 July 1955.

'Births, Deaths & Marriages Online'. *Te Kāwanatanga o Aotearoa: New Zealand Government*. www.bdmhistoricalrecords.dia.govt.nz

'Refugees Displaced by World War II'. National Archives of Australia. www.naa.gov.au/explore-collection/immigration-and-citizenship/migrant-stories/refugees/refugees-displaced-world-war-ii

'Register of Medical Practitioners'. *New Zealand Gazette*, 9 January 1913.

Remember.org. 'Hahn'. https://remember.org/unite/hahn.htm

Stolpersteine Hamburg. 'Auguste Friedburg 1879', 2023. www.stolpersteine-hamburg.de/en.php?MAIN_ID=7&BIO_ID=1157

Trust CH. Chilton St James School: School Records. National Library, Wellington, 2008.

NEWSPAPERS AND PERIODICALS

Ashburton Guardian
Auckland Star
Bay of Plenty Times
Clutha Leader
Colonist
Daily Telegraph
Dominion
Evening Post
Evening Star
Gisborne Herald
Hastings Standard
Hawera & Normanby Star
Hawke's Bay Herald
Manawatu Standard
Marlborough Express
Mataura Ensign
New Zealand Gazette
New Zealand Herald
Oamaru Mail
Otago Daily Times
Otago Witness
Otaki Today
Outlook
Poverty Bay Herald
Stratford Evening Post
Sydney Morning Herald
Taihape Daily Times
Taranaki Herald
The Argus
The Guardian
The Press
The Sun
Wanganui Chronicle
Woodville Examiner

Secondary sources

BOOKS AND CHAPTERS

Aldis, Stkadman. 'The Present Development of Women's Education in New Zealand'. In *Women and Empire 1750–1939*, edited by Caroline Daley. London: Routledge, 2009.

Anderson, W. A. *Doctor in the Mountains.* Wellington: A. H. & A. W. Reed, 1965.

——. 'Constance Frost in New Zealand and Australia: A Trans-Tasman Look at Colonial Medicine'. In *New Countries and Old Medicine: Proceedings of an International Conference on the History of Medicine and Health, Auckland, New Zealand*, edited by Linda Bryder and Derek Dow. Auckland: Pyramid Press, 1994.

Atkinson, Paul, Sara Delamont, Alexandru Cernat, Joseph W. Sakshaug and Richard A. Williams, eds. *Oral History.* London: Sage, 2020.

Bade, James N., and James Braund, eds. *Out of the Shadow of War: The German Connection with New Zealand in the Twentieth Century.* Melbourne: Oxford University Press, 1998.

Barrett, John. *Cancer and Cure: A Doctor's Story.* London: Bachman & Turner, 1976.

Beaglehole, Ann. *A Small Price to Pay: Refugees from Hitler in New Zealand 1936–46.* Wellington: Bridget Williams Books, 2015.

Beatson, K. 'Rina Moore'. In *The Book of New Zealand Women — Ko Kui Ma Te Paupapa*, edited by Charlotte Macdonald, Merimeri Penfold, and Bridget R. Williams. Wellington: Bridget Williams Books, 1991.

Belich, James. *Paradise Reforged: A History of the New Zealanders from the 1880s to the Year 2000.* Auckland: Allen Lane, 2001.

Brookes, Barbara. *A History of New Zealand Women.* Wellington: Bridget Williams Books, 2016.

Brown, Diana. *The Unconventional Career of Dr Muriel Bell.* Dunedin: Otago University Press, 2018.

Brown, Harvey. *Pickerill: Pioneer in Plastic Surgery, Dental Education, and Dental*

Research. Dunedin: Otago University Press, 2007.

Brown, R. D. J. 'Funeral of Dr Marion (Whyte) Cameron'. In *First Church of Otago, and How It Got There*, edited by Arthur Louis Salmond. Dunedin: Otago Heritage, 1983.

Bryder, Linda. *A Voice for Mothers: The Plunket Society and Infant Welfare, 1907–2000*. Auckland: Auckland University Press, 2003.

——. *The Rise and Fall of National Women's Hospital: A History*. Auckland: Auckland University Press, 2014.

——, and J. S. Werry. *Doris Clifton Gordon (1890–1956)*. Auckland: Auckland Hospital National Women's Health, 2017.

Clark, Margaret. *Beyond Expectations: Fourteen New Zealand Women Write about Their Lives*. Wellington: Bridget Williams Books, 2017.

Clayton, Jim. *The History of Anaesthesia in Dunedin Hospital*. Dunedin: Deptartment of Anaesthesia and Intensive Care, Dunedin Hospital and Otago Medical School, 2006.

Coney, Sandra. 'Health'. In *Women Together: A History of Women's Organisations in New Zealand*, edited by Anne Else. Wellington: Wellington Historical Branch, Department of Internal Affairs and Daphne Brasell Associates Press, 1993.

Creese, Mary R. S, and Thomas M. Creese. *Ladies in the Laboratory III: South African, Australian, New Zealand, and Canadian Women in Science; Nineteenth and Early Twentieth Centuries: A Survey of Their Contributions*. Lanham: Scarecrow Press, 2010.

Curtin, Jennifer. 'New Zealand: A Country of Firsts in Women's Political Rights'. In *The Palgrave Handbook of Women's Political Rights*, edited by Susan Franceschet, Mona Lena Krook and Netina Tan. London: Palgrave Macmillan, 2019.

Daley, Carolyn, and Deborah Montgomery, eds. *The Gendered Kiwi*. Auckland: Auckland University Press, 1999.

Daniell, Christine. *A Doctor at War: A Life in Letters, 1914–43*. Masterton: Fraser Books, 2001.

Edmond, Lauris, and Carolyn Milward, eds. *Women in Wartime: New Zealand Women Tell Their Story*. Wellington: Government Printer, 1986.

Frank, Miriam. *My Innocent Absence: Tales from a Nomadic Life*. London: Arcadia Books, 2010.

Frank, Tim. 'Bread Queues and Breadwinners: Gender in the 1930s'. In *The Gendered Kiwi*, edited by Carolyn Daley and Deborah Montgomerie. Auckland: Auckland University Press, 1999.

Fry, Ruth. *It's Different for Daughters: A History of the Curriculum for Girls in New Zealand Schools, 1900–1975*. Educational Research Series, no. 65. Wellington: New Zealand Council for Educational Research, 1985.

Galbreath, Ross, and Todd Corporation. *Enterprise and Energy: The Todd Family of New Zealand*. Wellington: Todd Corporation, 2010.

Gill, M. *Himalayan Hospitals: Sir Edmund Hillary's Everest Legacy*. Nelson: Craig Potton, 2011.

Gluckman, Ann. *Identity and Involvement: Auckland Jewry, Past and Present*. Palmerston North: Dunmore Press, 1990.

Gordon, Doris. *Backblocks Baby-Doctor: An Autobiography*. Wellington: Whitcombe & Tombs, 1955.

——. *Doctor Down Under*. Wellington: Whitcombe & Tombs, 1957.

Grant, Susannah. *Vision for the Future: A Centennial History of St Margaret's College, Dunedin 1911–2011*. Dunedin: St Margaret's College, 2010.

Green, Ann. *Virtue Leads, Fortune Follows: A Short History of the Shand Family from Scotland to New Zealand*. Rotorua: Self-published, 2013.

Gregory, Elizabeth, Elizabeth Wilson, John Malcolm and Muriel Bell. *Good Nutrition: Principles and Menus*. Wellington: Government Printer, 1956.

Grenville, Anthony, and Swen Steinberg, eds. *Refugees from Nazi-Occupied Europe in British Overseas Territories*. Leiden: Brill Rodopi, 2020.

Guthrie, Margaret W. *An Enduring Savour*. Porirua: MWG Pub., n.d.

——. *Different Stars for Different Times: Memoirs of a Woman Doctor*. Auckland: Self-published, 2014.

Hadden, Bruce. *Eye Surgeons and Surgery in New Zealand*. Auckland: Wairau Press, 2012.

Hanron, N. *The Hanrons: Background to the Hanron Family in Ireland, India and New Zealand*. Unpublished family monograph, 1994.

Harris, Beryl. *A Dame We Knew: A Tribute to Dame Cecily Pickerill*. Wellington: Self-published, 2014.

Hercock, Fay. *Alice: The Making of a Woman Doctor, 1914–1974*. Auckland: Auckland University Press, 1999.

Hercus, Charles, and Gordon Bell. *The Otago Medical School Under the First Three Deans*. Edinburgh and London: E. & S. Livingstone, 1964.

Hill, Bartha Finna. *Teaching Hundreds to Heal Millions: The Story of Dr Beryl Howie, Medical Missionary in India*. Auckland: Daystar Books, 2013.

History of National Women's Hospital. Auckland: Auckland District Health Board, 2010.

Host, Emily Olga. 'Emily H. Siedeberg-McKinnon'. In *Women Doctors in New Zealand: An Historical Perspective, 1921–1986*. Auckland: IMS NZ, 1990.

Hughes, Beryl, and Sheila Ahern. *Redbrick and Bluestockings: Women at Victoria, 1899–1993*. Wellington: Victoria University Press, 1993.

Hughes, Christina. *Key Concepts in Feminist Theory and Research*. London: Sage, 2002.

Ip, Manying. *Home Away from Home: Life Stories of Chinese Women in New Zealand*. Auckland: New Women's Press, 1990.

Jones, Dudley William Carmalt. *Annals of the University of Otago Medical School, 1875–1939*. Wellington: A. H. & A. W. Reed, 1945.

Kelly, Michael. *Carry On: A Biography of John Wilson*. Wellington: Wilson Family, 2012.

Lives Remembered: 'Exile in New Zealand', vol. 7. Vienna: Nationalfonds der Republik Österreich für Opfer des Nationalismus, 2022.

Lockyer, David R. *Beyond the Splendours of the Sunset — To the One Satisfying Goal: A Biography of Margaret Barnett Cruickshank, M.B., Ch. B., University of N.Z., 1897*, edited by Daphne Mackenzie. Christchurch: David R. Lockyer, 2014.

Macdonald, Charlotte, Merimeri Penfold and Bridget R. Williams, eds. *The Book of New Zealand Women — Ko Kui Ma Te Kaupapa*. Wellington: Bridget Williams Books, 1991.

Mackay, D. K. *An Appetite for Wonder: Cawthron Institute 1921–2011*. Nelson: Cawthron Institute, 2011.

Maclean, Hester. *Nursing in New Zealand: History and Reminiscences*. Wellington: Tolan Printing Company, 1932.

Mangere Bridge School Centennial Record 1889–1989. Auckland: Mangere Bridge School Centennial Committee, 1989.

Maxwell, Margaret D. *Women Doctors in New Zealand: An Historical Perspective, 1921–1986*. Auckland: IMS NZ, 1990.

McLaglan, Eleanor Southey Baker. *Stethoscope and Saddlebags: An Autobiography*. Auckland: Collins, 1965.

McIlraith, Jill, ed. *The Goods' Train Doctors: Stories of Women Doctors in New Zealand 1920–1993*. Dunedin: New Zealand Medical Women's Association, 1994.

Monnais-Rousselot, Laurence, and David Wright, eds. *Doctors beyond Borders: The Transnational Migration of Physicians in the Twentieth Century*. Toronto: University of Toronto Press, 2018.

Montgomerie, Deborah. 'Man-powering Women: Industrial Conscription during the Second World War'. In *Women in History 2: Essays on Women in New Zealand*, edited by Barbara Brookes, Charlotte Macdonald and Margaret Tennant. Wellington: Bridget Williams Books, 1992.

——. *The Women's War: New Zealand Women, 1939–45*. Auckland: Auckland University Press, 2001.

Morrison, Elizabeth Jamieson. *Dr. Margaret Barnett Cruickshank, MD: First Woman Doctor in New Zealand.* Wellington: Whitcombe & Tombs, 1923.

National Council of Women of New Zealand. *A New Earth: Pioneer Women of New Zealand.* Wellington: National Council of Women of New Zealand, 1975.

Nolan, Melanie. '"Keep New Zealand Home Fires Burning": Gender, Welfare and the First World War'. In *New Zealand's Great War*, edited by John Crawford and Ian McGibbon. Auckland: Exisle Publishing, 2007.

Nye, Edwin. *Medical Research in Otago, 1922–1997: As Portrayed by 75 Years of the Proceedings of the University of Otago Medical School.* Dunedin: Otago Medical School Research Society, 1998.

Page, Dorothy. *Anatomy of a Medical School: A History of Medicine at the University of Otago, 1875–2000.* Dunedin: Otago University Press, 2008.

——. 'Dissecting a Community: Women Medical Students at the University of Otago, 1891–1924'. In *Communities of Women: Historical Perspectives*, edited by Barbara Brookes and Dorothy Page. Dunedin: Otago University Press, 2002.

——. 'The First Lady Graduates: Women with Degrees from Otago University, 1885–1900'. In *Women in History 2: Essays on Women in New Zealand*, edited by Barbara Brookes, Charlotte Macdonald and Margaret Tennant. Wellington: Bridget Williams Books, 1992.

Paul, Diane B., John Stenhouse and Hamish G. Spencer, eds. *Eugenics at the Edges of Empire: New Zealand, Australia, Canada and South Africa.* Cham, Switzerland: Palgrave Macmillan, 2018.

Parry, Gordon. *Otago Medical School 1875–1975: An Historical Sketch.* Dunedin: University of Otago Medical School, 1975.

Platts-Mills, John. *Muck, Silk and Socialism: Recollections of a Left-wing Queen's Counsel.* Wedmore, UK: Paper Publishing, 2002.

Preston, Frances I. *Lady Doctor, Vintage Model.* Wellington: A. H. & A. W. Reed, 1974.

Rice, Geoffrey. *Black Flu 1918: The Story of New Zealand's Worst Public Health Disaster.* Christchurch: Canterbury University Press, 2017.

——, and Linda Bryder. *Black November: The 1918 Influenza Pandemic in New Zealand.* Christchurch: Canterbury University Press, 2016.

Rothwell, Jillian. *Against All Odds: The Dramatic Story of Escape from the Horrors of Nazi-Occupied Vienna to a Life in New Zealand.* Auckland: David Ling, 2020.

Sanerivi, Lafi. 'Samoa'. In *Examination Systems in Small States: Comparative Perspectives on Policies, Models and Operations*, edited by Mark Bray and Lucy Steward. Educational Development in the Small States of the Commonwealth. Commonwealth Secretariat, 1998.

Sargison, Patricia A. *Notable Women in New Zealand Health, Te Hauora Ki Aotearoa: Ōna Wāhine Rongonui.* Auckland: Longman Paul, 1993.

Scott, John H. *Without Parade or Fuss: A Biographical Memoir of John Halliday Scott, M.D.* Christchurch: Pandamonium Publishing, 1996.

Shand, Carol. *Things I Remember or Was Told: A Memoir.* Wellington: Writes Hill Press, 2022.

Smyth, H. *Rocking the Cradle: Contraception, Sex, and Politics in New Zealand.* Wellington: Steele Roberts, 2000.

Sparrow, Margaret. *Abortion Then and Now: New Zealand Abortion Stories from 1940 to 1980.* Wellington: Victoria University Press, 2010.

Tennant, Margaret. *Across the Street, Across the World: A History of the Red Cross in New Zealand 1915–2015.* Wellington: New Zealand Red Cross, 2015.

——. 'Missionaries of Health: The School Medical Service During the Inter-war Period'. In *A Healthy Country: Essays on the Social History of Medicine in New Zealand*, edited by Linda Bryder. Wellington: Bridget Williams Books, 1991.

Weisz, George. *Divide and Conquer: A Comparative History of Medical Specialization*. Oxford: Oxford University Press, 2005.

Whitford, Patricia. *Woodward Questions*. Self-published, n.d.

Wright-St Claire, Rex Earl. *Historia Nunc Vivat: Medical Practitioners in New Zealand, 1840 to 1930*. Christchurch: Cotter Medical History Trust, 2016.

THESES AND JOURNAL ARTICLES

Anderson, Kathleen. 'Beyond the Pioneer Woman Doctor: A Study of Women Doctors in Auckland 1900–1960'. MA thesis, University of Auckland, 1992.

Armstrong, John. 'Doctors from "the End of the World": Oral History and New Zealand Medical Migrants, 1945–1975'. *Oral History Society* 42, no. 2 (2014): 41–49.

——. 'The "Common-Health" and Beyond: New Zealand Medical Specialists and the International Medical Network, 1945–85'. *Health and History* 14, no. 1 (2012): 165–86. https://doi.org/10.5401/healthhist.14.1.0165

Baird, Barbara. 'Abortion and the Limits of the Personal Becoming Political'. *Australian Feminist Studies* 33, no. 95 (2018): 129–46. https://doi.org/10.1080/08164649.2018.1498735

Barker, Ailsa. 'Teologi, Studi Biblika, Dan Misi'. *Indonesian Journal of Theology* 5, no. 1 (2017): 99–131. https://doi.org/10.46567/ijt.v5i1.36

Barrington, J. M. 'The United Nations and Educational Development in Western Samoa during the Trusteeship Period 1946–1961'. *International Review of Education / Internationale Zeitschrift Für Erziehungswissenschaft / Revue Internationale de l'Education* 19, no. 2 (1973): 255–61.

Belgrave, Michael. 'A Subtle Containment: Women in New Zealand Medicine, 1893–1941'. *New Zealand Journal of History* 22, no. 1 (1988): 44–55.

Bertram, Christiane, Wolfgang Wagner and Ulrich Trautwein. 'Learning Historical Thinking With Oral History Interviews: A Cluster Randomized Controlled Intervention Study of Oral History Interviews in History Lessons'. *American Educational Research Journal* 54, no. 3 (2017): 444–84.

Borrie, J. 'Marion King Bennie Cameron' [obituary]. *New Zealand Medical Journal* 96, no. 741 (1983): 773.

Brookes, Barbara. 'A Corresponding Community: Dr Agnes Bennett and Her Friends from the Edinburgh Medical College for Women of the 1890s'. *Medical History* 52, no. 2 (2008): 237–56.

——, Claire Gooder and Nancy De Castro. '"Feminine as Her Handbag, Modern as Her Hairstyle": The Uptake of the Contraceptive Pill in New Zealand'. *New Zealand Journal of History* 47, no. 2 (2013): 208–31.

Bryder, Linda. '"Lessons" of the 1918 Influenza Epidemic in Auckland'. *New Zealand Journal of History* 16, no. 2 (1982): 97–121.

——, and J. S. Werry. 'Pulmonary Tuberculosis in Wellington: A Radiological Investigation Among Office and Factory Workers and Secondary School Children'. *New Zealand Medical Journal* 43 (1944): 73–81.

Buchler, Marie Stringer. 'An Analysis of 20,319 Obstetrical Case Records of the New Zealand Obstetrical and Gynaecological Society'. PhD thesis, University of Otago, 1938.

Burgess, Sonya, Elizabeth Shaw, Katherine A. Ellenberger, Louise Segan, Anastasia V. Castles, Sinjini Biswas, Liza Thomas and Sarah Zaman. 'Gender Equity within Medical Specialties of Australia and New Zealand: Cardiology's Outlier Status'. *Internal Medicine Journal* 50, no. 4 (2020): 412–19. https://doi.org/10.1111/imj.14406

Christie, M. 'Child Welfare Work in Western Samoa'. *Appendix to the Journals of the House of Representatives* (1926): 38–41.

Cooke, Nancy. 'A Remarkable Woman: Margaret Barnet Cruickshank'. *New Zealand Genealogist* 51, no. 382 (2020): 60–63.

Daley, Caroline. 'Colonial Helpmeets, Carnival Queens and Beauty Contestants: Multiple

Femininities in Twentieth-century New Zealand'. *New Zealand Journal of History* 51, no. 1 (2017): 164–83.

Dalziel, Raewyn. 'The Colonial Helpmeet: Women's Role and the Vote in Nineteenth-century New Zealand'. *New Zealand Journal of History* 11, no. 2 (1977): 112–23.

Delahunt, B., and A. J. Campbell. 'Evolution of the Degree Doctor of Medicine at the University of Otago'. *New Zealand Medical Journal* 115 (2002): 135–36.

'Dr. Constance Frost' [obituary]. *New Zealand Medical Journal* (1920).

'Emma Gertrude Atmore' [obituary]. *New Zealand Medical Journal* 58 (1959): 398–99.

'Eva Ruth Seelye'. *New Zealand Medical Journal* 124, no. 1328 (2011): 138–39.

Gleeson, Kate. 'The Other Abortion Myth: The Failure of the Common Law'. *Journal of Bioethical Inquiry* 6 (2009): 69–81. https://doi.org/10.1007/s11673-008-9131-4

Hercock, Fay. 'No Talents Wasted . . . No Time Misspent: An Account of the Early Life and Career of Alice Mary Bush'. MA thesis, University of Auckland, 1988.

'Helen McCreanor (née Young)' [obituary]. *New Zealand Medical Journal* 89 (1979): 402–03.

Hercus, Charles, and Eleanor Southey Baker. 'Statistical Study of the Incidence of Goitre Amongst the School-Children of Canterbury and the West Coast'. *New Zealand Medical Journal* (1921): 116–21.

Heslop, B. F., R. Molloy, H. J. Waal-Manning and N. M. Walsh. 'Women in Medicine in New Zealand'. *New Zealand Medical Journal* 77, no. 491 (1973): 219–29.

Heslop, Barbara. 'For Better or for Worse? Women Doctors at the End of the Decade'. *New Zealand Medical Journal* (1987): 176–79.

Horsley Family. 'Life in 1900: Dr. Alice Horsley, Auckland's First Woman Doctor'. *Journal of the Auckland Historical Society* 32 (n.d.): 29–30.

Hunter, A., and B. Quin. 'Dr Alice Mary Bush' [obituary]. *New Zealand Medical Journal* (1974).

'Joan Chappel' [obituary]. *New Zealand Medical Journal* (2021).

Jones, R. W. 'Doris Gordon: Foundation of a Legacy'. *New Zealand Medical Journal* 129, no. 1437 (2016): 71–76.

'Kathleen Anuei Pih-Chang' [obituary]. *New Zealand Medical Journal* (1991).

Le Couteur, C. Elizabeth. 'Dentist, Doctor, Dean: Professor Sir Charles Hercus and His Record of Fostering Research at the Otago Medical School, 1921–1958'. PhD thesis, University of Canterbury, 2013.

Leng, C. H. 'Health Status and the Development of Health Services in a Colonial State: The Case of British Malaya'. *International Journal of Health Services* 12, no. 3 (1982): 397–417.

Luxford, Sarah. 'Passengers for the War? The Involvement of New Zealand Women in Employment During the Great War 1914–1918'. MA thesis, Massey University, 2005.

McLellan, B. 'Doctor Gertrude Atmore: Beloved Physician'. *Otaki Historical Journal* 10 (1987): 40–41.

'Ngaire Margaret Walsh (née McKerrow)' [obituary]. *New Zealand Medical Journal* 95 (1982): 52.

Nolzen, Armin. 'The Nazi Party and Its Violence Against the Jews, 1933–1939: Violence as a Historiographical Concept'. *Yad Vashem Studies* 31 (2003): 245–86.

O'Regan, R. 'Hilda Fleischl' [obituary]. *New Zealand Medical Journal* 2 (1962).

Pickles, Katie. 'Empire Settlement and Single British Women as New Zealand Domestic Servants during the 1920s'. *New Zealand Journal of History* 31, no. 1 (2001): 22–44.

Porritt, Arthur. 'The History of Medicine in New Zealand'. *Medical History* 11, no. 4 (1967): 334–44. https://doi.org/10.1017/S0025727300012485

Rice, Geoffrey. 'Christchurch in the 1918 Influenza Epidemic: A Preliminary Study'. *New Zealand Journal of History* 13, no. 2 (1979): 109–37.

Roach, R. T. 'The Brave and Modest Charles Atmore'. *Otaki Historical Journal* 34 (2012): 18–20.

Robinson, R. G. 'The Otago Medical School, 1875–1975'. *British Medical Journal* 1, no. 5954 (1975): 378–82.

Runciman, W. B. 'Lessons from the Australian Patient Safety Foundation: Setting up a National Patient Safety Surveillance System — Is this the Right Model?'. *Quality & Safety in Health* 11, no. 3 (2002).

Samuel, Raphael. 'Local History and Oral History'. *History Workshop Journal* 1, no. 1 (1976): 191–208. https://doi.org/10.1093/hwj/1.1.191

Sargison, Patricia A. '"Essentially a Woman's Work": A History of General Nursing in New Zealand, 1830–1930'. PhD thesis, University of Otago, 2001.

Sherwood, V. 'Dr. Constance Helen Frost: General Practitioner, Bacteriologist, Pathologist'. *Prospect* 14 (2015): 32–36.

Sparrow, Margaret. 'The Contraceptive Practice of One Thousand Abortion Patients'. *New Zealand Medical Journal* 95, no. 722 (1982): 885–87.

Stein, John. 'Marianne Fillenz (1924–2013)' [obituary]. *Physiology News* (2013): 53. https://doi.org/10.36866/pn.93.53

Sulkunen, Irma. 'An International Comparison of Women's Suffrage: The Cases of Finland and New Zealand in the Late Nineteenth and Early Twentieth Century'. *Journal of Women's History* 27, no. 4 (2015): 88–111. https://doi.org/10.1353/jowh.2015.0040

Troughton, D., R. Troughton and M. Laigesen. 'Beryl Overton Howie' [obituary]. *New Zealand Medical Journal* 126, no. 1370 (2013).

Wong, Eva. 'Kathleen Anuei Pih-Chang' [obituary]. *New Zealand Medical Journal* (1991).

Yang Yuan, Sylvia. '"Kiwis" in the Middle Kingdom: A Sociological Interpretation of the History of New Zealand Missionaries in China from 1877 to 1953 and Beyond'. PhD thesis, Massey University, 2013.

ONLINE AND OTHER SOURCES

Adams, Margie, John Adams and Jenny Schurer. 'Daphne Phyllis Adams (née Morrison)'. *Early Medical Women of New Zealand* (blog), 23 May 2020. www.earlymedwomen.auckland.ac.nz/2020/05/23/daphne-phyllis-adams-nee-morrison

Anderson, Kathleen. 'Alice Woodward Horsley'. *Te Ara — the Encyclopedia of New Zealand*, 1996. https://teara.govt.nz/en/biographies/3h36/horsley-alice-woodward

Anderson, W. A. 'Constance Helen Frost'. *Te Ara — the Encyclopedia of New Zealand*, 1996.

——. 'New Zealand Medical Women's Association, 1921–2003'. New Zealand History — Nga Korero a Ipurangi o Aotearoa, 1993. https://nzhistory.govt.nz/women-together/new-zealand-medical-womens-association

ASMS Toi Mata Hauora. 'Demographic and Attitudinal Change in the New Zealand Specialist Workforce'. ASMS Research Brief, 2016.

Brookes, Barbara. 'Emily Siedeberg, New Zealand's First Woman Doctor'. *Corpus* (blog), 3 April 2017. https://corpus.nz/emily-siedeberg-new-zealands-first-woman-doctor

Bryder, Linda. 'Gordon, Doris Clifton'. *Te Ara — the Encyclopedia of New Zealand*, 1998. https://teara.govt.nz/en/biographies/4g14/gordon-doris-clifton

Christchurch City Council Libraries. 'Dr Margaret Cruickshank'. Christchurch City Council Libraries — Ngā Kete Wānanga-o-Ōtautahi, 2024. https://my.christchurchcitylibraries.com/dr-margaret-cruickshank

Clarke, Eric. 'Marianne Fillenz (1950)'. Somerville College Report, March 2012. https://issuu.com/somervillecollege/docs/somerville_college_report_2012-13/106

Cooke, R. 'Patients First: The Proud Tradition of Taumarunui Hospital'. Taumarunui Hospital Reunion Committee, 2005.

Cronin, Monica. 'The Great Women of Anaesthesia: Emily Hancock Siedeberg

McKinnon'. Geoffrey Kaye Museum of the Australian and New Zealand College of Anaesthetists, 8 June 2017. www.geoffreykayemuseum.org.au/the-great-women-of-anaesthesia-emily-hancock-siedeberg-mckinnon

Department of Physiology, Anatomy & Genetics. 'Marianne Fillenz'. www.dpag.ox.ac.uk/women-in-physiology-anatomy-genetics/marianne-fillenz

——. 'Marianne Fillenz Memorial Lecture Series'. www.dpag.ox.ac.uk/named-lectures/marianne-fillenz-lecture

Dunedin Multidisciplinary Health & Development Research Unit. 'The Dunedin Study'. https://dunedinstudy.otago.ac.nz/studies/assessment-phases

Faculty of Medical and Health Sciences History. 'Students'. https://fmhs-history.blogs.auckland.ac.nz/admissions

Fraenkel, Jon. 'Pacific Islands and New Zealand — Samoa'. *Te Ara — the Encyclopedia of New Zealand*. https://teara.govt.nz/en/pacific-islands-and-new-zealand/page-4

Fruean, Adel. 'Papalii Dr. Viopapa Atherton'. *Samoa Observer*, 2024. www.samoaobserver.ws/category/article/41849

Geoffrey Kaye Museum of Anaesthetic History. 'Lives of the Fellows: Margaret Stuart Smith (Riddell)'. 2007. www.geoffreykayemuseum.org.au/fellows/home/margaret-stuart-smith

Goodman, Lucy. 'Maire Jean Smith (née Tait)'. *Early Medical Women of New Zealand* (blog), 23 May 2020. www.earlymedwomen.auckland.ac.nz/2020/05/23/maire-jean-smith-nee-tait

Harris, Norma. 'Norma Beatrice Benson'. *Early Medical Women of New Zealand* (blog), 29 September 2020. www.earlymedwomen.auckland.ac.nz/2020/09/29/norma-beatrice-benson

Heritage New Zealand Pouhere Taonga. 'Hospital: 19 Buffalo Beach Rd, Mercury Bay, Whitianga'. 11 March 2018. www.heritage.org.nz/list-details/4631/Listing

Heslop, Helen, and Hilary Heslop. 'Obituary of John Herbert Heslop'. Royal Australasian College of Surgeons, 2014. www.surgeons.org/about-racs/about-the-college-of-surgeons/in-memoriam/obituaries/john-herbert-heslop

Holocaust Centre of New Zealand. 'Frank Monk'. www.holocaustcentre.org.nz/uploads/1/2/2/4/122437058/frank_monk_1.pdf

Hughes, Beryl. 'Margaret Barnet Cruickshank'. *Te Ara — the Encyclopedia of New Zealand*, 1996. https://teara.govt.nz/en/biographies/3c41/cruickshank-margaret-barnet

Hunter, Kate. 'Women's Mobilization for War (New Zealand)'. *1914–1918-Online International Encyclopedia of the First World War*, 2015. https://doi.org/10.15463/IE1418.10768

Institut Terezínské iniciativy. 'Erich Hahn'. 2 April 2014. www.holocaust.cz/databaze-obeti/obet/91804-erich-hahn

Irving, Esther. 'Sylvia Gytha de Lancey Chapman'. *Te Ara — the Encyclopedia of New Zealand*, 1998. https://teara.govt.nz/en/biographies/4c17/chapman-sylvia-gytha-de-lancey

Kennedy, Amanda. 'Ada Paterson (1880–1937)'. *The Northern Cemetery. Dunedin's Buried History*, 2022. www.northerncemetery.org.nz/biography/?id=43

Labrum, Bronwyn. 'Kathleen Mary Gertrude Todd'. *Te Ara — the Encyclopedia of New Zealand*, 2000. https://teara.govt.nz/en/biographies/5t15/todd-kathleen-mary-gertrude

Legal Helpdesk Lawyers. 'R v Wald | 28 October 1971'. *Legal Helpdesk Lawyers* (blog), 27 October 2014. https://legalhelpdesklawyers.com.au/2014/10/28/r-v-wald-28-october-1971

Legal Information Institute. 'R. v. Davidson'. www.law.cornell.edu/women-and-justice/resource/r_v_davidson

Leichter, Jill. 'Emily Siedeberg'. *Jewish Online Museum* (blog). www.jewishonlinemuseum.net/emily-siedeberg

Ludhiana CMC Board USA. 'Beloved Professor Remembered'. *Ludhiana CMC US Review*, 2013.

Lynch, Nora. 'Mabel Aileen Christie (née Hanron)'. *Early Medical Women of New Zealand* (blog), 22 May 2020. www.earlymedwomen.auckland.ac.nz/2020/05/22/mabel-aileen-christie-nee-hanron

Lythgoe, D. 'A Study of Annandale Families — Dr John Atherton', 2021. https://annandale.one-name.net/getperson.php?personID=I2156&tree=annandale

Mackay, Patricia. *Melbourne: Encyclopedia of Australian Science and Innovation.* www.eoas.info/biogs/P004343b.htm

Manawatu Heritage. 'Otaki Sanatorium'. 2021. https://manawatuheritage.pncc.govt.nz/item/e5ecc592-c713-4fb5-955f-f7f330b44feb#tab-item-description

'Microbiology Memoirs: The History of the Microbiology Department'. *The Inside Story*, 28 April 2017. https://otagomicrobes.com/category/The-inside-story/?order=asc

Ministry for Culture and Heritage. 'Margaret Cruickshank'. 8 November 2017. https://nzhistory.govt.nz/people/margaret-cruickshank

Murray, David. 'Emily Siedeberg's House'. *Built in Dunedin* (blog), 25 July 2016. https://builtindunedin.com/2016/07/25/emily-siedebergs-house

New Zealand WW100. 'Restored Memorial to WW1 Medics Rededicated'. 13 October 2016. https://ww100.govt.nz/restored-memorial-to-ww1-medics-rededicated

Otago Bulletin Board Uni News. 'Rising to the Challenge — First Pacific Graduate Paves the Way'. 2019. www.otago.ac.nz/otagobulletin/news/otago709868.html

Richardson, A. 'Profiles: A Woman of the Pacific'. *University of Otago Magazine*, 2019.

Royal Australasian College of Surgeons. 'Barbara and John Heslop Medal'. www.surgeons.org/about-racs/about-the-college-of-surgeons/awards-lectures-prizes/awards/distinguished-awards/barbara-and-john-heslop-medal

Royal College of Paediatrics and Child Health. 'About the College History'. www.rcpch.ac.uk/about-us/history-and-archive/history

Royal College of Pathologists of Australasia. 'History of the College'. www.rcpa.edu.au/About/History-of-the-College

Royal College of Physicians. 'John Donal McCreanor'. https://history.rcplondon.ac.uk/inspiring-physicians/john-donal-mccreanor

Royal Society. 'Alice Woodward Horsley'. *150 Women in 150 Words, Royal Society Te Aparangi.* www.royalsociety.org.nz/150th-anniversary/150-women-in-150-words/1867-1917/alice-woodward-horsley

——. 'Emily Siedeberg'. *Royal Society, Te Aparangi* (blog). www.royalsociety.org.nz/150th-anniversary/150-women-in-150-words/1867-1917/emily-siedeberg

Sargison, Patricia A. 'Emily Hancock Siedeberg'. *Te Ara — the Encyclopedia of New Zealand*, 1996. https://teara.govt.nz/en/biographies/3s16/siedeberg-emily-hancock

Selway, Michaela. 'Diana Manby Mason (née Shaw)'. *Early Medical Women of New Zealand* (blog), 27 July 2024. www.earlymedwomen.auckland.ac.nz/2024/07/27/diana-manby-mason-nee-shaw

——. 'Emily Hancock Siedeberg-McKinnon'. *Early Medical Women of New Zealand* (blog), 9 March 2021. www.earlymedwomen.auckland.ac.nz/2021/03/09/emily-hancock-siedeberg-mckinnon

——. 'Ina Burnman Moody (née Dugleby)'. *Early Medical Women of New Zealand* (blog), 12 May 2024.

——. 'Kathleen Pih-Chang (Bi Zhen-Wah)'. *Early Medical Women of New Zealand* (blog), 4 March 2024. www.earlymedwomen.auckland.ac.nz/2024/03/04/kathleen-pih-chang-bi-zhen-wah

——. 'Meon Carolyn (Carol) Shand'. *Early Medical Women of New Zealand* (blog), 24 April 2023. www.earlymedwomen.auckland.ac.nz/2023/04/24/meon-carolyn-carol-shand-biography

——. 'Miriam Frank'. *Early Medical Women of New Zealand* (blog), 4 November 2021. www.earlymedwomen.auckland.ac.nz/2021/11/04/miriam-frank

——. 'Moana Maru Gow (née Anderson)'. *Early Medical Women of New Zealand* (blog), 3 June 2021. www.earlymedwomen.auckland.ac.nz/2021/06/03/moana-maru-gow-nee-anderson-biography/#_ftn6

Taylor, Rennae. 'Eleanor Southey Baker-McLaglan (née Baker)'. *Early Medical Women of New Zealand* (blog), 30 May 2021. www.earlymedwomen.auckland.ac.nz/2021/05/30/eleanor-southey-baker-mclaglan-nee-baker

——. 'Emma Gertrude Atmore (née Applegate)'. *Early Medical Women of New Zealand* (blog), 3 October 2021. www.earlymedwomen.auckland.ac.nz/2021/10/03/emma-gertrude-atmore-nee-applegate

——. 'Florence and Teresa Craig'. *Early Medical Women of New Zealand* (blog), 27 July 2021. www.earlymedwomen.auckland.ac.nz/2024/07/27/florence-and-teresa-craig

——. 'Hilda Berdach Fleischl (née Barber)'. *Early Medical Women of New Zealand* (blog), 16 May 2024. www.earlymedwomen.auckland.ac.nz/2024/05/16/hilda-berdach-fleischl-nee-barber

——. 'Joan Eleanor Walton (née Robertson)'. *Early Medical Women of New Zealand* (blog), 28 September 2021. www.earlymedwomen.auckland.ac.nz/2021/09/28/joan-eleanor-walton-nee-robertson

——. 'Patricia Mackay (née Wilson)'. *Early Medical Women of New Zealand* (blog), 14 July 2024. www.earlymedwomen.auckland.ac.nz/2024/07/14/patricia-mackay-nee-wilson

——. 'Rina Winifred Moore (née Rōpiha)'. *Early Medical Women of New Zealand* (blog), 16 May 2024. www.earlymedwomen.auckland.ac.nz/2024/05/16/rina-winifred-moore-nee-ropiha

Te Whatu Ora Health New Zealand. 'Helen Rarity McCreanor'. 31 October 2016. www.ccdhb.org.nz/about-us/history/wellington-hospital-smo-archive/appointments-made/1961–1980/medical-admin-clinical-support-services/pathology/mccreanor-helen-r

Tennant, Margaret. 'Ada Gertrude Paterson'. *Te Ara — the Encyclopedia of New Zealand*, 1996. https://teara.govt.nz/en/biographies/3p13/paterson-ada-gertrude

'The War at Home'. New Zealand History — Nga Korero a Ipurangi o Aotearoa, 17 May 2017. https://nzhistory.govt.nz/war/first-world-war-overview/defending-our-shores

Thomas, P. 'The Samoan Women's Health Committees: A Study of Community Vulnerability and Resilience'. Otago University, 2014. http://devnet.org.nz/sites/default/files/Thomas%20Paper%20for%20Devnet%20Conf%202014%20for%20NZDEVNET%20website.pdf

Timaru District Council — Te Kaunihera ā-Rohe o Te Tihi o Maru. 'Dr Margaret Barnett Cruickshank'. 16 September 2021. www.timaru.govt.nz/community/our-district/hall-of-fame/category-three/dr-margaret-cruickshank

University of Otago Ōtākou Whakaihu Waka. 'A Woman of the Pacific'. www.otago.ac.nz/otagomagazine/issue50/profiles/a-woman-of-the-pacific

——. '"Influenzial" Career'. www.otago.ac.nz/otagomagazine/issue44/features/influenzial-career

——. 'Scholarships and Prizes'. www.otago.ac.nz/humannutrition/study/scholarships-prizes

Wellington City Council Me Heke Ki Poneke. 'Ewart Hospital Nurses' Home (Former)'. 20 April 2017. https://wellingtoncityheritage.org.nz/buildings/1-150/59-ewart-hospital-nurses-home-former

Williams, Susanna. 'Jewish Doctors in New Zealand 1933–1945'. Holocaust Centre of New Zealand, September 2008. www.holocaustcentre.org.nz/uploads/1/2/2/4/122437058/jewish_doctors_in_new_zealand_1933_-1945_2.pdf

Acknowledgements

Many people helped in the preparation of this book and we extend our thanks to:

The biography writing team who conducted interviews, recorded oral biographies and prepared biographies for the website: Rachel Bergin, Rennae Taylor, Lucy Goodman, Dr Nora Gillies, Professor Dawn Elder, Professor Cindy Farquhar, Michaela Selway and Dr Daniel Beaumont. The book writing team of Michaela Selway, Dr Daniel Beaumont, Rennae Taylor, Professor Dawn Elder and Professor Cindy Farquhar.

Researcher Dr Claire Gooder, who assisted in the early stages of the project, including ethics approval and providing training on oral histories.

Associate Professor Sue Crengle, University of Otago, who advised and supported the applications for funding and the ethics application with the University of Auckland.

Professor Barbara Brookes, who supported us throughout this project, particularly with grant applications and with advice during the drafting of the book.

University of Otago staff, particularly Dr Richard German, Sciences and Health Sciences; Chris Smith, curator of the W. D. Trotter Anatomy Museum; and Hocken Library staff.

The staff of the National Library and the Alexander Turnbull Library.

Professor Manyip Ip, who prepared the biography for Dr Lucy Chung and allowed us to draw on a published biography of Dr Kathleen Pih.

Geoff Farquhar and Claire Farquhar, for providing feedback during the process.

The Maurice and Phyllis Paykel Trust, Medical Protection Society, University of Auckland and the Community and Heritage Fund of the Lotteries Grant Board for funding the website and the biographical research.

Dr Wendy Hadden for her generous funding of the publishing of this book.

The School of Medicine at University of Auckland for enabling this project by agreeing to this research.

Massey University Press, which has been supportive and helpful from the first enquiry. We are particularly grateful to the publisher, Nicola Legat, for her expertise.

The many, many individuals, including the medical women graduates, their family members and their friends and colleagues, who gave their time generously, providing information and photos. We thank you all.

About the authors

Professor Cynthia (Cindy) Farquhar is the daughter of an early medical woman (Meredyth Gunn; 1952). Cindy trained in medicine and graduated from the School of Medicine at the University of Auckland in 1981. She trained in obstetrics and gynaecology in New Zealand and London and is the Postgraduate Professor of Obstetrics and Gynaecology at the University of Auckland. She has been the recipient of several research awards, most recently the Beaven Medal in 2024.

Michaela Selway is a PhD student in early medieval history at the University of Tübingen, Germany. She received her Master of Arts in History from the University of Auckland in 2020 and has worked as a historical researcher for the Early Medical Women of New Zealand project since that time. Her doctoral research is supported by the Studienstiftung des deutschen Volkes research scholarship for academic excellence.

Index

MASSEY
UNIVERSITY
PRESS

First published in 2025 by Massey University Press
Private Bag 102904, North Shore Mail Centre
Auckland 0745, New Zealand
www.masseypress.ac.nz

Design by Kate Barraclough

A catalogue record for this book is available from the National Library of New Zealand

Printed and bound in Malaysia by 1010 Printing Asia Limited

ISBN: 978-1-99-101698-0
eISBN: 978-1-991309-11-2